# Medical Statistics

2nd Edition

## An A–Z Companion

# Medical Statistics

## 2nd Edition

## An A–Z Companion

Filomena Pereira-Maxwell
MBBS  MSc Clinical Tropical Medicine  MSc Medical Statistics
Washington, USA

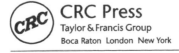

**CRC Press**
Taylor & Francis Group
Boca Raton  London  New York

CRC Press is an imprint of the
Taylor & Francis Group, an **informa** business

CRC Press
Taylor & Francis Group
6000 Broken Sound Parkway NW, Suite 300
Boca Raton, FL 33487-2742

International Standard Book Number-13: 978-1-4441-6734-4 (Paperback)
International Standard Book Number-13: 978-1-1380-9959-3 (Hardback)

**Visit the Taylor & Francis Web site at**
**http://www.taylorandfrancis.com**

**and the CRC Press Web site at**
**http://www.crcpress.com**

*To the memory of my parents,*
*Pedro and Nazareth*

# Contents

# Preface

*Motivation:* This *A–Z Companion* is intended primarily for medical students and health care professionals seeking to deepen their understanding of the role of medical statistics in answering pertinent questions in the medical and public health fields. It is my hope it will also be useful to those with a more solid background in medical statistics and epidemiology. The book seeks to provide explanations for terms frequently encountered by readers of the medical literature and by researchers, in such a way as to clarify their meaning and applicability, and show the inter-dependency between various important concepts. It aims to establish a connection between the proper treatment of data generated by research investigations and the ability to rely on study results to make impactful and consequential medical decisions. Included terminology relates to research methodology in the context of clinical and epidemiological investigations.

*Background:* The need for a collection of concise explanations of terms frequently encountered in medical journals became apparent during critical appraisal workshops organized by the North Thames Research Appraisal Group (NTRAG) in the UK, and led to the first edition of the present text, published in 1998. Much has changed since then, and many more excellent texts are now available that address the needs of the medical and allied professions, as well as of researchers and statisticians. Adding to the rather ubiquitous concepts of normality, randomization, standard errors, *P*-values, risk, study design, to name just a few, terms such as meta-analysis, overdispersion, multilevel modelling, cluster randomized trials, Bayesian inference and many others are more often seen in the medical literature, and an understanding of these concepts remains of central importance to the practices of critical appraisal of scientific evidence and evidence-based medicine and public health. Another development of the last 20 years has been the proliferation of collaborative efforts and networks aiming to standardize the reporting of research methods and findings, and systematize the best evidence under useful clinical guidelines. Umbrella organizations such as EQUATOR, GRADE and Cochrane have played an important role in this regard.

*Cross-referencing between terms:* This book has been structured as a dictionary, with substantial cross-referencing between the various entries (shown as **bolded** terms). It is hoped this will decrease the need for unnecessary repetitions. The intention with this presentation style is more to provide a 'word cloud' that reinforces the interrelation between concepts and methods, than a prompting for the constant back and forth between definitions. The reader will be the judge of the cross-reference checking that needs to be done. Connections between various terms are reinforced also by inviting the reader to consider additional entries for related material and for comparing and contrasting definitions. It is hoped the recognition of patterns of meaning and connection will help solidify fundamental concepts and principles in a clear and enduring way.

*Order of terms:* The placement of terms in the A–Z is based on word-by-word alphabetic order that considers hyphenated terms as two separate words. Two-word terms such as cause–effect and *P*-value should be searched on the basis of the first word of the term, and only then the second word. A few examples:

- All-subsets model selection before Allocation;
- Cross-validation before Crossover design;
- Effect-measure modification before Effective sample size;
- $F(x)$ at the end of section F.
- $H_1$ before Half-life;
- *HR* before $h(t)$;
- Likelihood ratio test before Likelihood ratios;
- $Log_{10}$ after Log odds but before Logarithmic scale;
- Logarithmic transformation before $log_e$;
- N-of-1 trial before Natural history of disease;
- *P*-value before PACF, PAF and Paired data;
- $S(t)$ before Stacked bar chart.

*Structure of terms:* Some terms such as post-test odds and log-linear model are hyphenated, others are not (pretest odds, pretreatment measurement). This reflects orthographic and style conventions and rules and long-standing usage by authors. The reader is encouraged to look up alternative wordings whenever a term is not first encountered (e.g. if looking for loglinear model, look for log-linear model and follow the rule above to find the term after Log likelihood ratio instead of after Logit transformation). Also, in looking up cross-referenced bolded terms, one or more terms may need to be looked up. For example, 'retrospective cohort study' makes reference to Retrospective study and Cohort study; 'chi-squared test statistic' directs the reader to the terms Chi-squared test and Test statistic.

*References and illustrative examples:* Textbooks and articles consulted are listed as Core and additional references. Their mention under the various entries serves to inform the reader who requires additional or more specialized information, and equally importantly to recognize a source of information that was included in the A–Z. These references include a mix of texts that appeal to a non-statistical audience (many of which are listed as Core references) and more specialized texts that may need to be consulted in addition. A significant number of concepts, methods and terms is illustrated with mostly examples from the medical literature. Sources for illustrative examples are listed separately in the References section.

*Filomena Pereira-Maxwell*
*Washington, DC*

# Acknowledgements

Firstly, my thanks to Dr. Joanna Koster, Senior Publisher at CRC Press/Taylor & Francis Group, who commissioned the writing of the *A–Z Companion* and patiently supported its various revisions through completion. Thanks also to Julia Molloy for assistance with obtaining permissions for the various illustrative examples.

My sincere thanks to the team led by Paul Bennett for their invaluable help and support through the production phase, and the quality of their work. I would like to thank Dr. Ruth Maxwell (copy editing) for her steadfast commitment to this project and Paul Bennett for his kind and competent support while supervising the entire process.

Professors Martin Bland and Basant Puri, and Dr. Simon Day, have all reviewed the text at different stages and made significant contributions with their comments, edits and suggestions. They have my gratitude and appreciation. Any errors in the text are the sole responsibility of the author.

I also want to reiterate my thanks to Professors Stephen Evans (who first suggested this project to me over 20 years ago) and Richard Morris for their helpful assistance with reviewing the first edition of the *A–Z*. Former colleagues at Barts and The London School of Medicine and Dentistry (Queen Mary University of London) and NTRAG (North Thames Research Appraisal Group) also provided helpful assistance and encouraging support. Richard Harris, former NTRAG project manager, played a crucial role in finding a publisher for the *A–Z*'s first edition. My continued gratitude to Richard and to Georgina Bentliff, formerly Director of Medical and Health Science Publishing at Hodder Arnold.

Thanks also to my husband Ray and to family and friends for kind words of encouragement along the way.

Lastly, but certainly not least, my thanks to the authors of the texts consulted during the writing of the *A–Z*, sources of knowledge and wisdom, to the researchers and experts whose work was used to illustrate concepts and methods, and to the reader, source of motivation and ever-present guiding star.

# Symbols

α     Lower case Greek letter alpha. See **alpha, intercept, Cronbach's alpha**.

β     Lower case Greek letter beta. See **beta, regression coefficient**.

Δ     Upper case Greek letter delta. See **Glass's Delta**.

ε     Lower case Greek letter epsilon. See **autoregressive model** (error term), **residuals**.

η     Lower case Greek letter eta. See **eta squared** ($\eta^2$), **prognostic index**.

κ     Lower case Greek letter kappa. See **kappa statistic**.

λ     Lower case Greek letter lambda. See **rate**.

μ     Lower case Greek letter mu, represents the population **mean**.

ν     Lower case Greek letter nu, represents **degrees of freedom** or *df*.

π     Lower case Greek letter pi, represents the **prevalence** or **proportion** in the population with a given characteristic or disease.

ρ     Lower case Greek letter rho. See **Spearman's correlation coefficient**.

σ     Lower case Greek letter sigma, represents the population **standard deviation**.

Σ     Upper case Greek letter sigma, represents summation (e.g. in the formula for the **mean**).

τ     Lower case Greek letter tau. See **Kendall's correlation coefficient**.

χ     Lower case Greek letter chi. See **chi-squared** ($\chi^2$) **distribution, chi-squared** ($\chi^2$) **test**.

ω     Lower case Greek letter omega. See **omega squared** ($\omega^2$).

!     See **factorial**.

∞     Symbol for infinity (e.g. minus infinity, $-\infty$, or plus infinity, $+\infty$).

√     The **square root** of a quantity, as in **standard deviation** [=√(**variance**)].

Cf.     Compare and contrast.

## 2 × 2 table

See **two-by-two** (2 × 2) **table**.

# A

## ABI

Abbreviation for **absolute benefit increase**.

## Abscissa

The value on the horizontal or $x$-axis for a datum point that is plotted on a two-dimensional graph. An individual or **study unit** is identified on such a graph by its coordinates, i.e. by the point of intersection between the value of the abscissa and the value of the **ordinate**.

## Absolute benefit increase

Or its abbreviation, ABI. An alternative way of expressing **treatment effect** when the outcome of interest is a *favourable* ('good') rather than an adverse outcome. It is calculated as an absolute difference, i.e. the probability of a good outcome in the treatment, intervention, or protective exposure group (assumed to have experienced a larger proportion of good outcomes) *minus* the same probability in the control group. The absolute risk reduction (ARR) conveys a similar idea when analysing adverse outcomes (see **absolute risk difference**). Cf. **absolute risk increase (ARI)**, **relative benefit increase (RBI)**. See also **absolute effect**, **measures of effect**.

## Absolute change

As opposed to relative change or percentage change from baseline. See **change scores**.

## Absolute dispersion

The extent of **variability** or dispersion displayed by a set of measurements. Absolute dispersion is usually calculated from the square of the differences between the values of a **quantitative variable** (typically, a continuous variable) and its **mean** (see **variance**). The frequently used **standard deviation** (the square root of the variance) measures absolute dispersion, and is expressed in the same units as the individual measurements. The corresponding measure of **relative dispersion** is the **coefficient of variation** (also known as coefficient of dispersion), a unit-less measure expressed as a fraction or percentage. For a meaningful assessment of its magnitude, a measure such as the standard deviation must be presented with the value for the mean. See also **measures of dispersion**.

## Absolute effect

The **magnitude** and **direction** of a **measure of effect**, which expresses in *net* terms the estimated effect of a given treatment or exposure. Measures of absolute effect are calculated as differences between risks and rates (or between means, although the terminology is not often used with quantitative outcomes). The absolute risk reduction and the absolute risk increase (both **absolute risk differences**) are examples of measures of absolute effect, as is the **absolute benefit increase**. This is in contrast to measures of **relative effect** such as the excess relative risk, which gives absolute effect as a fraction of baseline risk or rate, and to simple ratios such as the risk ratio, which measures the **strength of association** between treatments and outcomes, or exposures and disease. See also **standardized difference**, **effect size**. Absolute effect measures are sometimes expressed as the **absolute value** of the difference; direction of effect must nonetheless be stated.

## Absolute frequency

See **frequency**.

## Absolute risk

A term that is used somewhat inconsistently to mean both **risk** (in a single exposure or treatment group) and **absolute risk difference** or **attributable risk** (as opposed to **relative risk** or **risk ratio**).

## Absolute risk difference

Or simply, risk difference (RD). Often referred to as **attributable risk** and **absolute risk increase (ARI)** in the context of **observational studies**, and as **absolute risk reduction (ARR)** in the context of **clinical trials** and other **intervention studies**. In **comparative studies**, the absolute risk difference (ARD) is the difference in the **risk** of a given **outcome** or event (such as the occurrence of a particular disease or adverse disease outcome) between **exposed** and unexposed, or between the **control** and **treatment groups**. As opposed to the **risk ratio**, which only expresses the relative effects of treatments and exposures (e.g. *twice as many* patients died on treatment A compared to treatment B), the ARD measures the *net* risk decrease (or increase) from baseline. Treatment effects can therefore be expressed in absolute, net terms (likewise, with regard to detrimental and protective exposure effects). Using the example above, one is able to state how many deaths could be prevented (among the controls) by adopting treatment B instead of treatment A. The ARD is used to compute the **number needed to treat**, which conveys a related concept. From Table 2.b (Contingency table), p. 72:

$$ARD = risk_0 - risk_1 = \frac{c}{c+d} - \frac{a}{a+b}$$

where $risk_0$ is the risk of the event in the control or unexposed group (baseline risk) and $risk_1$ is the risk in the treatment, intervention or protective exposure group. In this instance, the absolute risk difference may be referred to as an absolute risk reduction, or it may be expressed as *risk_1 minus risk_0*, a difference which will likely have a negative sign (see **attributable risk** for harmful exposures). The example in Box A.1 illustrates these concepts.

---

### BOX A.1

Based on data from ISIS Collaborative Group (1988). Randomized trial of intravenous streptokinase, oral aspirin, both or neither among 17,187 cases of suspected acute myocardial infarction: ISIS-2. *Lancet* **332**: 349–60.

In this **multicentre trial**, over 17,000 patients suspected of having an acute myocardial infarction (AMI) were randomized to receive one of the four treatment alternatives mentioned above. This example concentrates on the comparison of all patients receiving aspirin (160 mg/day for 1 month) *vs.* all those not receiving aspirin, regardless of any other concomitant treatments. The results are (for vascular mortality at 5 weeks):

| | No. who died (%) | | ARD | *P*-value |
|---|---|---|---|---|
| **Aspirin** | 804/8587 (9.4%) | | | |
| | | | 0.024 (2.4%) | <0.000 01 |
| **No aspirin** | 1016/8600 (11.8%) | | | |
| | **95% CI for ARD** | **RR** | **RRR** | **NNT** |
| | 1.5% to 3.4% | 0.80 | 20% | 42 (1/0.024) |

*Interpretation:* The ARD is 0.024 or 2.4%. This indicates that for each 1000 patients receiving aspirin following a probable diagnosis of AMI, as opposed to not receiving aspirin, an average of 24 deaths may possibly be prevented.

See explanation of other estimates under the relevant entries (RR, **relative risk**; RRR, **relative risk reduction**; NNT, **number needed to treat**; CI, **confidence interval**; *P*-value). WALD (2004) gives further discussion of the ISIS-II trial.

---

In studies where length of **follow-up** varies among participants, **rates** and **rate differences** are calculated. Both are expressed in units of the reciprocal of time. See also **measures of effect**, **measures of impact**, **absolute value**.

## Absolute risk increase

Or its abbreviation, ARI. An alternative terminology for the **absolute risk difference** or **attributable risk**, which is calculated as the risk of an adverse outcome in the treatment, intervention, or detrimental exposure group (assumed to have a larger proportion of 'bad' outcomes) *minus* the risk in the control group. Cf. **absolute risk reduction (ARR)**, **absolute benefit increase (ABI)**, **relative risk increase (RRI)**. See also **absolute effect**, **measures of effect**.

## Absolute risk reduction

Or its abbreviation, ARR. An alternative terminology for the **absolute risk difference**, which is calculated as the risk of an adverse outcome in the control group *minus* the risk in the treatment, intervention, or protective exposure group (assumed to have a smaller proportion of 'bad' outcomes). Cf. **absolute risk increase (ARI)** or attributable risk, **relative risk reduction (RRR)**. See also **absolute effect, measures of effect**.

## Absolute value

The value of any given number irrespective of its sign, i.e. of whether it is a negative or a positive number. For example, the absolute value of both '−4.5' and '+4.5' is 4.5. Absolute values thus represent the distance any given number is from zero. Symbolically, $|-4.5| = |+4.5| = 4.5$ (and $|0| = 0$). **Absolute effect** measures are sometimes expressed as absolute values, which avoids negative sign differences and can make calculations more straightforward (see notation in STRAUS *et al.*, 2010). Nonetheless, direction of effect must always be stated. It should be noted that the meaning of 'absolute' in the term 'absolute risk difference' still refers to it being a *net*, rather than a proportional or *relative*, difference. In addition, it may also be expressed by its absolute value, which gives a non-negative sign (or a zero) difference, irrespective of which risk ($risk_0$ or $risk_1$, see **absolute risk difference**) is larger.

## Accelerated failure time models

A class of **parametric survival models** (exponential, Weibull, log-normal, log-logistic, and gamma) that includes an *acceleration parameter*. The assumed distribution of a model-derived quantity that includes the latter determines the specific type of model. Accelerated failure time (AFT) models predict 'time to failure' or **survival time** (on a logarithmic scale). For any given individual, time may be accelerated or decelerated (or neither), depending on the value of the acceleration parameter. Exponentiating the **regression coefficients** from an AFT model gives *time ratios* (rather than hazard ratios), which express the relative time delay between the categories of a binary predictor, or for each unit increase in a quantitative predictor. In addition, the effect of changes in the predictors, measured in *time units*, increases with predicted failure time, so that the absolute time delay increases with predicted time to failure (and predicted time to failure increases or decreases depending on whether the relevant regression coefficient has a positive or negative sign). AFT models may be specified also as predicting survival probability (i.e. the **survival function**, or $[S(t)]$), which sometimes is computationally more straightforward. Cf. **Cox regression** and (parametric) **proportional hazards models**, where the **hazard ratio** between any two exposure or treatment groups (or values of a continuous covariate) is assumed to remain constant over time. See CLEVES, GOULD & MARCHENKO (2016) for further details.

## Accrual period

The period of time during which **eligible** patients or healthy individuals are identified and recruited into a research study. See also **follow-up period**.

## Accuracy

In the context of **clinical measurement**, the quality of a measured value being close to its true value. Cf. **measurement error, measurement bias**. See also **precision, diagnostic odds ratio** (diagnostic accuracy), **calibration** (predictive accuracy).

## ACES

An acronym often seen in the context of clinical trials, which stands for **active control equivalence study**.

## ACF

Abbreviation for **autocorrelation** function. See also **correlogram**.

## Active control equivalence study

Or its acronym, ACES. A **clinical trial** that seeks to demonstrate a *similarity* of effect between interventions, drug therapies in particular. Comparisons are usually against **active control** groups rather than **placebo control** groups. **Sample size** calculations may be based on required **precision** rather than required **power**, as the goal may be to estimate the difference, or rather, the equivalence between the treatments, within a relatively narrow margin of uncertainty (POCOCK, 1983). In addition, the difference or effect to be estimated is likely of small magnitude, which affects the power of statistical tests unless sample size requirements are increased. An active control equivalence study is often conducted as a **non-inferiority trial**, i.e. a study that seeks to demonstrate a given experimental treatment to be *no worse* or not inferior (by a clinically important amount) to a standard or established treatment for a given target disease. This is in contrast to trials evaluating true **equivalence**, as described above (i.e. non-inferiority *and* non-superiority), and **superiority** of effect. This type of assessment is usually carried out when the objective is to find safer or cheaper alternatives of equal (non-inferior) **efficacy** to established treatments, which may be costly or ill-tolerated by some patients. Sackett, in HAYNES *et al.* (eds., 2006), argues in favour of non-inferiority trials over equivalence trials, and of using **one-sided** significance testing and estimation to analyse results, as being more consistent with the clinical question at hand. **Two-sided** statistical significance and estimation are still, however, generally recommended. **Null hypotheses** and **type I** and **II errors** are stated differently in equivalence trials: as a difference between the treatments being compared equal to or greater than some specified magnitude, as the mistake of failing to reject an inferior treatment (which is thus accepted as equivalent or non-inferior), and as the mistake of failing to accept a treatment as equivalent or non-inferior. **Intention-to-treat analysis** may be problematic if used as an approach to data analysis in dealing with **protocol breaches**, as results will be biased in the direction of the null value, which in this context is the **alternative hypothesis**. See also **bioequivalence study**, **Bayesian inference**. Cf. **superiority trial**. See SENN (2008) and MACHIN & CAMPBELL (2005) for further discussion and additional details. PIAGGIO *et al.* (2006) give reporting guidelines under the **CONSORT statement**.

## Active control group

A **control group** to whom an **active treatment** is administered. **Clinical trials** increasingly make use of active treatments for the control group, as opposed to **placebos**, and **active control equivalence studies** in particular, since their aim is to assess whether any two treatments (commonly, pharmaceutical drugs) have comparable effect.

## Active treatment

A pharmacological product or some other actual **treatment** or intervention which, as opposed to a dummy treatment or **placebo**, has some type of direct biological effect. See also **active control group**, **active control equivalence study**.

## Adaptive designs

In the context of **clinical trials**, adaptive designs allow for changes to the initial **study design**, whereby emerging data from a trial in progress inform the necessary course corrections, i.e. how the study should proceed henceforth. Typically, changes will not be effected once a trial is underway, but adaptive designs use the results from **interim analyses** to alter certain aspects of the design, commonly, the **hypothesis** under study, which **treatment arms** to retain and/or add to the trial, treatment **allocation** probabilities, and **sample size** requirements. Adaptive designs are seldom used outside of pharmacological research. See CHOW & CHANG (2008; 2011) for a full discussion. See also **sequential designs**.

## Adaptive seamless Phase II/III design

A **clinical trial** that seeks to combine the objectives of **Phase IIB** and **Phase III** efficacy trials. Competing experimental treatments are compared with each other and a **control** treatment, and the least effective (or least promising) experimental **treatment arms** are dropped early. This is usually a two-stage design, the first stage often referred to as the *learning stage*, while the second is referred to as the *confirmatory stage*. See CHOW & CHANG (2008; 2011) for further details.

## Additive effects model

As opposed to **multiplicative effects** model. A statistical **model** in which the combined effect of two or more **predictor variables** is calculated as the sum of their individual effects. In other words, the predicted outcome (on the **arithmetic scale**) is a linear function of the predictors in the model. **Linear regression** models with untransformed outcome variables are in this category, as are regression models that predict *untransformed* **risk** (for example, a **generalized linear model** for a binary outcome in which the **link function** is *identity*). In the latter case, **regression coefficients** represent **risk differences**, as opposed to models such as derived by logistic regression, which predict a transformation of the outcome variable, with regression coefficients representing the log of the **odds ratio** between, for example, different categories of a predictor variable or different levels of an exposure. The choice of an additive model is not equivalent with the underlying relationship being additive, i.e. with absence of **biological interaction**. See HILLS (1974) and ROTHMAN (2012) for further discussion.

## Adjusted estimate

As opposed to **crude estimate**. An estimate of **exposure effect** in an **observational study** that is computed after taking into account factors other than the exposure (known as **confounding factors**), which are unequally distributed between the exposure groups, and may explain, in part, an effect or an association that is observed. For example, a difference in crude mortality rate between two populations could simply reflect a different age structure, the older population experiencing a higher overall death rate. After age **standardization**, any remaining differences may then be attributed to factors other than age. Methods such as **stratification** and **multiple** or multivariable **regression** may also be employed to obtain adjusted estimates. These are less **biased** than unadjusted, crude estimates. See Box C.2 (Confounding), p. 70, for an example. In the context of **randomized trials**, adjusted estimates are sometimes obtained to assess the extent to which chance differences between treatment groups, with respect to relevant **prognostic factors**, affect estimates of **treatment effect**. These prognostic imbalances do not, however, reflect systematic differences between groups, but rather, the vagaries of a random **allocation** process, a more common occurrence in smaller trials (POCOCK, 1983; ROTHMAN, 2012). See also **adjusted treatment mean**, where adjustments are made also for **variance** reduction in the quantitative outcome variable.

## Adjusted *r*-squared

See **r-squared** ($r^2$).

## Adjusted treatment mean

In the context of **analysis of covariance**, this term refers to the estimated **mean** response in each of the treatment groups being compared in a **clinical trial** or other experiment, after an adjustment has been made for **covariates** included in the analysis (FAIRFIELD SMITH, 1957). The latter are often **baseline measurements** for the **outcome variable**, but may also be any variable that is strongly associated with the outcome variable. Where there are baseline imbalances between treatment groups (as may happen by chance in small randomized trials, and also in nonrandomized studies), estimates of **treatment effect** thus obtained will be **unbiased** (or less biased). HUITEMA (2011, p. 126) defines adjusted means as "…adjusted to the level that would be expected if all group covariate means were equal to the grand covariate mean…" (the overall covariate mean for all subjects). Where the covariate is not associated with the treatment factor, these adjustments can still reduce the **random error** component of response variability, thus increasing the **power** of **significance tests** and **precision** of **confidence intervals**, but should be specified in advance of the analysis. The proportion of total variability in the outcome variable that is explained by a treatment factor whose effect has been adjusted, is equivalent to the square of the **partial correlation coefficient**. See also **change** (study of), **adjusted estimate**.

## Adverse reaction

A hazardous reaction to a medical treatment, commonly, but not restricted to, a pharmaceutical drug. The occurrence of adverse reactions is an important outcome in **clinical trials** and post-marketing **Phase IV studies**. See STRAUS *et al.* (2010) for discussion of the critical evaluation of evidence of harm in both clinical trials and observational studies. POCOCK (1983) discusses the monitoring and evaluation of side-effects when conducting clinical trials, and implications for study validity and data analysis. WALLER & EVANS (2003), and COLEMAN, FERNER & EVANS (2006) provide in-depth discussion of issues around **pharmacovigilance**. See also SENN (2008), ROTHMAN (2012).

## Aetiological fraction

A term commonly used as synonym for **attributable fraction**. However, Greenland, Rothman & Lash, in ROTHMAN, GREENLAND & LASH (eds., 2012), make a distinction in that, under a given **exposure**, there will be a fraction of the **cases** that would still have occurred through a different **causal mechanism** in absence of the exposure of interest, and thus, unless this fraction is known, an aetiological fraction cannot truly be estimated.

## Aetiology

The cause(s) of a disease. See causality (**causal mechanism, component cause, cause-effect relationship**) for further discussion.

## $AF_{exposed}$

Abbreviation for **attributable fraction (exposed)**.

## $AF_{population}$

Abbreviation for attributable fraction (population), or **population attributable fraction (PAF)**.

## Age-specific rate

The **rate** or frequency of occurrence of an event among persons in a defined age group. Cf. **crude rate, standardized event rate**.

## Aggregate data

Data that have been summarized according to one or more factors, and are therefore available as **summary measures**, as opposed to individual observations. An example of aggregate data is provided in the data summaries for each of the **primary studies** included in a **meta-analysis**, where the aggregate (each individual study), not the individuals in each study, is the **study unit**. Another example arises from **clustered designs**, when measurements or observations made within each cluster are summarized and these summaries then analysed using standard methods. Again, the cluster, not the individuals within each cluster, is the study unit or unit of observation and analysis. A variation on this is where **repeated** or **serial measurements** are made, with the individual, not each separate measurement, as the cluster or study unit. Where observations are clustered but individual-level data are still available, more complex statistical methods may also be employed in their analysis that take the **hierarchical** structure of the data into account. Examples include **multilevel modelling** and **longitudinal analysis**. Cf. **individual participant data (IPD)**.

## Aggregation bias

Synonym for **ecological bias**.

## Agreement

In the context of **clinical measurement**, a term that refers to the extent of concordance between assessments made by different persons, different methods, different tools or at different times, when evaluating the same feature on the same group of individuals, or on the same **study units**. The term 'concordance' is usually employed in reference to **categorical** assessments on a **nominal** or **ordered nominal** scale. Two main areas are of interest: the accuracy of **diagnostic tests**, and the reliability of assessments that are made not in reference to a 'gold standard' (see **kappa statistic**). **Calibration** (accuracy), **method comparison** (repeatability and reproducibility) and **reliability** studies are carried out to evaluate agreement with regard to **quantitative measurements**. See ALTMAN (1991), BLAND (2015), and KIRKWOOD & STERNE (2003). MACHIN & CAMPBELL (2005) give details of the design of observer agreement studies (reproducibility/reliability). See also **misclassification, measurement bias, measurement error**.

## AIC

Abbreviation for **Akaike's information criterion**.

## Akaike's information criterion

Or its abbreviation, AIC. A statistic that is used in comparing competing **models** and, in particular, models that are not nested. With **nested models**, the **Wald** and **likelihood ratio tests** are usually employed. For any given parametric model, it is calculated on the basis of its **log likelihood**, $LL$, evaluated at the **maximum likelihood estimates** or MLEs for its parameters, and number of **parameters**, $k$ (AGRESTI, 2007):

$$AIC = -2LL + 2k$$

The model with the lowest value for AIC offers the best trade-off between simplicity and fit, i.e. **parsimony**. In the case of parametric survival models, the number of parameters of the assumed distribution of survival times is also taken into account (CLEVES, GOULD & MARCHENKO, 2016). For nested models (CLAYTON & HILLS, 1993), AIC is a direct comparison measure:

$$AIC = \textit{(reduction in deviance)} -2 \times \textit{(increase in number of parameters)}$$

where the **deviance statistic** reflects the difference in log likelihood between any given model and the corresponding saturated model (and 'reduction in deviance' is the difference between the deviances of the two nested models). Here, positive values for AIC reflect a good trade-off between increased complexity and improved fit or **predictive** ability. The opposite is true for negative values for AIC. See also **Bayesian information criterion (BIC), Mallow's $C_p$**.

## All-subsets model selection

A method for selecting explanatory or **predictor variables** to be included in a **regression model**. This method is considered preferable to **stepwise regression** (although previously less employed due to computational limitations). For a given set of outcome and predictor variables, all possible models are compared on the basis of a statistic, **Mallow's $C_p$**. As with stepwise methods, automated variable selection is better suited to the fitting of **predictive**, rather than **causal** or explanatory, models. The alternative terminology 'best-subsets' is also commonly used.

## Allocation

In the context of **clinical trials** and other intervention studies, the assignment of **study units** (usually, patients) to the different **treatments** being compared. Ideally, treatment allocation should be carried out at **random** and using **concealment** strategies, in order to prevent **selection bias** and **confounding**. **Simple randomization** is commonly used, which allocates new patients to the alternative treatments in a trial with equal probability. Other methods used with **adaptive designs** aim to bias the allocation probabilities as the trial progresses, while still maintaining an element of randomness. Greater **comparability** between treatment groups (with respect to the distribution of **prognostic factors**) may be achieved through **stratified randomization** and **minimization**. **Restricted randomization** and the **biased coin method** aim to produce treatment groups of equal or similar sizes. **Cluster randomization** is employed when whole groups, rather than individuals, are assigned to the interventions being compared in a **community trial**. See POCOCK (1983), ALTMAN (1991), BLAND (2015), SCHULZ & GRIMES (2002a), and FLEISS (1999) for further details. See also **blinding**.

## Allocation bias

See **concealment** of allocation, **selection bias**.

## Alpha

Or $\alpha$. The probability of making a **type I error** when carrying out **significance testing**. See also **significance level, nominal significance level, sample size** (required). Cf. **beta** or $\beta$.

## Alpha-coefficient

Synonym for **intercept**. See also **beta-coefficient**.

## Alternative hypothesis

Or $H_1$. As opposed to the **null hypothesis** ($H_0$), the alternative hypothesis for a **significance test** states that differences between groups, and associations between factors, do indeed exist. To ensure adequate **power** when calculating the required **sample size** for a study, researchers should also specify the magnitude of such differences and associations that would be considered of sufficient **clinical** and public health **significance**. See also **one-sided test, two-sided test**.

## Analysis of covariance

Or its acronym, ANCOVA. A statistical method that is an extension of **analysis of variance**. ANCOVA produces **adjusted treatment means** for the different groups being compared in a study, by allowing the inclusion of relevant **covariates** (commonly, **baseline measurements** for the **outcome variable**) in the analysis (COCHRAN, 1957). ANCOVA is often employed in the study of **change**, where before–after measurements have been taken. Where there are baseline imbalances between the groups being compared (as may happen by chance in small trials), ANCOVA produces estimates of **treatment effect** that are less biased (or **unbiased**, if the study is a randomized controlled trial) when compared to the analysis of 'post-treatment' measurements or the analysis of 'change score', which, under these circumstances, may lead to underestimation or overestimation of effect (VICKERS & ALTMAN, 2001). In addition, this approach reduces the **variance** in the 'after' or 'post-treatment' outcome variable, leading to greater **precision** of estimated effects and greater **power** for significance testing. ANCOVA may be carried out using **multiple linear regression**, with **dummy variables** representing the **treatment groups**. This is illustrated with the example in Figure A.1, which is discussed in the paper by VICKERS & ALTMAN: the vertical distance between the two parallel

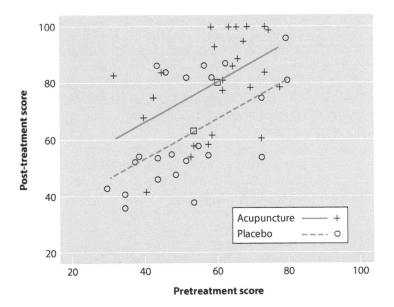

**Figure A.1** Graphical display of an analysis of covariance: effect of acupuncture *vs.* a placebo needle on pain from rotator cuff tendonitis, with adjustment for pretreatment pain score (*higher scores reflect a better outcome*). Squares show mean values for each of the two groups and the vertical distance between the regression lines gives the estimated treatment effect. (Reproduced from Vickers A, Altman D (2001). Analysing controlled trials with baseline and follow up measurements. *Br Med J* **323**: 1123 (with permission).)

lines is the estimated treatment effect of acupuncture *vs.* placebo needle after adjusting for baseline or pretreatment pain score. Covariates are assumed to have a **linear relationship** with the quantitative outcome, and data **transformations** may be necessary to this end. See also **model** (Box M.1, p. 219, for the equation that relates 'post-treatment pain score' to the two predictors, 'pre-score' and 'treatment group'), **efficiency**, **regression to the mean** (also, RTM in comparative studies), **interaction**. See HUITEMA (2011) for a full presentation. SENN (1995; 2006) addresses the issue of validity of ANCOVA in the study of change.

## Analysis of variance

Or its acronym, ANOVA. A statistical method that partitions the total **variance** of a given **quantitative variable** (commonly, a **continuous** variable on an **interval/ratio** scale) into different components, with regard to one or more other variables or factors with which it is associated. A common application of ANOVA is in comparing two or more groups with respect to their **mean** value for a quantitative **outcome variable**. In this regard, ANOVA is an extension of the independent samples *t*-test, which is used when there are just two groups. ANOVA partitions the total variance of the outcome variable into a *between-groups* and a *within-groups* component. The within-groups component is the **residual** or random error component, which cannot be attributed to systematic differences between the groups in regard of the factor (or factors) being analysed. The **significance test** for differences between groups is based on the comparison of these two components of response variability, under the assumption that no differences exist (null hypothesis). If the **null hypothesis** is true, there is no difference between within- and between-groups variance (also termed within- and between-groups **mean squares**), and the ratio between the two is equal to 1. This is known as the **F-test** or variance-ratio test. Depending on **study design**, **one-way** (see Box O.3, p. 246) or **two-way ANOVA** may be used. More complex designs may also be analysed with ANOVA. ANOVA may be carried out using **regression analysis**, with **dummy variables** representing the **comparison groups**. As with the *t*-test, validity **assumptions** for ANOVA are the **Normal distribution** (in each group) of the quantitative outcome, and **homoscedasticity**, although the test does show some **robustness** to moderate non-normality, especially where samples sizes are not too small. ANOVA may be used also to estimate the variance components for the **intraclass correlation coefficient**. See ALTMAN (1991), BLAND (2015), KIRKWOOD & STERNE (2003). See also **Kruskal-Wallis test**, **repeated measures ANOVA**, **analysis of covariance (ANCOVA)**.

## Analytical study

As opposed to **descriptive study**. A study that investigates the relationship between an **outcome** (such as developing a given disease or experiencing its complications) and an **exposure** (such as risk and protective factors, pharmacological drugs and other forms of treatment, behaviour-change interventions, etc.), seeking to draw **inferences** from the data at hand. An important goal of these studies is to unveil **causal relationships** where they exist, so that public health policies and clinical guidelines may be developed and implemented. Examples of analytical studies are **clinical trials**, **cohort studies** and **case–control studies**. **Cross-sectional studies** may also be analytical, but are usually less appropriate for drawing causal inferences.

## Ancillary statistic

A **statistic** is ancillary to a given **parameter** of interest in a parametric **model** if it does not provide information on the true value of the parameter, and its **sampling distribution** also does not depend on the parameter. As stated by GHOSH, REID & FRASER (2010), *conditioning* on ancillary statistics incorporates **frequentist** and **Bayesian** approaches to **inference**, and can affect the quality of the inference made (for example, the **precision** of estimates) in a number of situations. When the ancillary statistic provides complementary information, it is jointly referred to with the estimated parameter as a 'sufficient statistic', i.e. the ancillary statistic is used to recover information that was lost in the data reduction process that produces summaries or **estimates**. An example is **person-time at risk** as an ancillary to an estimated **rate**. Conditioning on ancillary statistics makes it possible to eliminate **nuisance parameters** from the distribution of a test statistic, as when conditioning on the **marginal totals** of a 2 × 2 contingency table when carrying out **Fisher's exact test**. This is particularly helpful when dealing with small **sample sizes**. Unconditional methods require large samples.

## ANCOVA

Acronym for **analysis of covariance**.

## Anecdotal evidence

A type of evidence that arises from observations made in the course of everyday occurrences and experiences (from **case series**, for example), and not in the context of scientifically designed and conducted **experimental** and **observational studies**. Such evidence is rarely considered adequate for determining **clinical guidelines** and public health policies, but is where study hypotheses often originate. See also **hierarchy of evidence**.

## ANOVA

Acronym for **analysis of variance**.

## Antagonism

As opposed to **synergism**. A type of **biological interaction** in which the joint effect of two factors that can affect a particular outcome is smaller than the sum of their separate effects. In other words, the presence of one factor reduces (or even negates) the effect of the other. An example would be strong immunity and the presence of an infectious agent, a situation that may be termed *causal* antagonism, where the effect of the agent might be more severe in a person with lower immunity. *Preventive* antagonism arises from a situation where one factor blocks the protective effect of another factor, as is sometimes the case with drug interactions. See Greenland, Lash & Rothman, in ROTHMAN *et al.* (eds., 2012), for a full discussion.

## Antedependence model

An extension of the **autoregressive** and **transition models** with lagged responses, or of the **autocorrelation model** for autoregressive errors. It allows a different parameter to be specified for each time point or occasion over the length of a time series or longitudinal period (SKRONDAL & RABE-HESKETH, 2004).

## Antilog

A value that has been **back-transformed** from a **logarithmic scale** to the **arithmetic scale** through the **exponentiation** function. See also **logarithmic transformation**, **geometric mean**.

## APACHE score

Acronym for Acute Physiology and Chronic Health Evaluation score (KNAUS *et al.*, 1985). A **severity of illness classification** system, which was developed as a means to provide an initial severity stratification of patients admitted to the intensive care unit (ICU), based on patient's age and chronic health status, and a number of physiological measurements pertaining to the acute illness (and measured within 24 hours of admission), specifically: pulse, mean blood pressure, body temperature, respiratory rate, PaO2 or A-aDO2 (depending on value of FiO2), arterial pH, haematocrit, white blood cell count, serum creatinine, serum sodium and serum potassium, in addition to the Glasgow Coma Score (GCS) (for the APACHE II score). The total APACHE II score is the sum of age points, chronic health points, and the total acute physiology score. The overall score lies between 0 and 71 for APACHE II, 0 and 299 for APACHE III, and 0 and 286 for APACHE IV, a zero score being the lowest risk of death. In the US, APACHE scores have been incorporated into **logistic regression models** to predict mortality based on data from large series of consecutive ICU patients (KNAUS *et al.*, 1991). APACHE scores have been used for clinical decision-making and **case mix** assessment. Other ICU severity of illness and prognostic scoring systems include the Simplified Acute Physiologic Score (SAPS), the Mortality Prediction Model (MPM) and the Sequential Organ Failure Assessment score (SOFA). See also VINCENT & MORENO (2010); **composite score**, **risk score**, **prognostic index**, **predictive model**.

## Approximation

The application of statistical methods based on a given **probability distribution** to data that are more accurately described by a different probability distribution. For example, the **Poisson** and **binomial distributions** (discrete distributions) are frequently approximated by the **Normal distribution** (continuous) for easier computation of **significance tests** and **confidence intervals**. A common application is the **chi-squared ($\chi^2$) test**, which is based on the extent to which observed ($O$) and expected ($E$) frequencies in each cell of a **contingency table** differ. Given a table's **marginal totals** (and an unrestricted sampling scheme) and the assumption that the **null hypothesis** is true, the observed frequency in each cell is from a Poisson distribution with parameters defined by the expected frequency. This may be approximated by a Normal distribution (with mean $E$ and standard deviation (SD) $\sqrt{E}$), if $E$ is not too small. As the **test statistic** ($X^2$) is based on the square of these $O$ *vs.* $E$ differences, it then follows a $\chi^2$ **distribution** with the appropriate number of **degrees of freedom**. **Non-parametric** tests may also be based on Normal approximations. A distinction should be made between the **sampling distribution** of an **estimate**, which may be approximated by a Normal distribution, and the distribution of a set of measurements, which may have an approximately Normal distribution (ALTMAN, 1991).

It is the former that provides the basis for the tests and methods described above. The validity of these approximations depends on **sample sizes** and **expected** numbers or **frequencies**. See also **central limit theorem, large sample method, continuity correction.**

## AR

Or AR($p$), i.e. $p$th-order **autoregressive model**; alternatively, model for autoregressive error process with AR($p$) disturbance.

## Arcsine square root transformation

A **variance-stabilizing** transformation for **proportions** in which the inverse sine ($\sin^{-1}$) or arcsine (arcsin) is the link function. This allows the use of **parametric methods** of analysis, normally employed in the analysis of quantitative data. The **logit** transformation, as obtained through **logistic regression**, is however more commonly used. See FLEISS (1999) for an illustrative example. See also **complementary log-log** transformation, **probit** transformation, **transformations.**

## ARD

Abbreviation for **absolute risk difference.**

## Area under the curve

A **summary measure** used in the analysis of **serial measurements**, and also in the analysis of quantitative measurements as **diagnostic tests**. In the latter context, the area under the curve or AUC is the area below the **ROC** (receiver operating characteristic) **curve** (Figure R.1, p. 319). Plotting ROC curves for different diagnostic tests enables a comparison of their diagnostic accuracy to be made: the greater the AUC the better the diagnostic test at correctly identifying individuals with, and without, a given condition. The AUC can thus be interpreted as the probability of correctly identifying the diseased and the non-diseased individual, given that one is presented with two individuals randomly selected from a population, where one is diseased and the other is not (HANLEY & McNEIL, 1982). See also **net benefit**; MALLETT *et al.* (2012), HALLIGAN, ALTMAN & MALLETT (2015). When analysing serial measurements, the AUC may be used instead of the **mean** to convey the idea of response over time, especially when measurements have not been made at equal time intervals, or even when some measurements, but not the last, are missing. Figure A.2 shows the diastolic blood pressure (DBP) measurements for two subjects over a period of 2 h following the administration of a hypotensive drug. Subject 2 appears to be slightly less responsive to the drug, and the AUC confirms that on average, over the 120-minute period, the DBP for subject 1 was lower by about 4 mmHg. ALTMAN (1991) gives the following formula for calculating an approximate AUC:

$$\text{AUC} = \frac{1}{2}\sum_{i=0}^{n-1}(t_{i+1} - t_i)(y_i + y_{i+1})$$

where the sigma notation, $\Sigma$, represents summation, $n + 1$ are the number of measurements (including the one at time 0), and the $y_i$s are the consecutive measurements at the

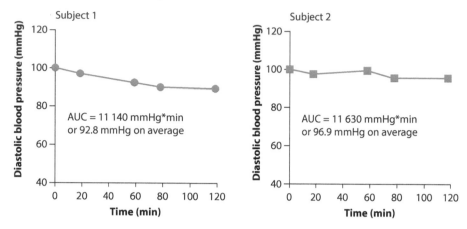

Figure A.2 Area under the curve: repeated (serial) diastolic blood pressure measurements for two individuals over a 2-hour period (drawn using Stata Statistical Software).

consecutive time points $t_i$s. The quantity ½ is applied as the AUC between any two consecutive measurements is the product of the time difference and the average of the two measurements. See also $C_{max}$, $T_{max}$; see Figures S.2a–S.2d, p. 330 (Serial measurements).

## ARI

Abbreviation for **absolute risk increase**.

## ARIMA

Acronym for **autoregressive integrated moving average** model. See **autoregressive model**.

## Arithmetic mean

See **mean**.

## Arithmetic scale

As opposed to **logarithmic scale**. A **measurement scale** in which equal-sized increments represent fixed absolute differences in the value of a **measurement** or **measure of effect**, as opposed to fixed proportional differences. The magnitude of a measurement value on the arithmetic scale is a true representation of its distance from zero, and the magnitude of a ratio on the arithmetic scale is a true representation of its distance from 1.

## ARMA

Acronym for **autoregressive moving average** model. See **autoregressive model**.

## ARMAX

Acronym for **autoregressive moving average** model with exogenous **predictor variables**. See **autoregressive model**.

## ARR

Abbreviation for **absolute risk reduction**.

## Array

An ordering of numerical **data** in an ascending or descending manner.

## Ascertainment bias

Synonym for detection bias, and sometimes also used as synonym for **assessment bias**. See **selection bias**.

## Assessment bias

A type of **bias** that may arise when measuring **outcomes** or responses, often due to lack of **blinding** (on the part of those making assessments) as to the treatment received by a patient in a **clinical trial**, or as to an individual's **exposure** status in a **cohort study**. **Response bias** on the part of study participants may be also largely due to lack of blinding. Both are more likely to occur when evaluation of the outcome of interest requires a subjective judgement. A possible solution is for a third party who is not aware of treatments given or received (or of exposure statuses) to make these assessments. Assessment bias may also occur in **case–control studies**, if those assessing exposure status are also aware of disease status. Assessment and response bias are special types of **information bias**.

## Association

A relationship between events, characteristics, or measurements that are not **independent**. Such a relationship may or not be **causal**. The variables in question may have a positive association if they change in the same **direction** (e.g. homocysteine levels and risk of heart disease), or a negative association if they change in opposite directions (e.g. vitamin D levels and risk of cancer). In addition, a steady increase or decrease in the values of one variable with increasing values of another variable often indicates the existence of a **linear trend**. At other times, the association will have a more complex pattern that may be described by a U-shaped or J-shaped curve, for example (see **non-linear-relationship**). Cross-tabulations and graphical methods should always be used for a visual assessment. The **strength** and **significance** of an association may be measured using a number of statistical methods and tests, such as **correlation** and the **chi-squared test**, or **modelled** using **regression analysis**, although this is probably best indicated when causality may be reasonably inferred and an effect can be estimated. Whatever the methodology employed, it is important to evaluate the extent to which the finding of an association could be due to the presence of **confounding** and other **biases**. A distinction should be made between association and **agreement**, as it can be shown that a perfect association may exist in the total absence of agreement. See also **measures of association.**

## Assumptions

Conditions required for the validity of many **significance tests** and methods of **estimation**. Many of these tests and methods are termed **parametric** since they assume a given **probability distribution** for the data being analysed. Common assumptions are: a **Normal distribution** for quantitative variables, **independence** of observations (i.e. observations come from different **study units**, and are not **repeated measurements** or assessments), a **linear relationship** between two variables that are associated, constant **variance** or **homoscedasticity**, etc., depending on the statistical method being used. For example, the independent samples *t*-test (which is carried out to compare two groups with respect to their mean value for a quantitative variable) assumes the variable in question to have similar variance in the comparison groups. In the presence of heteroscedasticity, test results may be incorrect, especially with small **samples sizes**. **Transformations**, **non-parametric methods**, **bootstrapping** and methods based on the calculation of **robust** standard errors may all be used when required assumptions cannot be met.

## Asymptotic method

Or **large sample method**. A method that provides a good **approximation** and valid results provided **sample sizes** are sufficiently large.

## Attack rate

In the context of **epidemiological studies** and, in particular, the study of outbreaks and **epidemics**, the attack rate measures the **cumulative incidence** of a disease among the **exposed**, as given by:

$$Attack\ rate = \frac{number\ of\ people\ exposed\ who\ are\ also\ affected\ by\ the\ index\ disease}{total\ number\ of\ people\ exposed} \times 100\%$$

Thus, the attack rate is not truly a **rate**, but a proportion, or **risk**. For example, if 240 children in a school are exposed to a particular pathogen, and 8 of them develop the corresponding illness, the attack rate is then $(8/240) \times 100\% \simeq 3.3\%$. See also **case-fatality rate**.

## Attributable fraction (exposed)

Or proportional attributable risk. The proportion of **cases** among the exposed that is attributed to the **exposure**. In other words, the attributable fraction ($AF_{exposed}$) expresses the **attributable risk** or **absolute risk increase** (i.e. the risk difference, exposed *minus* unexposed) as a fraction of the **risk** in the exposed, and thus **measures the impact** of exposure among the *exposed*. The attributable fraction is calculated as follows:

$$Attributable\ fraction = \frac{risk_1 - risk_0}{risk_1} = 1 - \frac{1}{RR}$$

where (from Table 2.a, p. 72) $risk_1$ is the risk among the exposed and $risk_0$ is the risk among the unexposed. The **population attributable fraction** (**PAF** or $AF_{population}$) measures the impact of a **risk factor** or exposure on a given *population*. The term 'attributable' implies **causality** or, at least, a clear, unconfounded association, and should be reserved for instances where the latter can reasonably be inferred. Where the **rate ratio** is a good approximation to the **risk ratio** (**RR**), it may be used to estimate the attributable fraction, as follows:

$$Attributable\ fraction = \frac{risk_1 - risk_0}{risk_1} = 1 - \frac{risk_0}{risk_1} = \frac{RR-1}{RR} \cong \frac{rate\ ratio - 1}{rate\ ratio}$$

In **case–control studies**, in which risks and risk differences may not usually be calculated, the formula $(RR-1)/RR$ allows the computation of the attributable fraction using the **odds ratio** as the measure of association (HENNEKENS, BURING & MAYRENT (eds.), 1987). With preventive exposures, the attributable fraction (with risk difference calculated as risk in control group *minus* risk in exposure or intervention group) is referred to as *preventable fraction*, **relative risk reduction** (**RRR**), or efficacy (Greenland, Rothman & Lash, in ROTHMAN, GREENLAND & LASH [eds., 2012]). See also **excess relative risk** (**ERR**), **measures of effect**.

## Attributable fraction (population)

Synonym for **population attributable fraction**. Also referred to as $AF_{population}$ or **PAF**.

## Attributable risk

Synonymous with **absolute risk difference** (**ARD**) or, more specifically, with **absolute risk increase** (**ARI**). This term is often used in the context of **epidemiological studies**, and sometimes, although incorrectly, as a synonym for attributable fraction. In contrast with clinical trials and intervention studies where treatments and preventive exposures are expected to decrease the risk of adverse outcomes (albeit with the possible occurrence of adverse reactions), **observational** epidemiological studies often focus on harmful or detrimental exposures that increase the risk of disease. The attributable risk is thus the risk difference, $risk_1$ minus $risk_0$ (risk in exposed *minus* risk in unexposed), and measures the excess risk in the *exposed* that is attributable to the exposure. **Exposure effect** is thus expressed in *net* or *absolute* terms. Additional **measures of impact** are the **attributable fraction (exposed)**, the **population attributable risk** (which measures the excess risk in the *study population* – or in a broader population – that is attributable to the exposure), and the **population attributable fraction**. Attributable fractions measure impact in relative or proportional terms.

## Attributable risk percent

Synonym for **attributable fraction**.

## Attrition

See **loss to follow-up**, **withdrawal**, **missing data**. Cf. **enrolment**.

## AUC

Abbreviation for **area under the curve**.

## Audit

A study that is conducted to evaluate the resources/logistics, processes, and/or outcomes of health care services and facilities. The concept of **case mix** is important when conducting audits. See AJETUNMOBI (2002) for a **critical appraisal** checklist.

## Autocorrelation

The **correlation** between the values of a given **variable** across its **observations** (HAMILTON, 1992), when these are ordered according to time or space. Autocorrelation is usually not observed with **independent** observations, but may be present when observations have been made on a time or space continuum, as is the case with **time series** and geographically indexed observations (see **spatial epidemiology**). Serial correlation within a time series may be modelled by employing **autoregressive** and **moving average** response models, or a combination. **Correlograms** displaying the autocorrelation (ACF) and partial autocorrelation or adjusted (PACF) functions may aid in measuring the correlation between present observation and previous observations (up to a given time-lag), and in identifying lags of response that may be useful predictors of present response (HAMILTON, 2012). When **regression analysis** involves additional **predictor variables**, i.e. variables exogenous to the series, the resulting errors or **residuals** may be autocorrelated, and therefore invalidate the assumption of independence that is central to **ordinary least squares** and other regression methods. The analysis of residuals from standard regression models may be useful in understanding the pattern of autocorrelation, as illustrated by HAMILTON with the use of time plots. The **Durbin–Watson statistic** is used to test for first-order autocorrelation [AR(1)] among regression *errors*. Inclusion of previously omitted predictors is sometimes sufficient to address the problem, if present. Autocorrelated errors or 'disturbances' may be further decomposed into a random component (the true residual), and a systematic component due to the underlying autoregressive or moving average process. **Correlograms** may be used to identify the appropriate lags of the errors (from a standard multiple linear regression analysis) that may be included as disturbances (see **autocorrelation model**). Figures A.3a and A.3b show correlograms of monthly locally transmitted malaria case counts, from the study by OSTOVAR *et al.* (2016) seeking to evaluate the influence of meteorological factors on malaria transmission in south eastern Iran. The strongest autocorrelation coefficient is at lag 1 for the unadjusted (ACF) analysis on A.3a ($r_1 \cong +0.6$), and lags 1 and 2 for the adjusted (PACF, adjusted for lower-order time-lags) analysis on A.3b ($r_1 \cong +0.6$, and $r_2 \cong -0.4$). These lags could possibly be used in fitting autoregressive *response* models to the data. The overall trend in the unadjusted analysis is for weaker correlation as time-lags increase. In addition, a cyclic pattern of positive and negative correlations may also be detected, meaning that instances in which high (or low) malaria case counts are associated with high (or low) counts an *x* number of months prior, alternate with instances in which high malaria case counts are associated with low counts (or vice-versa). This seems to be in line with the seasonal pattern of **cyclic variation** of malaria transmission. See also **cross-correlation** (Figures C.3a and C.3b, p. 85).

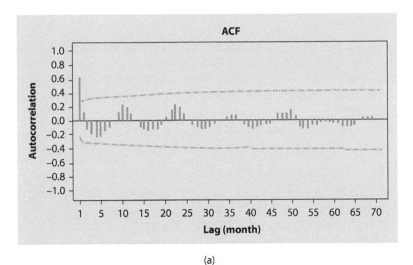

(a)

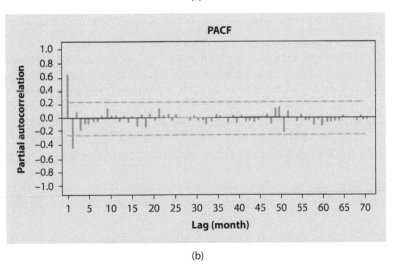

(b)

**Figures A.3a and A.3b** Autocorrelation (ACF) and partial autocorrelation (PACF) functions: correlogram of monthly locally transmitted malaria case count in the 6-year period (2002 cases in total) from March 2003 through March 2009 (Jalali calendar), in the Minab District, south eastern Iran. Graphs show autocorrelation coefficients at different time-lags. (Reproduced from Ostovar *et al.* (2016). Time series analysis of meteorological factors influencing malaria in south eastern Iran. *J Arthropod Borne Dis* **10**: 222–36 (with permission).)

## Autocorrelation model

A regression model for autocorrelated errors or **residuals**, and which includes autoregressive and/or moving average disturbances (e.g. ARMAX model). See also **autoregressive** (and **moving average**) **model**, which is a model that includes lagged values (or lagged errors) of the outcome variable or **time series**. See also **autocorrelation, correlogram, Durbin–Watson statistic, antedependence model**. Also, in reference to a model for continuous **longitudinal data**. See SKRONDAL & RABE-HESKETH (2004).

## Autoregressive model

Or **AR**($p$), i.e. $p$th-order autoregressive model. A **regression model** that assumes time **dependence** for the observations in a **time series**, where a previous value of the series is used as a predictor of present value, and the strength of **autocorrelation** between observations in the series depends on the time-lag between the same. Autoregressive models may be expressed in a number of ways. For example, a first-order autoregressive model [AR(1)] may take the following form (ARMITAGE, BERRY & MATHEWS, 2002):

$$Y_t = \rho Y_{t-1} + \varepsilon_t$$

where $Y_t$ is the value of the series at time $t$ after the mean value has been subtracted (thus, no constant), a coefficient $\rho$ (rho) that is constrained between –1 and +1 reflects stationarity (i.e. stable properties across all time points) for the series, $Y_{t-1}$ is the mean-subtracted value of the series at lag 1, and $\varepsilon$ (epsilon) represents random, uncorrelated 'white noise' errors. If normally distributed, these would be **Normal i.i.d.** errors or **residuals**. The serial correlation between observations is $\rho^p$, where $p$ is the lag or number of time units separating the observations. **ARMA**($p,q$) and **ARIMA**($p,d,q$) (**autoregressive *integrated* moving average** or Box–Jenkins) models include first- and higher-order autoregressive and **moving average** [**MA**($q$)] terms. Moving average terms are a function of past (up to lag $q$) and present errors, and are useful in detecting trends and changes. ARIMA models use differencing ($d$) to achieve stationarity for the time series. Differencing is the computation of first differences (the differences between consecutive observations), to be used in lieu of the original series. Second differences (between observations one and two lags apart) are sometimes also necessary. Seasonal ARIMA models may be fitted, and the simple ARMA model may be extended to include exogenous **predictor variables**; the general term for these models is **ARMAX**. See HAMILTON (2012) for further details and illustrative examples, including guidance in determining the order (i.e. appropriate lags) of a model. See also **correlogram, transition model, antedependence model, forecast**. Cf. **autocorrelation model**, i.e. models for autocorrelated errors (for example, ARMAX), which include autoregressive and/or moving average disturbances.

## Autoregressive moving average model

Or its acronym, ARMA; also, autoregressive integrated moving average model or ARIMA. See **autoregressive model**.

## Average

A general term for a **measure of central tendency**, usually taken to refer to the arithmetic **mean**, unless otherwise indicated. Other measures of central tendency include the **median, mode, geometric mean** and **harmonic mean**. See also **moving average, weighted average**.

## Back-transformation

The inverse process of a **transformation**. The inverse of **logarithmic transformation** is **exponentiation** or anti-logging. In the case of power transformations, the transformed variable, $x^*$, is calculated as $x^* = x^q$ (where $q$ is the power to which the values of variable $x$ are raised), and the inverse transformation is given by $x^*$ raised to power $1/q$, i.e. $x = (x^*)^{1/q}$ (HAMILTON, 1990). For example, the inverse transformation to the square power transformation $[x^* = x^2]$ is the square root transformation $[x = \sqrt{x^*}$, i.e. $x = (x^*)^{1/2}]$. When transformations are applied, data analyses are performed using the transformed variable(s), and back-transformation is applied to the **summaries** resulting from these analyses. A drawback of performing data analyses on transformed variables is the lack of meaning of back-transformed **confidence intervals** for differences between means, the exception being the logarithmic transformation and anti-logged confidence limits (see BLAND & ALTMAN, 1996b). See BLAND (2015) for an illustrative example and interpretation. See also **delta method**.

### Backward variable elimination

See **stepwise regression** (stepwise model selection).

### Balanced design

See **two-way ANOVA** (analysis of variance) for balanced design with and without replication. Cf. **unbalanced design**, in which the cross-classification of the two factors produces cells with an unequal number of observations.

### Balanced incomplete block design

An **incomplete block design** (also referred to by the abbreviation, BIBD) in which the **blocks** are of equal size, albeit smaller than the number of treatments under study. For example, in a **multiperiod crossover trial**, there will be fewer study periods than treatments, and therefore no patient or block receives all the treatments under study. Overall, each treatment is assigned an equal number of times, and every treatment pair sequence occurs the same number of times. See POCOCK (1983) and FLEISS (1999) for further details. Cf. **complete block design**.

### Balanced longitudinal data

Data that are **repeated measurements** over time, taken on each of the individuals or **study units** that comprise the study groups in a **longitudinal study**. Measurements for all the individuals are taken at the same points in time, which are not necessarily equally spaced over time. See also **longitudinal data, serial measurements, repeated measures ANOVA.**

## Bar chart

A **graphical display** of the **frequency** or **relative frequency** of the different categories of a qualitative or **categorical variable**. The height of each bar is proportional to the frequency of the category it represents. It is good practice to separate the bars on the chart, since the 'values' on the **x**-(horizontal) **axis** are simply labels given to these categories, and have no numerical meaning, although some ordering or ranking may be implied (cf. **histogram**). The bar chart in Figure B.1 shows the relative frequency of women wishing to receive epidural anaesthesia at their next delivery, according to whether they received it or not at the present delivery. See also **pie chart, stacked bar chart**. A different utilization of bar charts (the **error bar chart**) is discussed under **dotplot**.

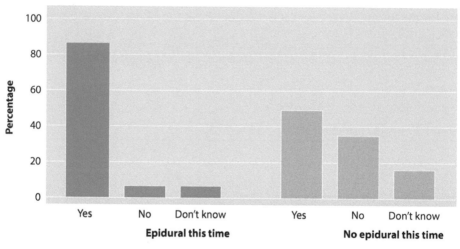

**Figure B.1** Bar chart: percentage of women wishing to receive epidural anaesthesia at next delivery according to whether it was used at present delivery. (Reproduced from Findley I, Chamberlain G (1999). ABC of labour care: Relief of pain. *Br Med J* **318**:927 (with permission).)

## Bartlett's test

A **significance test** that is an extension of the **F-test** and is carried out to compare the **variances** of more than two **populations** with respect to a given measurement (as estimated from the different groups in the study sample). The test is sensitive to non-normality, so **Levene's test** may be a better alternative whenever the measurement in question does not display a **Normal distribution** in the populations being compared. Both tests may be carried out to evaluate the assumption of **homoscedasticity**, or equality of variances, that is a requirement of **parametric tests** such as **analysis of variance**. Care should be taken when interpreting the test's results, as a small **P-value** could be indicative of non-normality rather than unequal variances.

## Baseline characteristics

In the context of **clinical trials** and other comparative studies, this term refers to the distribution of important **prognostic** (or risk) **factors** other than the treatment (or exposure) under evaluation, in each of the different **comparison groups**. Examples are age and gender distribution, average duration of symptoms, disease staging or spectrum of disease severity, comorbidity, concomitant treatments, and additional exposures, including socioeconomic indicators. In small **randomized controlled trials** imbalances may occur due to chance, and may be evaluated by comparing **crude** and **adjusted estimates** of treatment effect. Even with comparable groups, adjustments for baseline characteristics may still be of value in improving the **precision** of estimates of **treatment effect**, if baseline characteristics are strongly associated with a quantitative outcome (POCOCK, 1983). Significance testing for differences in baseline characteristics, however, is unnecessary (SCHULZ & GRIMES, 2002b). Baseline variables that are to be adjusted for in this manner should be specified in advance of the analysis. Sackett, in HAYNES *et al.* (eds., 2006), discusses the importance of prognostic balance in clinical trials, and how it may be achieved through alternative **allocation** strategies to simple randomization. In **observational studies**, baseline imbalances mainly arise due to **confounding**, i.e. they can be systematic rather than random occurrences. These imbalances should be adjusted for by employing appropriate methods (e.g. **stratification** and **multivariable regression**), which may be used also with clinical trials. Cf. adjustments for **baseline measurements** on the **outcome variable**. See also **comparability**; POCOCK *et al.* (2002).

## Baseline hazard function

Or $h_0(t)$. See **hazard rate**/hazard function [$h(t)$].

## Baseline measurements

Measurements taken before the start of a treatment or intervention. These baseline or pretreatment measurements may be included in an **analysis of covariance** or **linear regression model**, and will contribute to reducing the **random error** component of variance in the outcome variable and to increasing the **precision** of estimates of **treatment effect** (see **adjusted treatment mean**). See also **change** (study of), **before–after comparison**, **regression to the mean** (also, RTM in comparative studies), **baseline characteristics**.

## Baseline survival function

Or $S_0(t)$. This function is sometimes given in statistical analysis output in place of the **cumulative baseline hazard function**, $H_0(t)$. The relationship between these two functions parallels that between the survival function, $S(t)$, and the cumulative hazard function, $H(t)$. Thus, $S_0(t) = \exp[-H_0(t)]$. The baseline survival function may be used to compute the probability of surviving time $t$, the **survival function**, based on the linear predictive function ($\eta$) from the **Cox regression** model, as given by ALTMAN (1991):

$$S(t) = S_0(t)^{\exp(\eta)}$$

or equivalently,

$$S(t) = e^{-H(t)} = \exp[-H_0(t) \times \exp(\eta)]$$

## Bathtub curve

Or **failure** rate curve. A curve that depicts the **hazard function** (i.e. the conditional failure rate or force of mortality over time) as having three phases or periods: an early phase (also referred to as the 'infant mortality' period) during which the failure rate declines from a relatively high level, to remain fairly constant at a lower level throughout the intermediary period, which is then followed by the 'wear out' period of increasing failure rate. Given the constancy of the rate in the middle portion of the curve (in which failures are expected to take place at random), time to failure is modelled on the basis of the **exponential distribution**. This pattern is typical of the relationship between age and **overall mortality rate** in human populations, as shown in Figure B.2 (ENGELMAN, CASWELL & AGREE, 2014) with the Siler three-component competing risks model (SILER, 1979). It depicts the additive hazards that result from the action of three different hazard models, each of which dominates during prematurity, maturity or senescence. The age-related types of mortality are known as endogenous, exogenous or residual, and senescent. See also **U-shaped curve**.

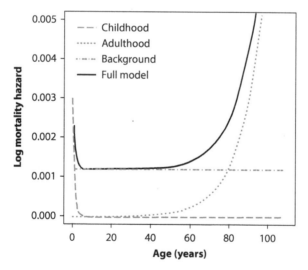

**Figure B.2** Bathtub curve: the three-component Siler model of mortality hazard as a function of age. (Reproduced from Engelman M *et al.* (2014). Why do lifespan variability trends for the young and old diverge? A perturbation analysis. *Demogr Res* **30**: 1367–96 (with permission).)

## Bayes' factor

In the context of **Bayesian inference**, a **likelihood ratio** used in the calculation of **posterior** probabilities for the **null hypothesis**. The factor is the ratio of two **likelihoods**: the likelihood of the data given the null hypothesis (**NH** or $N_0$) *vs.* the likelihood of the data given the **alternative hypothesis** ($H_A$ or $H_1$). The calculations parallel those for diagnostic

**post-test probabilities**, and require the statement of a **prior** probability (which must be accurate) from which the prior **odds** are calculated and multiplied by the factor to give the posterior odds. Unlike the ***P*-value** of **frequentist inference**, the resulting posterior probability makes a direct statement regarding the probability of the null hypothesis being true. Bayesian inference uses comparative rather than single probabilities to measure evidence, and thus eliminates the need to include outcomes other than what was observed (GOODMAN, 2008) (cf. 'the probability of a result of equal *or greater* magnitude if NH were true' in frequentist inference). By extension, any two given models for the same observed data may be compared in this way, which results in the calculation of a posterior probability for each of the competing models, or directly, through Bayes' Factor (*BF*), what is equivalent to the **likelihood ratio test**. In addition to probability values for the null hypothesis, *predictive p-values* may also be obtained, which give the probability of future data being more extreme given the present model. See also **credible interval (CrI)**, **Bayesian information criterion (BIC)**; GREENLAND (2008), SPIEGELHALTER, ABRAMS & MYLES (2004).

## Bayes' theorem

A mathematical equation that gives the **conditional probability** of an event, i.e. the probability that an event will occur *given* that some other event or condition is also present, by relating this unknown probability to the conditional probability of this other event *given* the occurrence of the first event. All quantities on the right-hand side of the equation must be known:

$$\mathrm{Prob}(B \; given \; A) = \frac{\mathrm{Prob}(B) \times \mathrm{Prob}(A \; given \; B)}{\mathrm{Prob}(A)}$$

This formula derives from the interchangeability of the **probability** that both events will occur, i.e. Prob(A *and* B) being the same as Prob(B *and* A), which under the *multiplicative rule* of probability results in Prob(A) × Prob(B *given* A) = Prob(B) × Prob(A *given* B) (KIRKWOOD & STERNE, 2003). The practical implication of the above is that it makes it possible to calculate, for example, Prob(B *given* A), provided one has knowledge of Prob(B), Prob(A) and Prob(A *given* B). These equivalences form the basis for the calculation of the probability of disease given the results of relevant **diagnostic tests**. For example, if we know the probability of testing positive among the truly diseased (**sensitivity**), the probability of disease (estimated by its **prevalence**), and the probability of a positive test result (for instance, the percentage testing positive at a given lab, $[(a + b)/(a + b + c + d)]$, from Table 4, p. 191), we can then calculate the probability of being diseased if the test is positive, i.e. the **positive predictive value** or **post-test probability** of disease for a positive test result. SPIEGELHALTER, ABRAMS & MYLES (2004) and BLAND (2015) provide an illustrative example of these calculations, which are simplified here in terms of Prob(A). See also **Bayesian inference**, **likelihood ratios**.

## Bayesian inference

An approach to statistical **inference** that is based on **Bayes' theorem**. Unlike **frequentist inference**, which is based solely on the data collected in a research study, the starting point for Bayesian inference is a prior belief about the value of the **parameter** (or parameters) to be estimated. This prior belief is usually expressed as a range of likely values, as opposed to a single value, the distribution of which is termed **prior distribution**. The second step is the calculation of the **likelihood function** for the sample **estimate** (as in frequentist inference), which corresponds to Prob(A *given* B) in the equation under 'Bayes' theorem', if we take Prob(A) as the probability or **frequency distribution** of the observed data, and Prob(B) as the probability of the parameter, i.e. the prior distribution. Through Bayes' theorem, these different components are integrated to produce a **posterior distribution** for the values of the parameter, from which a range of credible values may be constructed. The posterior (or joint posterior) distribution is therefore the **probability distribution** of the parameter (or parameters) *given* the sample data [Prob(B *given* A)], as follows (KIRKWOOD & STERNE, 2003):

$$\text{Prob}(\textit{model parameter given data}) = \frac{\text{Prob}(\textit{data given model parameter}) \times \text{Prob}(\textit{parameter})}{\text{Prob}(\textit{data})}$$

The prior belief may be an estimate of the overall **prevalence** of disease, if the usefulness of a **diagnostic test** is being evaluated, or it may be an estimate of **treatment** or **exposure effect** that was obtained from a previous study. The weight given to the prior belief depends on the **precision** with which it is estimated. For very vague prior beliefs, Bayesian and frequentist approaches yield comparable results. The posterior distribution may be used to obtain, for example, a 95% **credible interval (CrI)**, which is interpreted as having 95% probability of containing the true value of the parameter (cf. interpretation of **confidence intervals**). **Bayes' factor** is used to calculate the posterior probability of the null hypothesis being true, and to compare alternative models for the data observed. KIRKWOOD & STERNE point out the usefulness of Bayesian inference when carrying out **interim analyses** (specifically, where treatment effects have not been clinically significant), and also in the analysis of **equivalence trials**. See also BLAND (2015), CLAYTON & HILLS (1993), GREENLAND (2008), and SPIEGELHALTER, ABRAMS & MYLES (2004), ARMITAGE, BERRY & MATHEWS (2002).

## Bayesian information criterion

Or BIC. A statistic that is used in comparing competing **models**, and in particular models that are not **nested**. It is interpreted in a similar way to **Akaike's information criterion (AIC)**, but models with greater complexity are penalized more so for their lack of **parsimony**, i.e. for improving **fit** at the expense of simplicity. ARMITAGE, BERRY & MATHEWS (2002) point out that with large sample sizes, the criterion may be used to approximate **Bayes' factor (BF)**, with BIC $\cong -2 \log BF$.

## BC

Abbreviation for bias-corrected **confidence interval**; and $BC_a$, abbreviation for bias corrected and accelerated confidence interval. See **bootstrapping**.

## Before-after comparison

An estimate of **treatment effect** that is obtained by comparing measurements on the same variable before an intervention and again, after the intervention. Studies using this type of design should nonetheless include a **control group** on whom before/after measurements are also made. This is due to the possibility of **placebo effects**, and also the fact that **regression to the mean** is likely to occur when measurements are subject to **measurement error**. Having a control group helps separate these effects from the actual treatment effect. In addition, a number of different approaches are available for the analysis of **change** from **baseline measurements**. See FLEISS (1999) for further details. Without a control group, before-after comparisons give rise to **paired data**. However, any comparisons thus carried out will have questionable **validity**.

## Begg and Mazumdar test

A test that is commonly used in conjunction with the **funnel plot**, and which provides a formal assessment as to the presence of **publication bias** in the results of a **meta-analysis** (BEGG & MAZUMDAR, 1994). As with **Egger's test**, the aim is to evaluate whether the size of study estimates is related to study size, as results from smaller, poorer quality studies are often overestimated. The Begg and Mazumdar test is based on the calculation of a measure of **correlation (Kendall's tau**, $\tau$) between the estimates of effect and their standard errors (as a proxy for study size). A large **P-value** suggests no evidence of publication bias, or more generally, of small study effects. The test appears to have low **power** when the number of **primary studies** is small. See also **meta-regression**; Sterne, Egger & Davey Smith, in EGGER, DAVEY SMITH & ALTMAN (eds., 2001), STERNE et al. (2011), BLAND (2015).

## Bell-shaped distribution

A **continuous distribution** that is symmetrical about its centre and has a single peak or mode. Well-known examples are **Normal** and $t$ distributions. See Figure N.1 (Normal curve), p. 235.

## Berkson's fallacy

A type of **selection bias** that occurs in **case-control studies**, in particular hospital-based and practice-based studies, when the **exposure** of interest is itself an 'admittable' condition, and admission (or outpatient consultation) rates differ between **cases** and **controls**. The effect of this is to bias the estimate of **exposure effect**, which is then underestimated or overestimated, depending on whether cases or controls have the highest probability of being admitted independently of exposure. A spurious positive association between exposure and the case-control status with the lowest admission or referral rate will be observed where none exists. Stated differently, the case-control status with the lowest admission/ referral rate will show a spurious positive association with the admittable/referable exposure, even if exposure occurs independently of the conditions defining case and control status, and admission/referral rates for all conditions (i.e. the conditions defining the cases, the controls and the exposure) operate independently (ANDERSEN, 1990). Under these circumstances, the case-control status with the lowest admission rate will have a smaller proportion of unexposed individuals than it would have otherwise, and the status with the highest admission rate will have a larger proportion of unexposed than it would have otherwise. Unlike **confounding**, this type of bias cannot be corrected through use of statistical techniques of data analysis. See ANDERSEN (1990) and SACKETT (1979) for further details and examples. FEINSTEIN, WALTER & HORWITZ (1986) discuss how bias may still occur (in the form of a falsely elevated **odds ratio**) when controls are selected from the population, and how it may be avoided by selecting both cases and controls from the community (i.e. from the population), or if the rate of admission or hospitalization rate among controls is zero, in which case 'hospitalization' would no longer act as a **collider**. SNOEP *et al.* (2014) illustrate the structure of the fallacy through diagrams, both in regard to disease-disease associations (as discussed above), and also in the case of indirect exposure-disease associations via an admittable disease or condition other than those defining case and control status and which is associated with the exposure of interest. Use of **incident** (as opposed to **prevalent**) cases attenuates the bias in the latter case (SNOEP *et al.* also reserve the term 'bias' for associations involving incident cases). FLANDERS, BOYLE & BORING (1989) had previously considered the extent of bias when using incident cases. Bias is completely avoided by excluding those hospitalized due to other conditions (i.e. other than the conditions defining case and control status) from study participation.

## Beta

Or β. The probability of making a **type II error** when carrying out **significance testing**. See also **power, sample size** (required). Cf. **alpha** or α.

## Beta-binomial distribution

A **probability distribution** for **overdispersed** binomial outcomes, which show greater variability than is assumed under the **binomial distribution**. Overdispersion is often due to within-cluster or within-subject **dependence** in the number with the outcome of interest (or the number of occurrences of the outcome of interest). A **dispersion parameter** accounts for the related between-cluster, or between-subject, heterogeneity. The binomial distribution is a beta-binomial distribution with dispersion parameter equal to zero. See also **beta-binomial regression**; DIGGLE *et al.* (2002), AGRESTI (2013).

## Beta-binomial regression

An alternative to **logistic regression**, which may be used with **overdispersed** binomial outcomes. A **dispersion parameter** accounts for the extra-binomial variation. The beta-binomial model belongs to a class of models known as *conjugate mixture models*. Alternatively, **random effects** models (generalized linear mixed models) may be fitted, with the cluster-specific random term usually assumed to be normally distributed. For beta-binomial regression, it is assumed to have a beta distribution. See also **beta-binomial distribution**; DIGGLE *et al.* (2002), AGRESTI (2013).

## Beta-coefficient

Synonym for **regression coefficient**. Usually denoted as *b* or β, and subscripted to indicate the **predictor variable** for which it is estimated. Also, a standardized regression coefficient.

## Between-cluster variance

Also, between-cluster heterogeneity. See **intraclass** (intracluster) **correlation coefficient (ICC)**, **overdispersion**, **random effects**. Cf. **within-cluster variance**.

## Between-groups variance

See **analysis of variance (ANOVA)**, *F*-test. Cf. **within-groups variance**.

## Between-subject variance

Also, between-subject heterogeneity. See **intraclass** (intracluster) **correlation coefficient (ICC)**, **overdispersion**, **random effects**. Cf. **within-subject variance**.

## *BF*

Abbreviation for **Bayes' factor**.

## Bias

An error or distortion that can occur in all study designs (irrespective of sample size) in the form of **selection bias**, **information bias** and **confounding**. These are broad categories commonly used in the literature. HENNEKENS, BURING & MAYRENT (eds., 1987) stress the distinction between bias and confounding in that "Unlike bias, which is primarily introduced by the investigator or study participants, confounding is a function of the complex interrelationships between various exposures and disease." (p. 287). These biases are also referred to as systematic errors, as they stem from systematic patterns of sample selection, information collection and relationship between variables that cause study results to be consistently wrong in a given **direction**. Selection and information biases may be *non-differential*, if they affect the comparison groups in a similar manner, or *differential*, if they do not. Non-differential misclassification of exposure and disease status tends to distort an estimate of effect in the direction of the null value. See also SACKETT (1979), ANDERSEN (1990), GRIMES & SCHULZ (2002), and ROTHMAN (2012) for a comprehensive discussion of bias in analytical research. The presence of bias affects the **validity** of study results. See also **measurement bias**, **ecological bias**, **publication bias**. Cf. **accuracy**, lack of **precision**, **unbiased**.

## Biased coin allocation

A **random allocation** method that may be used concomitantly with **simple randomization** to ensure comparable group sizes during a sequential allocation of individuals to the different treatments being compared in a **clinical trial**. For example, in a trial comparing two treatment groups, this is achieved by assigning a **probability** of greater than one-half (i.e. >50%) that the next individual will be allocated to the group with the fewest members. At the times when the allocation process is succeeding in producing even-sized groups, simple random allocation is employed. The name derives from the fact that the toss of an **unbiased** coin has a probability of exactly one-half of landing heads-up or tails-up (assuming that the coin does not end up on its edge), whereas in the case of a biased coin, one side has a greater than one-half probability of landing face up. See also **block** or **restricted randomization**. See POCOCK (1983) for further details.

## BIBD

Abbreviation for **balanced incomplete block design**.

## BIC

Abbreviation for **Bayesian information criterion**.

## Bimodal distribution

As opposed to **unimodal distribution**. This term describes a **variable** whose **distribution** has two **modes**, i.e. two peaks. An example is shown in Figure B.3 (BINNIAN *et al.*, 2016 – data from the US National Health and Nutrition Examination Survey or NHANES, 2011–2012), with the distribution of total urinary NNAL in a representative sample of the US population aged 6 years and over, which includes 4831 non-smokers and 961 cigarette

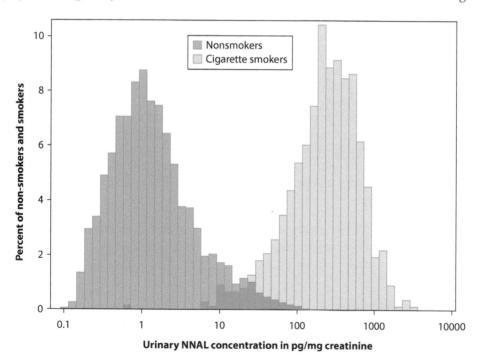

**Figure B.3** A bimodal distribution: total urinary NNAL concentrations in a representative sample of the US population (age ⩾6 years). The overlapping distributions for tobacco smokers and non-smokers are shown separately (NNAL is creatinine corrected and measured on a log scale) (NHANES, 2011–2012). (Reproduced from Binnian W *et al.* (2016). Assessing exposure to tobacco-specific carcinogenic NNK using its urinary metabolite NNAL measured in US population: 2011–2012. *J Expo Sci Environ Epidemiol* **26**: 249–56 (with permission).)

smokers. NNAL is a major metabolite of the tobacco-specific nitrosamine carcinogen NNK, and was detected in 62.2% of non-smokers, and 99.8% of smokers. Values are on average higher for smokers than for non-smokers. As in this example, a bimodal distribution is often indicative of the presence in the sample of two distinct **populations**, with respect to the variable or characteristic being examined. Other examples could be blood glucose levels in a sample that includes diabetics and non-diabetics, or testosterone levels in a sample that includes males and females, for which each of the groups/populations has a distinct distribution, with a different **average** or measure of location, and sometimes also spreading over a wider or narrower **range** of values.

## Binary variable

Or dichotomous variable. A **categorical variable** that takes only two possible values, for example, yes/no, dead/alive, or positive/negative. Such a variable may also result from the dichotomization of a quantitative variable. Binary data are commonly summarized as **proportions**, **risks** or **odds**, and may be analysed using statistical methods for these summary measures, including methods that rely on approximations to the **binomial distribution**. Binary outcomes may also be summarized as **rates**, where the number of occurrences of an event is related to the total **person-time at risk** of the sample of individuals being followed-up. See also **dummy variable**, **nominal variable**, **measurement scale**.

## Binomial distribution

Given an outcome that is a **binary variable** (for example, yes/no) where the probability of occurrence for one of the two possible outcomes (for example, 'yes') is $p$, the binomial distribution is the **probability distribution** followed by the number of 'yeses' (or, likewise, by the proportion of 'yeses'), out of $n$ number of **independent** trials. **Parameters** $n$ and $p$ define the binomial distribution. **Exact probabilities** may be calculated from its **probability mass function**:

$$\text{Prob}(X = r) = \frac{n!}{r!(n-r)!} p^r (1-p)^{(n-r)}$$

where $X$ is a binomial **random variable**, $r$ is the number of successes or 'yeses', and ! represents **factorials**. As the number of trials (or **sample size**) increases, the shape of the binomial distribution (a **discrete** distribution) **approximates** that of the **Normal distribution** (a **continuous** distribution), with **mean** $np$ and **variance** $np(1-p)$. (The approximation holds when both $np$ and $np(1-p)$ are >5.) The practical application of the above is that **estimation** and **significance testing** can be easily carried out with methods based on the properties of the Normal distribution. For example, if we take a sample of size $n$ (the number of 'trials') from a given **population** and estimate the **proportion** of individuals with a given outcome of interest to be $p$, a 95% **confidence interval** for this estimate can be easily calculated based on a Normal approximation to the **sampling distribution** of the estimate, provided the conditions stated above. This application may be extended to comparisons between groups: when comparing the proportions with a given outcome in each of two groups, the large sample **z-test** may be used. A **continuity correction** should be applied in these situations. For smaller samples, the calculations are more cumbersome,

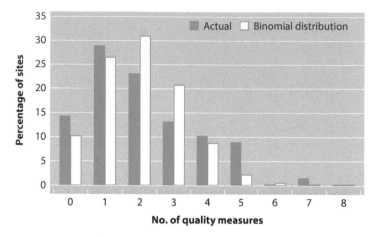

**Figure B.4** Empirical and theoretical binomial distribution, with parameters $n = 8$ and $p = 0.25$ (percentage of sites performing in top quarter for up to eight quality measures of HIV care). (Reproduced from Wilson IB *et al.* (2007). Correlations among measures of quality in HIV care in the United States: cross sectional study. *Br Med J* **335**:1085 (with permission).)

although easy to compute with a statistical analysis package, and involve the calculation of exact probabilities. When sample size is large and $p$ is small (for example, <0.05), the **Poisson distribution** may be used to approximate the binomial. See also **beta-binomial distribution**. Figure B.4 shows the empirical sampling distribution of the number of times sites scored in the top quarter of performance (the 'yes' outcome) for eight different quality measures (the trials) of HIV care, and the corresponding theoretical probability distribution (*number of participating sites*, or number of 'samples' on which sampling distribution is based = 69; $p = 0.25$; *number of trials* or 'sample size' = 8). A **chi-squared ($\chi^2$) goodness-of-fit test** did not find the two distributions to be significantly different, which suggested sites were in the top quarter of performance no more often than predicted by chance.

## Bioequivalence study

An early **clinical trial** aiming to compare the pharmacokinetics of different drugs or formulations, i.e. their distribution in different tissues and organs over a period of time. Subjects are often healthy volunteers, but in cases where the target disease affects the pharmacokinetics of a drug, actual patients may be studied. The **crossover design** is recommended for these studies as it provides better control for individual variability of response through **blocking**. See MACHIN & CAMPBELL (2005) and SENN (2002; 2008) for further details. See also **Phase I trial**, **active control equivalence study**; $C_{max}$, $T_{max}$, **AUC**.

## Biological interaction

Also, biologic interaction (ROTHMAN, 1974). In the context of disease **causation**, biological **interaction** is said to be present when two or more factors act in **synergistic** or **antagonistic** fashion to determine occurrence or prevention of disease. **Statistical interaction** relates to biological interaction, in that heterogeneity of **risk differences** and homogeneity of **risk ratios** both indicate an underlying biological interaction. Biological interaction is thus evaluated as a departure from **additivity** of **absolute effects** (however, additivity of effects does not necessarily imply absence of biological interaction, as interactions may be present that mutually cancel out). When estimates of effect are obtained from **multiplicative models** such as logistic regression and other generalized linear models, biological interaction cannot be evaluated by the simple inclusion of interaction or **product terms**, as the base model is no longer an expression of the independent actions of exposures or predictors, from which a departure may be measured. Such assessments can be misleading, in that any joint or interaction effects that subtract from the starting point of a multiplicative effect would seem to indicate antagonistic interactions, where synergistic interactions exist as evaluated from additivity. The choice of an additive (or multiplicative) model is not equivalent with the underlying relationship being additive (or multiplicative), i.e. absence (or presence) of biological interaction. See Greenland, Lash & Rothman, in ROTHMAN, GREENLAND & LASH (eds., 2012), and ROTHMAN (2012) for further discussion and illustrative examples. The authors also suggest methodology for evaluating biological interaction in **case–control studies** (where measures of absolute effect may not be obtained), and multiplicative regression models (such as **logistic**, **Cox** and **Poisson**), and discuss the evaluation of interaction in the context of public health interventions.

## Biological plausibility

The degree to which a research hypothesis fits in with accepted biological theories. Biological plausibility is considered a criterion for causal inference, although not always listed among the essential criteria. A notable exception is WALD (2004). In recent years, discussion of the role of **science-based medicine** has placed a new emphasis on the need for a solid understanding of biological processes alongside research that is carried out in accordance with sound scientific principles. See **cause–effect relationship**.

## Birth-cohort study

A **follow-up study** in which the common characteristic shared by the members of a **cohort** is time (commonly year) of birth. In Britain, for example, the Centre for Longitudinal Studies houses four such **prospective**, **longitudinal studies**, namely the 1958 National Child Development Study, the 1970 British Cohort Study, the Millennium Cohort Study and Next Steps. See also **cohort effect**.

## Birth rate

The number of live births occurring during a given time-period, in a given geographical region (such as a country), and over the total population size in the same region at the mid-point of the given time-period. The birth rate is often multiplied by 1000 to be given as a rate per 1000 of the relevant population. See also **demographic indicators**, **population pyramid**, **mortality rate**.

## Bivariate analysis

Data analysis that explores the relationship between any two variables, as, for example, a **scatterplot** examining the relationship between two continuous variables. In the context of regression analysis, such a relationship is sometimes referred to as **univariate**, an indication that the predicted outcome is being modelled by a single explanatory or predictor variable. Where two explanatory variables are involved, reference is made to bivariate (or bivariable) regression. The term 'bivariate' (as opposed to 'bivariable') may also indicate the joint analysis of two outcome variables. See also **multivariable analysis, multivariate methods**.

## Bland–Altman plot

In the context of **method comparison studies**, the Bland–Altman plot is a plot of the differences between measurements obtained by two different methods (on the *y*-axis), against the average of the two measurements (on the *x*-axis). The average of the two measurements gives the best estimate of the true value of what is being measured. The technique enables an assessment to be made of the extent of (dis)**agreement** between the methods in question. As shown in Figure B.5a, the **bias** or mean difference between the methods is represented on the plot as a solid horizontal line. When the plotted differences are randomly scattered around this line, their **mean** and **standard deviation** may be used to calculate **limits of agreement** between the methods. These are also marked on the plot, as dotted horizontal lines. If, on the other hand, there is greater scatter or variability of observed differences as the magnitude of the measurements increases, the calculations may be performed on

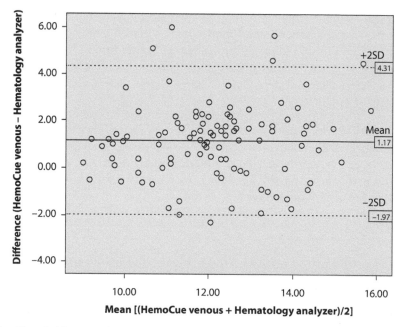

**Figure B.5a** Bland–Altman plot: extent of agreement (as *absolute differences*) between the HemoCue® haemoglobin-meter (using venous blood samples) and an automated haematology analyser in measuring haemoglobin levels in 108 pregnant women at Khartoum hospital, Sudan. (Reproduced from Adam I *et al.* (2002). Comparison of HemoCue® hemoglobin-meter and automated hematology analyser in measurement of hemoglobin levels in pregnant women at Khartoum hospital, Sudan. *Diagn Pathol* **7**: 30.)

the **logs** of the measurements, and the results **back-transformed** to the original scale. This approach gives a measure of relative or proportional agreement, rather than absolute differences, as above, so the limits of agreement now tell us that for any given individual, method A is expected to be within $x\%$ and $y\%$ of the measurement given by method B, as shown in Figure B.5b (SCHERPBIER-DE HAAN *et al.*, 2011). A regression-based alternative approach is given by BLAND & ALTMAN (1999). The example in Figure B.5a is a Bland–Altman plot from the study by ADAM *et al.* (2002) that compares haemoglobin measurements in 108 pregnant women using a portable meter (the HemoCue®) and a lab-based automated haematology analyser. Haemoglobin measurements are used to screen for maternal anaemia, an important cause of maternal and perinatal morbidity and mortality. With regard to the extent of agreement between these two methods (using venous blood samples), the authors concluded that "The mean difference with limits of agreement between the two readings was 1.17 (–1.97, 4.31) g/dl. [...] According to the previously pre-defined clinical acceptable limits of ± 1 g/dl, the 2 methods could not be considered as interchangeable." See also BLAND & ALTMAN (1986), ALTMAN (1991), BLAND (2015), and KIRKWOOD & STERNE (2003) for further discussion and illustrative examples. See also **difference** *vs.* **average plots**.

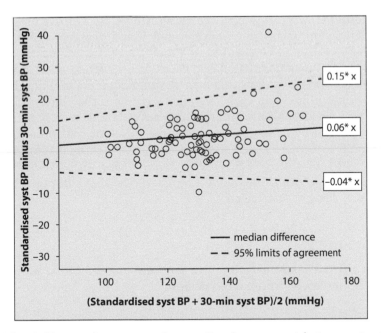

**Figure B.5b** Bland–Altman plot: extent of *proportional* agreement between standardized and 30-minute systolic office blood pressure measurements (OBPM), in 83 adult patients from two general practices participating in an academic research network in the Netherlands. Back-transformed results show that standardized OBP measurements were on average 6% above 30-minute OBP measurements, with 95% limits of agreement between -4% and 15% (i.e. 4% below and 15% above; in other words, standardized measurements were within 96% and 115% of 30-minute measurements for 95% of study participants). (Reproduced from Scherpbier-de Haan N *et al.* (2011). Thirty-minute compared to standardized office blood pressure measurement in general practice. *Br J Gen Pract* **61**: e590–7 (with permission).)

## Blinding

Or masking. In the context of **clinical trials**, whenever participants or researchers (single blind trial) or both participants and researchers (double blind trial) are kept unaware of treatments administered or received. Blinding reduces the occurrence of **assessment** and **response bias** (**information biases**). In trials comparing an active treatment with no treatment, **placebos** should be administered where possible to patients in the **control group**, as any effects observed in the **treatment group** could be, to some extent, attributable to a **placebo effect**. Blinding is not always feasible, as, for example, in some intervention trials, such as a trial comparing a medical treatment *vs.* a surgical procedure. In such cases, whenever possible, a third party should conduct the blind assessment of outcomes and responses (POCOCK, 1983). Cf. **concealment** of treatment **allocation**, in which various forms of masking are used to ensure the allocation of patients to a trial's comparison treatments is **unbiased** (SCHULZ, 2000).

## Block

A group of patients or healthy individuals sharing relevant characteristics and thought likely to respond in a similar way to a given form of treatment. In **clinical trials** and other **experimental studies** in which treatment **allocation** is carried out according to block or **restricted randomization** (**randomized block design**), blocks of size $x$ are formed (where $x$ is chosen to be equal to or a multiple of the number of treatments) to assign a total sample size of $n$ individuals to each of the different alternative treatments. All possible treatment permutations that include $x$ number of treatments and result in an equal number of assignments to each treatment group are then devised, and assigned at random. In **two-period** and **multiperiod crossover trials**, each patient is treated as a block. Permuted treatment sequences across the different trial periods are devised, and then randomly assigned to each study participant. Blocking is a form of **matching** that allows for control of sources of response variability. See ALTMAN (1991), POCOCK (1983), and FLEISS (1999) for illustrative examples. See also **complete block design**, **incomplete block design**, **restriction**.

## Block randomization

Synonym for **restricted randomization**. See also **randomized block design**; cf. **simple randomization/completely randomized design**.

## BMI

Abbreviation for body mass index, which is calculated as follows:

$$BMI = \frac{mass(kg)}{\left[height(m)\right]^2}$$

where 'kg' is kilograms, and 'm' is metres.

## Bonferroni correction

A correction used in the context of **multiple significance testing**, i.e. when several significance tests are carried out on the same body of data. The correction is applied by multiplying each **P-value** obtained by the number of tests performed. If, for example, two groups of patients are compared with respect to three different outcomes (for example, diastolic blood pressure, weight and fasting blood glucose) and a P-value of 0.04 (**statistically significant**, using the conventional cut-off point of 0.05) is obtained for each of these comparisons, the value for P becomes 0.04 × 3 = 0.12, which is no longer significant. The Bonferroni correction tends to give over-corrected P-values as it does not take into account the fact that the different tests being performed are not truly **independent** of each other (they are based on data from the same study units, after all). For this reason, this approach is generally unsuitable for the analysis of **repeated measurements**. In addition to the issue of **multiple outcomes** discussed above, problems also arise from multiple comparisons within different subgroups (**subgroup analyses**). A better use of the Bonferroni correction is in the planning stages of a study (and in particular, when calculating **sample size** requirements), when consideration of the number of tests likely to be performed should inform the **nominal significance level** for the individual tests to be carried out, in order to achieve the desired level of **power** at the desired overall significance level. The latter will be lower (i.e. higher probability of a **type I error**) than the nominal level(s) specified for the individual tests, but still acceptable for the hypotheses being tested. See also **Dunnett's correction, multiple-comparison procedures**. See ALTMAN (1991), BLAND (2015), and POCOCK (1983) for further discussion.

## Bootstrapping

An empirical method of calculating **confidence intervals** (**CI**), which is used in the absence of a suitable mathematical formula, or when the sample estimate of variability (commonly, the **standard deviation**) cannot be considered a reliable estimate of its value in the population. The computations are usually carried out using a statistical analysis package, by taking a very large number of '**samples**' (with replacement, and of the same size as the **study sample**) from the study sample itself. For example, to obtain a confidence interval for the **mean** of some variable of interest, the mean for each 'sample' is calculated. The confidence interval is based on the empirical **distribution** of these 'sample' means, and can be constructed by finding the 2.5th and the 97.5th **centiles** of this distribution (for a 95% CI). This is a simple, straightforward method that is, however, prone to **bias**. For more accurate interval estimates, methods that give bias corrected (BC) intervals and bias corrected and accelerated ($BC_a$) intervals are used instead (KIRKWOOD & STERNE, 2003). Bootstrapping may be used for interval estimation in connection with any other **parameters**, including regression coefficients, and provides a means for interval estimation when **non-parametric methods** are used. It may also be used to carry out resampling analysis as part of **model checking**. This provides an additional assessment of **sampling error**, i.e. the extent to which random variability could have influenced the results obtained (Greenland, in ROTHMAN, GREENLAND & LASH [eds., 2012]). HAMILTON (1992) contrasts bootstrapping and **Monte Carlo** simulation methods: whereas the former uses real data and resampling to derive an empirical **sampling distribution** for an estimate, against which the performance of **estimators** may be compared, the latter uses artificial data to assess the performance of estimators at 'discovering' the parameters of a prespecified model. **Jackknifing** is an alternative method for obtaining **standard error** and **bias** estimates, which, however, does not provide information about the shape of the sampling distribution of the estimate of interest.

## Box-and-whiskers plot

A **graphical display** of the **distribution** of an **ordinal** or **quantitative variable**, which is especially useful when the latter displays a **skewed distribution**. Box-and-whisker plots are also termed boxplots. Figure B.6 compares the distribution of NNAL, a major metabolite of the tobacco-specific nitrosamine carcinogen NNK, among male cigarette smokers, male waterpipe smokers and their non-smoking wives, in rural Egypt. On average, NNAL levels were higher for cigarette smokers, followed by waterpipe smokers, and they also displayed greater **variability** in these two groups. The distribution among non-smoking wives was positively skewed in both instances, and possibly reverse J-shaped among those exposed to waterpipe smoke. The 'box' represents the central 50% of the data, and is further divided in two halves by the **median**. The upper and lower boundaries of the box represent the upper and lower **quartiles** (see **interquartile range** or **IQR**). The 'whiskers' usually represent the minimum and maximum values of the variable in question, except when these are **outlying** observations, in which case the whiskers are made to represent the 'inner fences', i.e. values no further than 1.5 × IQR from the lower and upper quartiles. Outliers are marked individually outside of the range defined by the whiskers; those outside the 'outer fences' (further than 3.0 × IQR from the lower and upper quartiles) are usually identified using a

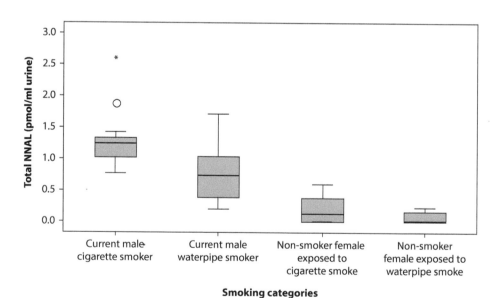

**Figure B.6** Box-and-whiskers plot: distribution of total urinary NNAL concentrations (in pmol/ml) among 26 male smokers (cigarette and waterpipe) from rural Egypt (Delta region) and 22 female non-smokers exposed to either type of environmental tobacco smoke (ETS). (Reproduced from Radwan G *et al.* (2013). Tobacco-specific nitrosamine exposure in smokers and nonsmokers exposed to cigarette or waterpipe tobacco smoke. *Nicotine Tob Res* **15**: 130–8 (with permission).)

different symbol. HAMILTON (1990) gives details on the construction of boxplots. See also **dot plot**, **stem-and-leaf plot**.

## Box–Cox transformation

A **normalizing transformation** for non-negative **quantitative variables**, which is given by the following equation: $Y = (X^{\lambda} - 1)/\lambda$ (BOX & COX, 1964). The value of $\lambda$ is estimated from the data through the method of **maximum likelihood**. As $\lambda$ approaches zero, the transformation becomes the **logarithmic transformation**, i.e. $Y = \ln X$, where $X$ refers to the variable on its original scale. See HAMILTON (2012) for an illustrative example of Box–Cox regression.

## Boxplot

Synonym for **box-and-whiskers plot**.

## Bradford Hill criteria

See **cause–effect relationship**.

## Breslow–Day test

A test of the assumption of homogeneity or constancy of **odds ratios** across the strata of a **confounding variable**. This test is equivalent to the **chi-squared ($\chi^2$) test for heterogeneity** that is usually employed with the **Mantel–Haenszel method** of stratification. HOSMER, LEMESHOW & STURDIVANT (2013) give the corrected formula for the **test statistic**, which also follows a $\chi^2$ distribution when the **null hypothesis** is true, with **degrees of freedom** equal to the number of strata *minus* 1. The test is also equivalent to the **likelihood ratio test** that would be performed for the relevant **product term(s)** in a **logistic regression** model. See also Deeks, Altman & Bradburn, in EGGER, DAVEY SMITH & ALTMAN (eds., 2001).

## Bryant–Day design

A two-stage **Phase II trial** design that incorporates toxicity considerations (which are usually the focus of attention of **Phase I trials**). MACHIN & CAMPBELL (2005) give details.

# C

## C

See **contingency coefficient**.

## $C_p$

See **Mallow's $C_p$**.

## C statistic

Synonym for **AUC** or area under the **ROC curve**.

## $\hat{C}$ statistic

Synonym for **Hosmer and Lemeshow goodness-of-fit statistic**.

## Calibration

A procedure by which measurements that were obtained by means of a method or tool that might be **biased** are compared against an accepted standard. A correction factor for the method or tool in question is derived from such an exercise, often by means of **regression modelling**. A calibration curve may be drawn, allowing the estimated true value for the measurement to be read off, given the value obtained with the biased method. See also **accuracy, measurement bias, method comparison studies**. The term is also used to refer to an assessment of the accuracy of a **predictive model**, as is the case when the **Hosmer and Lemeshow goodness-of-fit statistic** is computed to evaluate the predictive accuracy of logistic regression models. Cf. **discrimination**.

## Capture–recapture sampling

A method for estimating the size of a specific **population**, which is particularly useful when estimating the size of elusive groups such as the homeless, or when assessing the completeness of cancer registries (LAST (ed.), 2001; PORTA (ed.), 2014; EVERITT, 2006; EVERITT & SKRONDAL, 2010). The method is also known as 'capture-mark-recapture' or 'mark-release-recapture' sampling. The estimation is carried out in at least two stages. In the first stage, the initial 'capture', a sample of individuals belonging to the population of interest is obtained and marked for identification, and subsequently released back into the general population (the terminology stems from using such methods for counting animals or insects but the method is also used for human populations). At the following stage(s), an independent **sample** is taken from the general population, and the **proportion** of 'marked' individuals that is 'recaptured' is calculated. Assuming the proportion in the sample is a good estimate of the proportion in the general population, this gives a means of calculating the size of the population.

## Carry-over effect

In the context of **crossover trials**, a carry-over effect is said to have occurred when a treatment given in one of the trial periods continues to exert its effect into the following period(s). It is important to evaluate the extent to which the effect observed in the latter period (and attributed to the treatment given at this time) is a result of, or a response to, the treatment given in the previous period. Carry-over effects may give rise to **treatment–period interactions**, and may be prevented by inserting appropriate **wash-out periods** between treatments. For practical and clinical reasons, *active* wash-out periods are sometimes preferred, where the wait period to begin the next treatment is reduced, and measurement of relevant outcomes is delayed until a more suitable time. SENN (2002; 2008) comments on the **bias** that may be introduced by converting a crossover trial into a **parallel trial** using only data from the first period and discarding subsequent data. Issues around the control and evaluation of carry-over are discussed.

## Case

In the context of **epidemiological studies** and studies conducted in **clinical settings**, a case is an individual who has been identified as having a given disease or condition, according to specific **diagnostic** and **eligibility criteria**. The importance of correctly **classifying** study participants with regard to disease status is to avoid **information** and **selection biases**. In a **cohort study**, a given number of cases will arise over the **follow-up period** among the **exposure** groups being compared. Ideally, these cases should all be included in a **case–control study** based on the same **source population**. (However, the number of **controls** in the case–control study would not equal the number of non-diseased in the source population, as controls are normally sampled or selected from among those without the disease in question.) See also **case series**.

## Case–cohort sampling

See **case–cohort study**. Cf. cumulative sampling, **density sampling**.

## Case–cohort study

A **case–control study** in which **controls** are selected as a **random sample** of the entire **source population** from which the cases arose, at the start of the 'at risk' period. Exposure among controls reflects the exposure distribution among individuals in the source population. As with the **cumulative case–control design**, in a case–cohort study, the **odds ratio** (the **measure of association** between exposure and disease) gives an estimate of the **risk ratio** rather than the **rate ratio** (cf. **density case–control study**), as controls are sampled from the 'total *number* at risk' in the source population, rather than from its total **person-time at risk** (ROTHMAN, 2012). This is true for both rare and common diseases. Unlike the cumulative case–control design, the control group may include individuals who eventually develop the disease of interest and are included also as **cases**. ROTHMAN discusses the practicality rationale for carrying out case–cohort studies (as opposed to using a density-sampling design), and the circumstances under which **risk** in *each* exposure group may be estimated.

## Case–control study

An **analytical observational study** that aims to evaluate the relationship between a disease or **outcome** and one or more **exposures** or **risk factors**. This is achieved by selecting a group of people known to have the outcome or disease of interest – the **cases**, and comparing it with a group known not to have the outcome in question – the **controls** (commonly selected from the **source population** through **random sampling** or through some form of **matching**). All study participants are then assessed with respect to past exposure to the risk factor being investigated. The comparison between cases and controls with respect to distribution of exposure is typically expressed by the **odds ratio**, which may provide an estimate for the **risk ratio** or for the **incidence rate ratio**, depending on the manner in which controls are selected. Risks and rates in *each* exposure group cannot usually be estimated. MIETTINEN (1976) examines this issue and the assumption that the odds ratio provides an estimate of risk or rate ratio only if the disease in question is rare. Differential recall of exposure, and difficulties presented by the process of case and control selection, are potential sources of **bias** in this type of study (see **recall bias/assessment bias [information biases], detection bias/overmatching [selection biases]**). **Berkson's fallacy** is a known cause of spurious associations in hospital/practice-based studies. Proper control of **confounding** effects requires reliable information on potential confounders to be collected. The case–control design is particularly useful in the study of rare conditions and infectious disease outbreaks. Sometimes referred to as **retrospective studies**, since cases are usually patients who have already been diagnosed, case–control studies may also be conducted **prospectively**, i.e. using incident (newly occurring), rather than existing cases. See also **nested case–control study, cumulative case–control study, case–cohort study, density case–control study, case–crossover study**. See **chi-squared test, Mantel–Haenszel method, logistic regression** for data analysis methodology. See **matched case–control study** for individual matching of cases and controls. Cf. **cohort study**. ROTHMAN (2012), MACHIN & CAMPBELL (2005) and KIRKWOOD & STERNE (2013) provide additional details. For a comprehensive presentation, see SCHLESSELMAN (1982), BRESLOW & DAY (1980), HENNEKENS, BURING & MAYRENT (eds., 1987) and Rothman, Greenland & Lash, in ROTHMAN, GREENLAND & LASH (eds., 2012).

## Case–crossover study

A **case–control study** that combines features from both the case–control design and the **crossover design**. The main feature is the absence of a **control** series whose exposure pattern is to be evaluated and compared to that of the **cases**. As with patients in a crossover trial, cases act as their own controls, and the occurrence of the condition of interest is compared between periods of **exposure** and periods of absence of exposure. Similarly also to the crossover design, this design is only suitable in situations where exposure is intermittent, **exposure effect** is immediate and transient and the onset of the **outcome** is abrupt. Diseases or conditions that have an insidious onset are not suitable to be studied in this way. Statistical methods for matched or **paired data** are appropriate for the analysis of case–crossover studies. See MACHIN & CAMPBELL (2005) and ROTHMAN (2012) for further details.

## Case-fatality rate

The proportion of patients with a particular disease who die from it within a given period of time. The case fatality rate (not truly a **rate**, but a **risk**) reflects the **prognosis** for patients with the disease over the specified time-period. This term is more commonly used in the context of epidemics and acute illnesses that can rapidly lead to death. When studying chronic diseases, methods for the analysis of **survival times** are more appropriate as they take into account variable length of follow-up, **losses to follow-up**, and death from **competing causes**. See also **attack rate**.

$$\text{Case-fatality rate} = \frac{\text{number of fatal cases of a disease during a given time-period}}{\text{total number of cases of the disease during the same period}}$$

## Case-mix index

A measure of how **cases** admitted to a given hospital or ward, or seen at an outpatient or emergency facility, are distributed along the spectrum of disease severity for the disease in question. Consideration of case-mix is important in health outcomes and health economics research, and when conducting **audits**, especially when comparing different health facilities. For example, Hospital A may report a higher postadmission mortality rate for disease X compared to Hospital B only because it admits the more severe cases of this disease, whereas cases admitted to Hospital B have a more favourable **prognosis**. See also **severity of illness index**, **prognostic index**.

## Case–Morgan design

A two-stage **Phase II trial** design for trials estimating **survival probabilities**, which does not require prolonged suspension of **accrual** for the preliminary **interim analysis**. Correct specification of the distribution of **survival times** and accrual rate is necessary for the design to operate efficiently. Cf. **Simon designs** and other two-stage designs that monitor binomial probabilities, i.e. response proportions. See CASE & MORGAN (2003) for further discussion.

## Case series

A group of patients (**cases**) – often consecutive hospital admissions or outpatient visits over a period of time – diagnosed with a particular disease, who may have also received experimental treatments or undergone new interventions or procedures, but usually not as part of a **randomized controlled trial**. Observations based on the experience of a case series may raise questions and generate hypotheses that lead to properly designed and conducted clinical trials. See also **anecdotal evidence**, **hierarchy of evidence**.

## Catchment area

The geographical area that is served by a particular health facility. The concept of catchment area is important in **case–control studies**, in particular hospital and practice-based studies, as **controls** should be representative of those who would end up in the same facility as the **cases**, had they developed the disease in question. Catchment area (and therefore, **source population**) is not always easily defined, as in the case of first tier hospitals, which normally receive referrals from far beyond the immediate surrounding areas. In these situations, cases are often *individually* **matched** with neighbourhood controls living in close proximity to the cases, and therefore thought similar to the cases in a number of relevant ways.

## Categorical variable

A **variable** whose values represent different categories or expressions of the same feature rather than numerical counts or measurements. Examples are ethnicity, blood group and area of residence, also known as qualitative or **nominal variables**. A categorical variable with only two categories is termed **binary** or dichotomous (e.g. gender, survival status). Where the categories have an inherent ordering, the term **ordered categorical variable** is used. Continuous and discrete **quantitative variables** are also often **categorized**. Cf. **ordinal variable**, which normally results from the attribution of scores or ranks. Statistical methods for the analysis of categorical data include the **chi-squared test** and the **chi-squared test for trend**, **polytomous** and **ordered logistic regression**, and **log-linear modelling** for **contingency tables**. Additional methods may be used with binary outcomes. See AGRESTI (2007) for a comprehensive overview of the analysis of categorical data.

## Categorized continuous variable

A **continuous variable** that has been converted into an **ordered categorical variable** or a **binary variable** by dividing its range of values into a number of **classes** or levels, in accordance with **quantiles** of its distribution or some other appropriate choice of class **cut-offs**. A categorized variable may be included in regression models as **dummy variables**, with no assumption made as to the shape (linear or otherwise) of its relationship with the predicted outcome. The ease of interpretation of this approach is offset by the loss of information that takes place with categorization and by the loss of **efficiency** when a number of additional parameters (depending on the number of classes, i.e. dummy variables) must now be estimated. In addition, the 'assumption' of sudden changes in risk, for example, to coincide with class cut-off points may not fit the data accurately. Choice of cut-offs or class limits should be made in advance of data analysis, which can also facilitate comparability with similar research. Often, the attempt to identify optimal cut-off points leads to overestimation of effect and spurious statistical significance (ROYSTON, AMBLER & SAUERBREI 1999; ROYSTON, ALTMAN & SAUERBREI, 2005; NAGGARA *et al.*, 2011). See also **trend tests**, **fractional polynomials**.

## Causal mechanism

The mechanism through which causal factors **interact** to cause disease. For every case of disease, there may be a single sufficient cause – the presence of a single **risk factor** – or, more likely, a combination of factors, or the presence of one or more risk factors combined with the absence of other factors. The different factors that make up a causal mechanism or sufficient cause are termed **component causes**. Different cases of the same disease may be caused by different mechanisms. For example, although cigarette smoke is a component cause in a significant proportion of lung cancer cases, lung cancer also occurs among non-smokers, which suggests causal mechanisms not involving first-hand exposure are at work in these cases. Component causes that are involved in a large proportion of cases of a given disease are said to have a 'strong effect', as evidenced by the magnitude of **measures of association** (e.g. **risk ratio**, **odds ratio**). However, **strength of association** cannot be viewed separately from the actual **prevalence** of other component causes (Rothman *et al.*, in ROTHMAN, GREENLAND & LASH (eds., 2012); ROTHMAN, 2012). For example, among groups with occupational **exposures** that cause lung cancer, the effect of cigarette smoke might be weaker than in the general population. See also **cause–effect relationship**, **induction time**, **latency period**.

## Causal model

A **regression model** that is developed for the purpose of identifying **risk factors** with a possible direct causal link with the outcome of interest (i.e. with a clear, un**confounded** and **unbiased** association), usually, the occurrence of a disease or condition of interest, and of estimating the effects of the same. Here, careful consideration of any external knowledge of possible **causal mechanisms** and hierarchical relationships between the explanatory variables under consideration is necessary. Analysis is focused on the assessment of **biological interactions** rather than the inclusion of variables and statistical interaction terms that improve the predictive ability of the model. See also **cause–effect relationship**. Cf. **predictive model**.

## Causative factor

Synonym for **aetiological factor**. See **causal mechanism**, **component cause**.

## Cause–effect relationship

A term that describes the relationship between two (or more) factors that are **associated**, whenever it can be established that one of the factors causes the other through a given **causal mechanism**. Essential criteria for a causal relationship are: a small probability that the association is due to chance (or small probability of a **type I error**), the finding of an association not likely to be due to a **biased** assessment (due to the presence of **confounding**, **selection biases** or **information biases**), and the ability to demonstrate a **temporal relationship**, where cause precedes effect. These and a number of other non-essential criteria are often referred to as the 'Bradford Hill criteria'. Non-essential criteria should be viewed with caution, as they are not always applicable. One such criterion is the **strength of the relationship**. However, a rare **component cause** of a common disease will have a weak association with the disease in question, despite the fact that it participates in at least one of the causal mechanisms for this same disease. Other criteria are the existence of a **dose–response relationship**, the specificity ('uniqueness') of the association, evidence from animal experimentation, consistency with other studies and the **biological plausibility** of the hypothesis put forward. WALD (2004) includes biological plausibility among the set of essential criteria, and adds *reversibility*, i.e. a demonstrable reduction in incidence of disease following a reduction in the level of exposure, as providing further supporting evidence. ROTHMAN (2012) offers some discussion on the relevance of the non-essential criteria. Tugwell & Haynes, in HAYNES *et al.* (eds., 2006), give an overview of the topic, with special focus on the assessment of claims of causation in the context of a number of different **study designs**. See also HENNEKENS, BURING & MAYRENT (eds., 1987), GRIMES & SCHULZ (2002).

## Cause-specific rate

The **rate** or frequency of occurrence of an event (e.g. death) in reference to a particular **cause**. For instance, and for a given **population**, the overall **mortality rate** can be broken down into its components, the cause-specific mortality rates for causes such as cardiovascular disease, accidents, malignant disorders and infections, to name a few, reflecting the health status and susceptibilities of that particular population. Cf. **overall rate**. See also **crude rate**, **age-specific rate**, **standardized event rate**.

## CCF

Abbreviation for **cross-correlation** function. See also **correlogram**.

## CDA

Abbreviation for **confirmatory data analysis**.

## CDF

Abbreviation for **cumulative distribution function**.

## Censoring

In the context of **follow-up studies**, the **outcome** (e.g. death, likely measured as 'time to event') for a study participant is said to be censored if not observed within the duration of follow-up for that individual. This type of censoring is more correctly referred to as *right* censoring and may arise due to withdrawal of participation and loss to follow-up, death from a competing cause or simply because the study in question has come to an end before the outcome of interest has occurred in all participants. *Interval* censoring arises when the exact time at which the outcome occurs is not known, although the outcome is known to have occurred during a specific time interval. With *left* censoring, the outcome has in fact already occurred by the time an individual enters a study. Another situation that may give rise to left-censored observations is when measurements are below their limit of detection. Methods employed in the analysis of **survival times** are often indicated to analyse this type of data. Left-censored data may be analysed using **non-parametric methods** for ranked data (BLAND, 2015). Censoring may be *informative* or *non-informative*, depending on whether it is associated with greater probability of a particular outcome. It may also be *differential* or *non-differential*, depending on whether it affects all exposure groups equally. Informative censoring may be a source of **selection bias** (CLAYTON & HILLS, 1993), in particular if also differential. See also **truncation**, **missing data**. See CLEVES, GOULD & MARCHENKO (2016), and Greenland, in ROTHMAN, GREENLAND & LASH (eds., 2012), for a fuller discussion, including an important distinction between censoring due to **loss to follow-up** and due to **competing causes**.

## Centering (centring)

In the context of **regression analysis**, the shifting of the values of a **predictor variable** so that the **intercept** (the predicted value of the outcome variable when the value of all predictors equals zero) may be given a meaningful interpretation. The shifting may be done by subtracting the **mean** value for a given predictor from the value of each of its observations, or by subtracting an equally meaningful quantity in the variable's distribution such as a relevant quantile. The intercept now represents the predicted value of the **outcome variable** for a value of the predictor variable(s) other than zero (or the mean outcome if the centring was around the mean value of the predictor), and the values of the predictor variable(s) in question are now the differences between the original values and the quantity on which they are centered. Relationships between variables are not altered by centring because shifting, unlike rescaling, does not affect the spread or variability of observations. See ROTHMAN (2012), KIRKWOOD & STERNE (2003). Cf. **regression through the origin**.

## Centile charts

Figure C.1 shows **centiles** of respiratory rate by body temperature, for infants (<12 months), children aged 1 to <2 years, children aged 2 to <5 years, and older children up to age 16 years, from a study by NIJMAN *et al*. (2012) (infants under 1 month were not included). The centile curves give the expected range of variability of respiratory rate. For example, and although lower centiles are not shown, the range of values from the 25th to the 75th

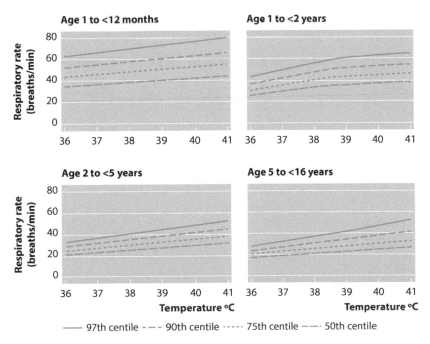

**Figure C.1** Centile chart: expected median and upper centiles of respiratory rate at different temperatures in children, by age group. (Reproduced from Nijman R *et al*. (2012). Derivation and validation of age and temperature specific reference values and centile charts to predict lower respiratory tract infection in children with fever: prospective observational study. *Br Med J* **345**: e4224 (with permission).)

centiles gives a 50% reference interval (at each value of body temperature), and the range of values from the 10th to the 90th centiles gives an 80% reference interval. The 97th centile gives the values below which (at each body temperature value) 97% of respiratory rates are expected to be found. Thus, only 3% of children will have respiratory rates equal to or greater than the value that corresponds to the 97th centile. This type of information can be a useful reference for health care professionals managing episodes of febrile illness in children. The authors have found, for example, that "…cut-off values at the 97th centile were more useful in detecting the presence of lower respiratory tract infection than existing respiratory rate thresholds". See also **reference interval**, **growth charts**. See BLAND (2015) and ALTMAN (1993) for additional details and methodology.

## Centiles

For a given **ordinal** or **quantitative variable** with observations sorted in ascending order according to the magnitude of their values, centiles (or, alternatively, percentiles) are the values of the variable that divide the data values in hundredths. Below each $x$th centile (from the 1st to the 99th), $x$% of the observations is found. For example, and for a given set of measurements, 10% of the observations have values below the value corresponding to the 10th centile. Special centiles are the **median** (50th centile), and the 25th and 75th centiles, also known as **quartiles**. The following numbers are height measurements (in feet) for a group of 13 people. The centiles of this distribution are shown in the row below the measurements:

5.2 5.2 5.3 5.3 5.4 5.4 5.5 5.6 5.6 5.7 5.8 5.9 6.1
    10th      25th         50th        75th   90th

See also **quantiles, tertiles, quintiles, deciles, reference interval, centile charts**.

## Central limit theorem

A theorem that states that when several **samples** of size $n$ are taken from a **population** and the mean for a given variable is computed for each sample, the **sampling distribution** of these means tends to follow a **Normal distribution** with **mean** equal to the population mean, $\mu$ (mu), and **variance** equal to the population variance, $\sigma^2$ (sigma squared), divided by $n$. This observation holds true even when the variable in question does not itself follow a Normal distribution, provided the **sample size** is sufficiently large, and provides justification for the many formulae based on the properties of the Normal distribution, which are used to calculate **confidence intervals** for sample **estimates** and to assess their **statistical significance**. Thus, methods based on **approximations** by the Normal distribution may also be used when the parameters of interest are **proportions** and **counts** (or **rates**), and their differences and ratios. See also **asymptotic** or **large sample method**.

## Central range

A range of values that encompasses a given percentage of the observations at the centre of the **distribution** of a set of measurements, and which is used as a descriptive **measure of dispersion** or **variability**. Central ranges may be constructed based on parametric or non-parametric methods. A 95% central range, for example, may be based on the standard deviation (mean ± 1.96 × SD), or it may be based on the relevant **centiles** of the variable's distribution (in this example, the 2.5th and 97.5th centiles). A 90% central range is *narrower* than the corresponding 95% central range, as it encompasses fewer observations. See also **reference interval, limits of agreement**. Cf. **confidence interval**.

## CER

Abbreviation for **control group event rate**.

## CFA

Abbreviation for confirmatory factor analysis. See **factor analysis**.

## CFD

Abbreviation for **cumulative frequency distribution**.

## Change (Study of)

A particular case that arises in the context of longitudinal or follow-up studies is where a 'pretreatment' or **baseline measurement** for the response variable is taken, as there is interest in measuring the change brought about by a given treatment or intervention. Different strategies may be used to analyse change from baseline. One may calculate a 'difference' or **'change score'** variable and use it in place of the 'post-treatment' response variable, or, alternatively, one may disregard the pretreatment measurement and focus the analysis on the comparison of post-treatment responses. The choice of approach is mainly determined by the degree of **correlation** between 'pre' and 'post' measurements, with analysis of change scores being more **efficient** where there is strong correlation (or stated differently, when the 'change score' variable shows less variability than the 'post' variable). When imbalances are present between **comparison groups** with regard to baseline levels of the measurement, the analysis of change scores will not adequately correct for these imbalances (due to the phenomenon of **regression to the mean**) and the result is a **biased** estimate of treatment effect. Here, the preferred approach is to retain the post-treatment measurement as the response variable, while adjusting for pretreatment or baseline measurements, what is also known as **analysis of covariance** or **ANCOVA** (see **regression to the mean in comparative studies**). In addition, ANCOVA has greater efficiency when compared to the analysis of change scores and the analysis of post-treatment measurements alone, since incorporating baseline measurements in the analysis reduces the **random error** component of variability in the **outcome variable** (the post-treatment measurements), which in turn leads to greater **precision** in the estimate of **treatment effect**. An index of relative efficiency for ANCOVA *vs.* 'post measurement' may be calculated from the correlation coefficient ($r$) between 'pre' and 'post' (FLEISS, 1999) (likewise, it may be calculated for ANCOVA *vs.* 'change score', based on the correlation between 'pre' and 'change'):

$$RE = \frac{100}{1-r^2}\%$$

As the correlation between 'pre' and 'post' increases, so does the efficiency of ANCOVA *vs.* 'post' (BLAND, 2015). The same is true with regard to ANCOVA *vs.* 'change' (using the correlation between 'pre' and 'change'). If the correlation between 'pre' and 'post' is high, ANCOVA will not be much more efficient than the analysis of 'change score'. If it is low (for example, <0.2), **analysis of variance (ANOVA)** of the post-treatment measurements is usually preferable to ANCOVA or change score analysis. Whenever the measurement in question is subject to significant **measurement error**, it is recommended that duplicate 'pre' and 'post' measurements be taken and each then averaged. See VICKERS & ALTMAN (2001), VICKERS (2001), and SENN (2008) for further discussion. See **Oldham plot**, under which the issue of correcting for regression to the mean when evaluating the correlation between amount of change and magnitude of initial measurement is addressed. SINGER & WILLETT (2003) discuss the necessity for more than two waves of data for change to be properly assessed. This allows true change to be differentiated from measurement error (and regression to the mean), and for the shape of individual trajectories of change to be adequately described. Thus, a study in which there are only two data waves (for example, a pretreatment and a post-treatment measurement) is better described as a **before–after comparison**, whereas studies generating three or more data waves are often referred to as **longitudinal studies** of change.

## Change scores

The difference between **baseline measurements** or scores and the corresponding **follow-up** scores. Change scores may be used to analyse the data generated in a **before–after** or in a **longitudinal study**, although it is sometimes preferable to simply incorporate baseline scores as **covariates**. When change scores are taken as the outcome variable, *absolute* and *relative* change may be calculated. However, as described by VICKERS (2001), relative change or *percentage change from baseline* is not the best option in terms of statistical **power**, even when change is proportional to the value of the baseline measurement. In addition, computing the percentage change from baseline will not correct for baseline imbalance. As pointed out by VICKERS, results may nonetheless be *expressed* as percentage change from baseline, if that is of interest, by using mean baseline and post-treatment scores, while carrying out significance testing and estimation through ANCOVA, 'change', or 'post' analysis. See **change** (study of), **before–after comparison**, **regression to the mean** (also, RTM in comparative studies), **Oldham plot**. See also VICKERS & ALTMAN (2001), SENN (2008).

## Chi-squared ($\chi^2$) distribution

The **probability distribution** that is followed by the square of a **standard Normal** random variable, and by extension, by the sum of $n$ independently distributed standard normal variables squared. The number of **degrees of freedom**, $\nu$ or $df$, is given by $n$, where $n$ is the **sample size** (see also calculation of $df$ for **contingency tables**). The shape of the chi-squared distribution changes with $\nu$, from very positively skewed at 1 $df$ to approximately Normal as the number of degrees of freedom increases, with **mean** $\nu$ and **variance** $2\nu$. The percentage points (**critical values**) of the $\chi^2$ distribution (with the appropriate number of degrees of freedom) provide the significance levels for the $X^2$ **test statistic** (Table 1; note that the critical values of the $\chi^2$ distribution with 1 $df$ – identified in **bold** – correspond to the square of the critical values of the standard Normal distribution for the same significance levels). See also **Poisson distribution**.

Table 1 Select percentage points of the $\chi^2$ distribution: values in the body of the table are the critical values of $X^2$, at different levels of statistical significance, according to the number of degrees of freedom

| Degrees of freedom | P-value or α | | | | |
|---|---|---|---|---|---|
| | 10% (0.1) | 5% (0.05) | 1% (0.01) | 0.5% (0.005) | 0.1% (0.001) |
| 1 | 2.71 | 3.84 | 6.63 | 7.88 | 10.83 |
| 2 | 4.61 | 5.99 | 9.21 | 10.60 | 13.82 |
| 5 | 9.24 | 11.07 | 15.09 | 16.75 | 20.52 |
| 10 | 15.99 | 18.31 | 23.21 | 25.19 | 29.59 |
| 30 | 40.26 | 43.77 | 50.89 | 53.67 | 59.70 |
| 60 | 74.40 | 79.08 | 88.38 | 91.95 | 99.61 |

Kirkwood BR & Sterne JA (2003): percentage points give two-sided P-values for 2 × 2 tables, Mantel–Haenszel $\chi^2$ test, and trend test (in each case, $df = 1$). For larger degrees of freedom, the concept of one- and two-sidedness does not apply.

## Chi-squared ($\chi^2$) test

A **significance test** that is carried out to compare two or more independent groups with respect to the **proportion** in each group with a given outcome, and to test for the presence of an **association** between two **categorical** or nominal **variables** (e.g. ethnicity and blood group) or between a nominal and an **ordered categorical variable** (e.g. oral cancer [binary] and amount of alcohol consumption). In the latter case, the chi-squared test for **trend** should be used as one variable is binary and the other is ordered categorical. When carrying out the chi-squared test, the **observed frequencies** (O) are displayed in a **contingency table**, and the **expected frequencies** (E) calculated. This is done for each cell in the table (for Table 2, p. 72, the cells are a, b, c and d). The test is based on the *differences between observed and expected frequencies* across the table cells: the larger the differences (and the test statistic), the smaller the **P-value** produced by the test and the greater the evidence to reject the **null hypothesis** of no difference or no association. (Note that the test is based on the frequencies, not the proportions themselves.) The **test statistic** ($X^2$) is calculated as follows (sigma, $\Sigma$, symbolizes summation across table cells):

$$X^2_{df} = \sum \frac{(O-E)^2}{E}$$

and is referred to tables of the $\chi^2$ **distribution** with the appropriate number of **degrees of freedom** (**df**) for an assessment of **statistical significance**. **Assumptions** for the chi-squared test are **independence** of the observations (i.e. each observation coming from a different individual), at least 80% of the cells with expected frequency >5, and all cells with expected frequency >1. When these assumptions cannot be met, other tests should be used, such as **McNemar's test** for paired proportions or **Fisher's exact test**. The latter is always a valid test for comparing independent groups. **Yates' continuity correction** should be subtracted from the test statistic when the $\chi^2$ test is applied to 2 × 2 tables. The **Mantel–Haenszel $\chi^2$ test** is a special application of the $\chi^2$ test that may be used in the presence of **confounding**. The **z-test** for the difference between two proportions is equivalent to the $\chi^2$ test on a 2 × 2 table. See also **chi-squared test for goodness-of-fit, chi-squared**

**test for heterogeneity, chi-squared test for trend**. An illustrative example is given in Box T.1 (p. 359).

## Chi-squared ($\chi^2$) test for goodness-of-fit

A test of how well a given **theoretical distribution** fits an actual or *observed* **frequency distribution** (i.e. a one-way table). As with the standard $\chi^2$ test, it is based on a comparison of observed *vs.* **expected frequencies**, this time in each class or category of the frequency distribution against the expected count or frequency under the theoretical distribution. **Degrees of freedom** for the test are calculated as the number of categories or classes (or discrete values) in the frequency distribution *minus* the number of parameters that must be estimated from the data (to give the parameters for the theoretical distribution, if necessary) *minus* 1. The larger the test statistic, the smaller the *P*-value, and the greater the evidence against the **null hypothesis** of no differences between observed and expected frequencies, i.e. the greater the evidence of a poor fit. See also **goodness-of-fit (GoF)**, **Hosmer and Lemeshow $X^2$ statistic**.

## Chi-squared ($\chi^2$) test for heterogeneity

A test that is used with the **Mantel–Haenszel method** to test for heterogeneity (i.e. statistical **interaction** or effect-modification) of treatment or exposure effect across the different **strata** of a **confounding variable**. This test is equivalent to the **Q test** that is used in the context of **meta-analysis**. The two tests differ in the way the stratum- or study-level components of the test statistic are weighted, using either Mantel–Haenszel or **inverse variance** weights (see **weighted average**). **Degrees of freedom** for the test are calculated as the number of strata *minus* 1. The larger the test statistic, the smaller the *P*-value, and the greater the evidence against the **null hypothesis** of a constant **exposure effect** across strata. See also **heterogeneity**, **index of heterogeneity ($I^2$)**, **Breslow–Day test**.

## Chi-squared ($\chi^2$) test for trend

An extension of the **chi-squared test** that is used to compare the **frequencies** (or **proportions**) in each of the $k$ levels or categories of an **ordered categorical variable**. The ordered data form a $2 \times k$ **contingency table** with two rows (for the **binary outcome**) and $k$ columns (one for each ordered category, in incremental order). The overall chi-squared statistic ($X^2$) for the contingency table may be calculated using the chi-squared test, with $k - 1$ **degrees of freedom**. This simply tests the **null hypothesis** of no differences between the categories, without taking their ordering into account. However, a trend effect may be present across the categories. To test for such a trend, we perform the chi-squared test for trend (always, with 1 degree of freedom). In addition, if there appears to be a trend, a chi-squared test with $k - 2$ degrees of freedom tests the hypothesis that no other differences, other than due to the trend effect, exist. Furthermore, if the groups are equally spaced, the trend may be said to be **linear**. With generalized linear models (as, for example, logistic regression models), a plot of the **log odds** of the outcome of interest (on the $y$-axis) *vs.* the ordered categories (coded either 1, 2, 3, etc., or expressed as the mean or median value in each exposure group, on the $x$-axis) provides a visual assessment of the existence of a trend (KIRKWOOD & STERNE, 2003). The $\chi^2$ test for trend may be significant even if the overall test is not. Though powerful for detecting linear trends, the test is weak for detecting non-linear relationships. The only sample size requirement for the test is that it be equal or greater than 30. **Kendall's tau** may be calculated as an alternative to the $X^2$ trend statistic (BLAND, 2015). See AGRESTI (2007) for further details. See also **trend** (test for), **dose-response relationship**; cf. **ordered logistic regression** (for ordered *outcome* variables).

## Child mortality rate

LAST (ed., 2001) give a child death rate and a child mortality rate definition. The former relates deaths in children 1 to 4 years of age in a given year to the number of children in that age group (rate per 1000 children 1 to 4 years old); the latter (UNICEF definition, also termed 'under-five mortality rate') relates annual deaths among children under 5 years of age to the number of live births (rate per 1000 live births) in the same year, and averaged over the past 5 years. It is noted that although the child mortality rate is easier to compute in many settings, it is not truly an age-specific rate as the denominator does not directly reflect the size of the population in the age group. See also **infant mortality rate**, **demographic indicators**. See also PORTA (ed., 2014).

## CI

Abbreviation for **confidence interval**.

## Class interval

In the following **frequency distribution** (IQ test results for 120 individuals), an interval such as 120–129 is termed a class interval. The size of a class interval is the difference between successive upper (or lower) **class limits**, which in this case is 10 IQ points. See also **categorized continuous variable**.

| IQ score | n |
|----------|-----|
| 100–109 | 42 |
| 110–119 | 34 |
| 120–129 | 26 |
| 130–139 | 12 |
| 140–149 | 6 |
| **Total** | **120** |

## Class limits

The minimum and maximum values of a **class interval**. For example, for the class interval 120–129 in the IQ example, the lower class limit is 120 and the upper class limit is 129. For a **continuous** measurement, the lower and upper limit of this class interval would be expressed as 120 and <130.

## Classification

The process of grouping people or items according to a shared characteristic, such as a diagnosis of disease. An example of classification in medical research are verbal autopsies, in which children who have died from an unidentified disease are diagnosed retrospectively based on the symptoms and signs exhibited during their fatal illness, according to information later relayed by parents or other care givers. Classification is often carried out through **diagnostic testing**, and through the use of classification rules or models derived from **discriminant analysis**. **Cluster analysis** provides another classification method, which is used to identify classifying categories or groupings when none has been specified *a priori*. See also **discrimination, misclassification, classification table; prognostic index, risk score, severity of illness index**.

## Classification table

A table displaying the '**diagnostic**' accuracy of the predicted probabilities from a **logistic regression** or other **discriminant model**. The layout of the table is similar to that shown in Table 4 (p. 191), with 'test' results (i.e. predicted probabilities) dichotomized by the choice of a **cut-off point**. The probability of misclassification (PMC) or expected error rate may be computed as a summary measure, and it may be estimated by the proportion (or percentage) of incorrectly classified observations (i.e. by the proportion that are **false positives** or **false negatives**). Classification tables aid in assessing accuracy of **classification**, while other measures and tests should be used preferably to assess **goodness-of-fit**. See HOSMER, LEMESHOW & STURDIVANT (2013) for further discussion and formula.

## Clinical epidemiology

A branch of medical research that is mainly concerned with clinical procedures and outcomes, and applies the standards of scientific enquiry to such pertinent problems as deciding which **treatments** to administer, determining the most effective doses of a pharmaceutical drug, evaluating the accuracy and usefulness of **diagnostic tests**, establishing **reference intervals** for biochemical, physiological and other clinical measurements, making predictions on likely **prognosis** based on choice of treatment and on patient and disease characteristics, etc. HAYNES *et al.* (eds., 2006) provide a comprehensive discussion of the subject. See ROTHMAN (2012) for an overview. See also **evidence-based medicine, critical appraisal**. Cf. **epidemiology**.

## Clinical guidelines

A set of precepts and recommendations for the management of patients with a given disease or condition, which are devised to ensure and promote high-standard quality of care in everyday practice. Clinical guidelines should be based on evidence stemming from sound research, and are a particular focus of health services research. See also **clinical epidemiology, evidence-based medicine, hierarchy of evidence, GRADE approach**. Haynes, in HAYNES *et al.* (eds., 2006), discusses the evaluation of quality improvement interventions.

## Clinical measurement

An evaluation made in a clinical or research setting, which provides a measure of a patient's condition and responses to treatments, and also of any and all factors and characteristics that may influence the same. Clinical measurement is subject to both **random** and **systematic error**, the former arising in large part due to natural biological variation. Systematic error, on the other hand, may be due to measurement tools and methods that consistently deviate in a given direction from the 'true' value of what is being measured. The **reliability** of measurements (or assessments) that are subject to random error (i.e. fluctuation) is evaluated through the computation of indices of reliability. These include the **intraclass correlation coefficient** and the **kappa statistic**. **Diagnostic performance** studies are carried out to evaluate the **accuracy** of diagnostic tests, and **calibration** and **method comparison** studies the extent of **measurement bias** between different methods or tools. These assessments are an important component of **clinical epidemiology**. See BLAND (2015) for an overview of issues relating to clinical measurement. POCOCK (1983) discusses steps that may be taken to reduce measurement errors and biases when conducting clinical trials, in order to ensure reproducibility. The discussion extends to clinical assessments and subjective patient responses. See also KIRKWOOD & STERNE (2003), ALTMAN (1991), and DUNN & EVERITT (1995). Additional discussion may be found under **misclassification, measurement error, measurement bias, regression dilution bias, regression to the mean, information bias**.

## Clinical significance

A **treatment** (or exposure) **effect** is said to be clinically significant if it is of sufficiently large magnitude as to impact on disease and other health-related outcomes to an important extent. A decision about clinical (or public health) significance requires a judgement as to what constitutes a large enough effect (see **minimally important difference** or **MID**). An effect that is **statistically significant** may nonetheless be too small to warrant any changes in treatment or other policies, in which case the same result cannot be considered to be clinically significant. The converse may occur, i.e. clinical significance without statistical significance. This last situation may be avoided by having **study samples** of appropriate **size**. **Confidence intervals** can help assess the clinical significance of study results (Box C.1, p. 69). See Sackett, in HAYNES *et al.* (eds., 2006), for further discussion. See also **negative study, positive study**.

## Clinical trial

A **comparative, experimental study** in which researchers intervene in the **natural course of a disease**, by administering drugs or other treatments/interventions to at least one of the study groups, after which patients' responses are measured or assessed and **treatment effects** estimated. The benchmark for clinical trials is the **randomized controlled trial (RCT)**. The term may also be used in reference to non-comparative studies (e.g. **Phase I** and **Phase II trials** for drug development), but often it is used to refer to the equivalent of a **Phase III trial** (see ARMITAGE, BERRY & MATHEWS, 2002). POCOCK (1983) discusses a number of issues relating to the design, conduct and analysis of clinical trials, including historical background, rationale, ethics and trial monitoring. MACHIN & CAMPBELL (2005) provide details of study designs for Phases I, II and III trials. Sackett, in HAYNES *et al.* (eds., 2006), offers detailed guidance on the planning, conduct, analysis and interpretation of therapeutic trials. Non-drug trials (surgical trials in particular) and ethical considerations are also discussed. SENN (2008) gives a comprehensive discussion of relevant issues, with special focus on drug trials. See also **equipoise, informed consent**, trial **phases**, trial **protocol, superiority trial, equivalence trial, non-inferiority trial, study design, sample size** (required), **placebos, compliance, multicentre trial, megatrial**. See **CONSORT statement** for reporting guidelines.

## Closed sequential plans

See **sequential designs**.

## Cluster analysis

A **multivariate method** (also known as unsupervised pattern recognition in artificial intelligence language) that is employed for the purpose of **classification**. Individuals who are 'close' together on the basis of their 'profiles' are classified as being in the same cluster or group. The groups into which individuals are to be classified are not known or defined *a priori*, rather, their recognition stems from the analysis itself. The term 'profile' refers to a set of measurements pertaining to a single individual. These may be **repeated measurements** on a single variable, measurements on a number of different variables, or a combination of both. An example are the set of facial trait and brain structure measurements in studies seeking to identify clinical subgroups (in terms of symptoms and severity) or subtypes of autism, on the basis of measurements obtained from 3D facial scans and structural brain MRIs. Cf. **discriminant analysis**, which classifies into *known* groups. See HAMILTON (2012) for further details and illustrative examples.

## Cluster randomization

A **random allocation** method that assigns all individuals in a given group or cluster (the **study unit**) to the same treatment or intervention. This is done mainly for practical reasons. For example, in a **community trial** on the relationship between vitamin C supplementation and incidence of influenza in school children, parents of children not receiving vitamin C may object to having other children in the same school receive a potentially beneficial intervention. If parents decide to give vitamin C to their children outside of trial **protocol**, this could result in contamination of the **control group**. **Sample size** calculations and data analysis will need to take into account the fact that the study unit is the cluster, not the individual. See MACHIN & CAMPBELL (2005) for an overview, and ELDRIDGE & KERRY (2012) for a comprehensive guide to the design, conduct, analysis and reporting of cluster randomized trials in health services research. Grieve (in ELDRIDGE & KERRY, 2012) discusses systematic reviews, cost-effectiveness analyses, process evaluation, and monitoring issues. See **clustered designs**, **clustered data**, **design effect**, **effective sample size**, **intraclass correlation coefficient** (**ICC**), **stepped wedge design**. See also **CONSORT statement**.

## Cluster randomized trial

Or its abbreviation, CRT. An **intervention study** in which treatment allocation is carried out by **cluster randomization**.

## Cluster sampling

A **sampling** method in which entire groups of people are treated as the **sampling units**, as opposed to **simple random sampling** in which individuals are the sampling units. Typically, entire households, communities, schools or general practices are sampled. When calculating **sample size** requirements for a study using a cluster sampling scheme, adjustments should be made to the formulae commonly used. The **effective sample size** of the study will be smaller than the total number of individuals in the study. See **clustered designs, clustered data, intraclass correlation coefficient (ICC)**.

## Clustered data

Or multilevel data. Data that arise from **clustered designs**, including those that generate **serial** and **repeated measurements**. The shared feature of these data is the lack of **independence** of within-cluster observations, which requires special methods to be used in their analysis. A straightforward approach is the calculation of **summary measures** within each cluster (the cluster being the **study unit**), a data reduction strategy that results in a single observation per cluster. These summaries may then be analysed using standard methods for independent or uncorrelated data. Advanced methods include **multilevel** or **random effects models**, and **repeated measures analysis of variance**, which allow the hierarchical structure of the data to be taken into account. KIRKWOOD & STERNE (2003) discuss additional approaches to the analysis of clustered data that include **generalized estimating equations (GEEs)** and use of **robust standard errors**, in addition to the limitations or disadvantages of the summary measures approach. Inclusion of cluster-level and individual-level characteristics in random effects models is also discussed. Clustering creates a **design effect** that should be taken into account in the planning stages of a study, when calculating **sample size** requirements. The **effective sample size** of a clustered design is reduced, as compared to a study of equal size in which the data are unclustered. Ignoring the effect of clustering is likely to cause spurious **precision** in the study results (small standard errors, narrow confidence intervals) and spurious **statistical significance** (small $P$-values). The magnitude of the design effect is determined in part by the **intraclass**, or more precisely, *intracluster* **correlation coefficient (ICC)**.

## Clustered designs

**Study designs** in which the **study units** are groups or clusters, each cluster comprising a number of individuals who share certain risk or prognostic factors. Intervention studies in which allocation is carried out by **cluster randomization**, and observational studies using **cluster sampling** schemes are common examples. A special case of the clustered design is where **serial** or **repeated measurements** are taken on a group of individuals, in which case the individual represents the cluster or grouping of repeated measurements (see **longitudinal study**). Clustering may also be a factor in studies in which individuals share family, geographic and socioeconomic membership, as individuals within each group may be reasonably expected to share many relevant characteristics, owing to a common genetic makeup, and to similar environmental exposures, including diet and other lifestyle behaviours. This type of study design gives rise to data with particular characteristics (**clustered data**), and which should be analysed using appropriate methodology. In addition, a **design effect** must be factored into **sample size** calculations, as clustering reduces the **effective sample size**. See also **intraclass correlation coefficient (ICC)**.

## Clustering

A disease distribution pattern in which multiple **cases** are identified, all closely linked with respect to time, person or place. This clustering may be mapped (disease mapping), which helps elucidate disease **causation**, as in, for example, the clustering identified during the 1980s of AIDS cases among certain high-risk groups. Clustering requires the utilization of special methods of statistical analysis. See also **spatial epidemiology, small area estimation**. See ARMITAGE, BERRY & MATHEWS (2002) for a comprehensive overview, and Hertz-Picciotto, in ROTHMAN, GREENLAND & LASH (eds., 2012), and ELLIOTT & WARTENBERG (2004) for an in-depth discussion.

## $C_{max}$

The highest concentration of drug (usually in the blood) for an individual subject over a specified length of time, following the administration of a medical treatment or some other intervention. See also **serial measurements, repeated measurements analysis, summary measures, $T_{max}$, area under the curve, bioequivalence study, Phase I trial**.

## Cochrane Collaboration

A non-profit organization named after Archie Cochrane, which aims to promote evidence-informed health decision-making by producing **systematic reviews** and other synthesized research evidence. According to their web site (www.cochrane.org; accessed 12/2016), "We gather and summarize the best evidence from research to help make informed choices about treatment. [...] (Established in 1993,) Cochrane is a global independent network of researchers, professionals, patients, carers, and people interested in health. Cochrane contributors – 37,000 from more than 130 countries – work together to produce credible, accessible health information that is free from commercial sponsorship and other conflicts of interest. [...]" TURNER *et al.* (2013) give an overview of the Cochrane Collaboration's contributions to the assessment of bias in systematic reviews of interventions. HIGGINS & GREEN (eds., 2008) give comprehensive guidance for the conduct of systematic reviews of interventions. See also **evidence-based medicine**.

## Coefficient

See **correlation coefficient, regression coefficient**.

## Coefficient of concordance

Usually denoted by $W$, the coefficient of concordance is a measure of the extent of **agreement** among a number of raters assigning **ranks** to individuals in a group, with respect to a given characteristic. $W$ is calculated as follows:

$$W = 12S/[m^2(n^3 - n)]$$

where $m$ is the number of raters, $n$ is the number of individuals being ranked, and $S$ is the sum of $d^2$ across all individuals, where, for each individual, $d$ = (sum of the ranks assigned by each rater) − [$m(n + 1)/2$]. $W$ can take any value from 0 to 1, with 1 indicating perfect agreement between raters. See also **kappa statistic**.

## Coefficient of determination

Synonym for **r-squared** ($r^2$) and $R^2$ (coefficient of multiple determination – see **multiple correlation coefficient**).

## Coefficient of dispersion

Synonym for **coefficient of variation**.

## Coefficient of variation

A measure of **relative dispersion** that is calculated as the ratio between the **standard deviation** and the **mean** of a set of measurements. It is sometimes used as a measure of the **repeatability** of a measurement method. In this context, the coefficient of variation (CV) is calculated by taking replicate measurements with the method in question (in respect of a variable of interest), and dividing the 'standard deviation of the measurement errors' (see **repeatability**) by the **mean** of *all* measurements, initial and repeated (see BLAND [2015] and BLAND & ALTMAN [1996c], for an alternative methodology based on a **logarithmic transformation** of the data). The CV is unitless and is sometimes multiplied by 100 and expressed as a percentage. This measure is most useful when the error of the method is proportional to the magnitude of the measurements, otherwise the standard deviation of the measurement errors (also known as 'standard error of measurement' or SEM) should be used.

## Cofactor

A **categorical variable** that is **adjusted** for when measuring the association between exposure and disease. See also **covariate**.

## Cohen's *d*

A standardized measure of the difference between two **means**, often employed in the context of **meta-analysis**. The common estimate of **standard deviation** (**SD**) is used as the scaling factor. See **standardized difference**, **standardized measures of effect**, **effect size**, **weighted average**. See also **Hedge's adjusted *g*** and **Glass's Delta** (Δ).

## Cohort

A group of individuals sharing some common characteristic, which is followed up in a research study for a specified length of time. In studies of **prognosis**, an 'inception cohort' of patients newly diagnosed, or in the early stages of treatment, can give a more accurate estimate of the true probability of **survival** (Guyatt, in HAYNES *et al.* [eds., 2006]). A distinction is made between closed or *fixed* cohorts (such as the study group in a clinical trial), where membership is closed off once participants have been selected (although the size of the group may decrease over time due to **failure**, withdrawals or losses to follow-up, but usually not due to a study participant leaving a given geographical area), and open or *dynamic* cohorts, where individuals are allowed to enter and exit the cohort throughout the duration of a study, through births, deaths, loss to follow-up and migration.

Dynamic cohorts do not allow for the calculation of risks, but **rates** may be calculated based on the **person-time** contribution of each person in the cohort. Fixed cohorts allow the calculation of **risks** if duration of **follow-up** is relatively short and follow-up is complete for all study participants. See also **birth cohort**, **cohort effect**, **cohort study** (general population cohort *vs.* special exposure cohort), **follow-up study**. ROTHMAN (2012) provides additional details and discussion.

## Cohort effect

A health-related pattern or trend manifested among members of a **cohort**, which differs from patterns seen in cohorts with different characteristics. This term is often used in reference to **birth cohorts**, each exposed to unique environmental, nutritional, socioeconomic and cultural factors, which interact to determine health status and disease susceptibility.

## Cohort study

An **analytical observational study** that is carried out to investigate the relationship between an **exposure** (**risk** or **preventive factor**) and one or more diseases or **outcomes**. In a cohort study, the exposure status of each member of the **cohort** is established at the outset of the investigation. Depending on the **prevalence** of the exposure being studied, exposure status may be determined subsequently to study group selection (*general population cohorts*), or it may be used as a selection criterion (*special exposure cohorts*) to ensure adequate numbers in all exposure categories (ROTHMAN, 2012). In the latter case, selection of controls may be carried out through some form of **matching** in order to minimize potential **confounding** effects. The ascertainment of exposure status establishes subcohorts, which will then be followed up for a given period of time, the '**follow-up period**' or 'time at-risk', during which the **incidence** of one or more diseases is measured in each of the subcohorts. Potential difficulties are the high cost and lengthy duration of investigations, as a relatively large number of study participants and sufficiently long follow-up periods are often required. **Censoring** and **losses to follow-up** (which may result in **selection bias**) and surveillance bias (see **information bias**) are potential sources of error with this study design. Cohort studies are sometimes termed **prospective**, although this term can also be applied to **case–control studies** that are conducted with newly-occurring cases of disease. In addition, cohort studies may be conducted **retrospectively** using existing data (from occupational records, for example). ROTHMAN (2012) points out that cohort studies may be viewed as case–control studies in which the **source population** is sampled in its entirety. Whether looking at newly arising or at existing data, cohort studies take place on a **longitudinal** time frame, which allows researchers to be sure that exposure has preceded disease by a reasonable length of time, based on knowledge of the average **induction time** for the exposure or component cause being studied. In cohort studies, **exposure effect** is usually estimated from **risk** and **rate** measures, depending on whether a uniform follow-up period allows for the calculation (in each subcohort) of risk measures – based on the total **number at risk**, or varying length of follow-up simply allows for the calculation of rate measures – based on the total **person-time at risk**. In addition to simple comparisons of risks and rates, **stratification** and **standardization**, **Poisson regression**, and methods for **survival analysis** are all frequently used in the analysis of data stemming from cohort studies. See Rothman, Greenland & Lash, in ROTHMAN, GREENLAND & LASH (eds., 2012),

HENNEKENS, BURING & MAYRENT (eds., 1987) and BRESLOW & DAY (1987) for a comprehensive presentation. See ROTHMAN (2012) and MACHIN & CAMPBELL (2005) for an overview. Cf. **case–control study, cross-sectional study**.

## Collapsibility

See **non-collapsibility**.

## Collider

A variable that is a *common effect* of two *distinct causes* (e.g. exposure and disease). Data analysis strategies commonly used to adjust for **confounders** (which, on the other hand, are *common cause* of exposure and disease) are not appropriate in this case, and may result in spurious **associations** between the causes in question. An example of a collider is 'hospitalization', which may result in **Berkson's fallacy** in hospital-based case–control studies. The 'causes' here are the disease defining case or control status and the exposure of interest, itself an 'admittable' condition. When controls are selected from the population, 'hospitalization' still acts as a collider, inflating or alternatively leading to a spurious positive association between the case disease and the exposure disease, unless the hospitalization rate among controls is zero (FEINSTEIN, WALTER & HORWITZ, 1986).

## Collinearity

In the context of **multiple** or **multivariable regression** analysis, collinearity is said to be present when there is perfect **association** between **predictor** or **explanatory variables** in a regression **model**. In other words, collinear predictors vary in concert, and fully account for each other's effect. More frequently, predictor variables are simply **correlated** or highly correlated, where a variable accounts only in part for another's effect (e.g. different socioeconomic variables). The presence of highly correlated variables in the same regression model is often unnecessary and produces large **standard errors** for the estimated **regression coefficients**, which reflects an undesirably high degree of uncertainty. This might wrongly suggest that neither variable is associated with the **outcome variable**, even when an association does exist. In addition, estimates of effect (the coefficients) will often be distorted, and thus are rendered meaningless. Their joint effect, however, may still give an accurate measure of effect for the underlying 'variable' that is doubly represented (KIRKWOOD & STERNE, 2003). **Exploratory analyses** should be performed prior to **model specification** and **model fitting** to help clarify the relationships between predictor variables, and between outcome and each of the predictors. See also **correlation matrix**.

## Community intervention trial

An **intervention study** in which entire groups or communities are assigned to one of a number of interventions being compared. All **eligible** members of a community are assigned the same intervention. The main purpose of community trials is similar to that of **field trials**, and that is to measure the effect of **exposure** to **preventive factors** in 'non-diseased' individuals. In contrast, individuals participating in **clinical trials** are usually diseased, and the outcome of interest is not prevention or occurrence of disease, but prevention or occurrence of an adverse disease outcome. Community trials are carried out preferentially to field trials if the **control group** is likely to become 'contaminated', with individuals in this group ending up experiencing the intervention under study. In this type of study, **cluster randomization** is the method utilized for treatment **allocation**, and the **clustered** nature of the **data** must be taken into account when calculating sample size requirements and analysing study results.

## Comparability

The degree of similarity between the **comparison groups** in a research study, with respect to relevant **baseline characteristics**. Comparability is a necessary condition for the internal **validity** of study results. Where it is lacking, **adjustments** are usually made at the data analysis stage to minimize the resulting **bias**. See POCOCK (1983) and Sackett, in HAYNES *et al.* (eds., 2006), for further discussion.

## Comparative study

A research study whose goal is to estimate **exposure** and **treatment effects** by comparing groups in which these factors are present or absent, or present in varying degrees, while all other relevant factors are kept as similar as possible, either by virtue of the **study design** (as in a **randomized controlled trial**, or a **cohort study** in which controls are selected through **matching**) or through the use of appropriate statistical techniques such as **stratification** (for example, to analyse the results from a **case–control study**). Paradoxically, the greater comparability that is achieved through matching in a case–control study can in turn be a source of **bias**. The term 'comparative study' is also used to refer specifically to analytical observational studies, as opposed to randomized trials (HILLS, 1974).

## Comparison group

In a **comparative study**, the **control** or comparison group is the group of individuals that provides a standard of comparison for the group that has the **exposure** under investigation, or is assigned the **active treatment**, experimental treatment or **intervention** in a trial. The expression 'comparison groups' is usually in reference to *all* study groups, i.e. all treatment or exposure groups.

## Competing cause

Or competing risk. A cause, other than the exposure or treatment under study, which results in the occurrence of the event of interest in a **follow-up study**, thus preventing an assessment to be made as to whether the same **outcome** would still have occurred in connection with the factor being investigated, or as to how long it would have taken for the event of interest to have been observed in connection with this same factor. When length of follow-up is relatively short, competing causes are less likely to be an intervening factor in the assessment that is underway of the relationship between exposure and disease (or adverse outcome), and **incidence** (or mortality) **risks** (including **attack rates** and **case-fatality rates**) may be calculated. However, the longer the follow-up period, the greater the probability that the outcome for some of the study participants will be **censored**, due to competing causes and also due to **losses to follow-up**. In these studies, disease occurrence and occurrence of adverse outcomes are usually measured as incidence or mortality **rates**, and methods for **survival analysis** give estimates of survival probability.

## Complement

For a fraction or **percentage** whose values range from 0 to 1 (or 0% to 100%), the complement is calculated as 1 *minus* the fraction (or 100 *minus* the percentage). For example, and in the context of **diagnostic testing**, the **false-positive rate** is the complement of **specificity**, and thus it is calculated as 100 − specificity%.

## Complementary log-log transformation

A **transformation** that can be applied to **proportions**, as an alternative to the **logit** transformation. Unlike the latter, this transformation is asymmetrical around $p = 0.5$. The complementary log-log transformation of a proportion ($p$) is $\ln[-\ln(1 - p)]$, where **ln** is the natural logarithm (that is, a logarithm to base $e$). This transformation is particularly useful in the analysis of results from toxicology and titration studies (involving the assessment of **dose–response relationships**), and in the analysis of grouped survival data where **proportionality of hazards** is assumed. See also **arcsine square root** transformation, **probit** transformation; AGRESTI (2013).

## Complete block design

A **study design** for an **experimental study** in which complete **blocks** are used to provide control for one or more sources of response variability (other than the factor or factors under study). A complete block is one that has size equal to, or a multiple of, the number of treatments under study (e.g. **randomized block design**), or equal to the number of trial periods, where the number of periods equals the number of treatments under study (e.g. **multiperiod crossover trial**). See also **Latin square**. Cf. **incomplete block design**.

## Completely randomized design

A **study design** for a **clinical trial** or other experimental study in which patient or **study unit** allocation to the different treatments or interventions is carried out by **simple randomization**. Cf. **randomized block design/restricted randomization**, **stratified randomization**.

## Compliance

The extent to which patients follow prescribed treatments regimens. Compliance is important not only in clinical practice, but also in the context of **clinical trials**. Lack of compliance is an important determinant of **effectiveness** as measured by **treatment effect**. POCOCK (1983) discusses factors affecting patient compliance, and strategies for measuring and improving it. See also Sackett, in HAYNES *et al.* (eds., 2006), and HENNEKENS, BURING & MAYRENT (eds., 1987). See **adverse reaction**, **concomitant treatment**, **pragmatic trial**, **intention-to-treat analysis**.

## Component bar chart

Synonym for **stacked bar chart**.

## Component cause

Each of the different factors that **interact** under a given **causal mechanism** or sufficient cause of disease. Component causes such as smoking, diet and occupational exposures are environmental or external, whereas others are genetic, i.e. they reflect a biological predisposition for a particular disease, as is the case with cystic fibrosis. Each component cause that is part of a specific causal mechanism plays a *necessary* role, which may be causative or preventive (ROTHMAN, 2012). However, there may be cases of the same disease in which any one of those same component causes does not play a role, as a different causal mechanism is involved. Component causes that are part of the same causal mechanism play different roles in the **natural history of disease**, with some *predisposing* an individual to the actions of subsequent or concomitant components (for example, genetic or hereditary factors; low immunity), while others *precipitate* the clinical manifestation of the disease (for example, a fall or an infection). As discussed under **causal mechanism**, the **strength of relationship** between individual component causes and disease must be evaluated in context. See also **induction time, latency period**.

## Composite score

A score that is computed by adding or averaging scores. The latter are given by each of the component subscales that form a composite scale. Subscales are often **Likert scales**, each measuring a different aspect or feature of the same trait, commonly, a **latent variable**. Examples are the intelligence quotient (IQ) score, made up of component verbal and performance scores, and the APGAR score, in which the component subscales measure heart rate, breathing, muscle tone, skin colouration and response to stimuli, all seeking to evaluate the vitality of a newborn. Methods suitable for **quantitative** and **ordinal data** are usually indicated in the analysis of composite scores. BLAND (2015) illustrates the construction of composite scales and the evaluation of their internal consistency. See also **Cronbach's alpha, factor analysis, principal components analysis**.

## Compound symmetry

See **correlation structure**.

## Concealment

More specifically, concealment of treatment **allocation**. In **clinical trials** and other intervention studies, knowledge of the next treatment assignment can influence those making decisions on the **eligibility** of prospective participants. Without concealed allocation, researchers might instead be influenced by their personal biases in favour or against a given treatment or intervention. This could result in patients being declared ineligible when they would not otherwise, or not being **enrolled** in the order in which they arrive at a study and therefore not receiving the assignment they would otherwise. Use of pre-enrolment **randomization lists** on which treatment identifiers are masked, or of other similarly suitable forms of concealed allocation, is therefore of great importance in preventing the **selection bias** and **confounding** that may result from lack of concealment. Concealment of allocation and **blinding** are related but separate concepts. As noted by SCHULZ (2000, Background section), "Allocation concealment should not be confused with blinding. Allocation concealment concentrates on preventing selection and confounding biases, safeguards the assignment sequence *before* and *until* allocation, and can always be successfully implemented. Blinding concentrates on preventing study personnel and participants from determining the group to which participants have been assigned (which leads to ascertainment bias), safeguards the sequence after allocation and cannot always be implemented." ALTMAN & SCHULZ (2001) make a similar statement. Details on methods and evaluation are given by SCHULZ & GRIMES (2002b). See also Haynes, Sackett & Guyatt, and Sackett & Haynes, in HAYNES *et al.* (eds., 2006).

## Concomitant treatment

In the context of **clinical trials**, an additional treatment (not one that is being studied) that is administered to a trial participant or self-administered. Where concomitant treatments reflect some breach of trial **protocol**, the usual approach in **pragmatic trials** is to still include those patients in the groups to which they were randomized, and consider the evaluation of treatment effect as an evaluation of 'real-world' **effectiveness** rather than **efficacy**. See also **intention-to-treat analysis**.

## Concordance

See **agreement**.

## Concurrent controls

As opposed to historical controls. See **controls**.

## Conditional failure rate

Synonym for **hazard rate**.

## Conditional logistic regression

A type of **logistic regression** that is appropriate for the analysis of **paired binary outcomes**. A common application of this method is the analysis of **case–control studies** where cases and controls have been individually **matched**. An example would be a study where the relationship between use of oral contraceptives and breast cancer is investigated in women aged 20–60 years. Women with breast cancer might be individually matched for age with a **control** since the risk of breast cancer also increases with age, thus making the comparison of cases and controls with respect to exposure more **efficient**. The method can be extended to situations where there is more than one control per case. Unlike **stratification** with application of the **Mantel–Haenszel method** to the matched design, conditional logistic regression allows the effects of other variables (other than age, in this example) to be controlled for. However, estimates of their effect cannot be interpreted in the usual ways (KIRKWOOD & STERNE, 2003). See also **conditional model**, **McNemar's test**, **matching**, **confounding**; AGRESTI (2007).

## Conditional model

A **regression** model that may be used in the analysis of **clustered** (including **longitudinal**) **data** and **paired data**. It includes two classes of models: **random effects** or generalized linear mixed models, in which cluster-specific or between-cluster random terms are introduced to account for data **dependence** (cf. **marginal model**), and conditional ML (**maximum likelihood**) models, such as obtained with **conditional logistic regression** for analysing matched case–control studies, which estimate within-cluster **fixed effects** (AGRESTI, 2007). See also **transition model**, **generalized linear model**; DIGGLE *et al.* (2002).

## Conditional probability

The **probability** of an event or **outcome**, given the presence of one or more factors. **Bayes' theorem** is often applied when working out conditional probabilities, as given by the equation below:

$$\text{Prob}(B \; given \; A) = \frac{\text{Prob}(B) \times \text{Prob}(A \; given \; B)}{\text{Prob}(A)}$$

It is important to note the two conditional probabilities (between A and B) are not generally equivalent, although equivalence holds when the two events are **independent**. Thus, using the **diagnostic test** result layout in Table 4, p. 191, and calling 'disease true', B, and 'diagnostic test positive', A, we can see that Prob(A *given* B) is given by $a/a+c$, the **sensitivity**, and Prob(B *given* A) is given by $a/a+b$, the **positive predictive value** or **post-test probability** of disease for a positive test result. See also AGRESTI (2007), in the context of **contingency tables**.

## Confidence interval

In the context of **estimation**, a confidence interval (CI) is a range of values within which the 'true' **population parameter** is believed to be found, with a given level of confidence. This is a frequently used definition of CIs, though more in line with **Bayesian inference** (see **credible interval**, **CrI**). Strictly speaking, under **frequentist inference**, a CI is one of a large number of CIs, all estimating the same population parameter, and all based on study samples of the same size, a given percentage of which will contain the true population parameter. The parameters of interest are **means**, **proportions**, differences between means and proportions, **regression coefficients**, **correlation coefficients**, **relative risk** measures, etc. The rationale for calculating CIs is the uncertainty that is always associated with **sample estimates** (see sampling distribution/error/variation). CIs (also termed 'interval estimates') provide a measure of the **precision** with which point estimates are calculated, and that is reflected in the width of the same.

Large **sample sizes** provide more precise, i.e. narrower, CIs. Different levels of confidence can be placed on a CI, so, for example, 90%, 95% or 99% CIs may be calculated. A 99% CI will be wider than the corresponding 95% CI. CIs are essential for assessing the **clinical significance** of study results (see Box C.1): the lower and/or upper boundaries of a CI may indicate the possibility of important treatment and exposure effects in **negative studies**, or of lack of effect in **positive studies**. Generally, the limits of a 95% CI are calculated as follows:

$$95\% \; CI = sample \; estimate \pm 1.96 \times SE$$

When computing the CI for a mean, the formula above applies if sample sizes are large. For smaller samples (roughly <30), the **standard error** (**SE**) of the estimate should be multiplied by the critical value of *t* (instead of 1.96); these critical values can be found in tables of the *t* **distribution** against the appropriate number of **degrees of freedom**.

---

### BOX C.1

From **Box A.1**, p. 3.

The 95% CI for the ARD (absolute risk difference) was 1.5 to 3.4%: for each 1000 AMI patients given aspirin, between 15 and 34 vascular deaths are believed to be prevented (at 5 weeks), with 95% certainty. Both limits are clinically significant and seem to justify a change in treatment policy, as these results are not likely due to chance ($P < 0.00001$) or bias.

---

Cf. **central range** and **reference interval** (which measure the variability around a mean, not the uncertainty around an *estimated* mean). See also **supported range, prediction interval**. See ALTMAN *et al.* (eds., 2000) for further details and formulae; see also GREENLAND *et al.* (2016).

## Confidence limits

The lower and upper boundaries of a **confidence interval**.

## Confirmatory data analysis

Or its abbreviation, CDA. An approach to statistical data analysis that seeks to draw **inferences (hypothesis testing, estimation, model fitting)** from the data generated in a research study. These differ from the kinds of analyses carried out under an **exploratory data analysis (EDA)**, where distributions and relationships are plotted and tabulated, but not formally quantified and tested. Studies often contain elements of both exploratory and confirmatory analyses.

## Confirmatory factor analysis

Or its abbreviation, CFA. See **factor analysis**. Cf. exploratory factor analysis (EFA).

## Confirmatory trial

A **clinical trial** that is conducted in accordance with a prestated **protocol** and, ideally, a sufficiently large **sample size**, and which aims to provide conclusive evidence regarding one or more research hypotheses that possibly result from observations made during a preceding **pilot trial**.

## Confounder

Or alternatively, confounding variable. See **confounding**. Cf. **collider**.

## Confounding

A **bias** or distortion that occurs when the comparison groups in an **observational study** differ in a systematic way, with regard to the distribution of important **risk factors** other than the factor (or **exposure**) under investigation. In the presence of confounding, **crude estimates** of **exposure effect** are likely to be biased and **adjusted estimates** should be calculated. Certain **study designs** are more prone to bias via confounding, in particular the **case–control** design, given the greater difficulty in collecting reliable information on potential confounders. In **randomized trials**, random treatment allocation often succeeds in making treatment groups comparable with regard to known and unknown **prognostic factors**. However, prognostic imbalances may still occur by chance, especially in small trials, which has the potential to distort the estimate of treatment effect. In observational studies (and also in experimental studies), strategies such as **restriction** (restricting the population being studied to one that is relatively homogeneous in respect of a potential confounder) and **matching** (in **cohort studies**, not in case–control studies) may be used at the study design stage. Regardless of how confounding arises in a study, adjustments should be made at the data analysis stage, through methods such as **stratification** (**Mantel–Haenszel method**), **standardization** and **multivariable regression**, provided reliable information on potential confounders has been collected. The example in Box C.2 illustrates some of the concepts above. See also Rothman, Greenland & Lash, in ROTHMAN, GREENLAND & LASH (eds., 2012); ROTHMAN (2012); GRIMES & SCHULZ (2002).

### BOX C.2

Based on data from Pérez Gutthann S *et al.* (1997). Hormone replacement therapy and risk of venous thromboembolism: population based case–control study. *Br Med J* **314**: 796–800.

In this population-based case–control study, 292 women admitted to hospital for a first episode of pulmonary embolism and deep venous thrombosis and 10,000 controls (randomly selected from the source cohort of 347,253 women aged 50–79 years and without major risk factors for venous thromboembolism (VTE) – UK General Practice Research Database, January 1991–October 1994) were investigated for exposure to hormone replacement therapy (HRT). The crude **odds ratio** (**OR**) estimate (without taking age into account) is calculated as follows:

*continued...*

*continued...*

|  | User | Non-user |
|---|---|---|
| **Cases** | 37[a] | 255[b] |
| **Controls** | 1179[c] | 8821[d] |
| **OR** | 1.09 i.e. $ad/bc = (37 \times 8821)/(255 \times 1179)$ | |

Following **stratification** by age, the results in each age group are:

|  | Age ≤60 | | Age >60 | |
|---|---|---|---|---|
|  | User | Non-user | User | Non-user |
| **Cases** | 26 | 50 | 11 | 205 |
| **Controls** | 1009 | 3440 | 170 | 5381 |
| **OR** | 1.77 | | 1.70 | |

**Note:** The analysis presented in the paper (Table 3) does not include 'past users' (12 cases and 375 controls that are included among the 'non-users' in the tables above). The crude OR is **1.1**, and the adjusted OR from multivariable logistic regression is **2.1**. The increased risk seemed to be restricted to first-year users, in particular, in the first 6 months (OR = 4.6; 95% CI: 2.5–8.4).

*Interpretation:* These adjusted OR estimates show that age has confounded the association between hormone replacement therapy and idiopathic venous thromboembolism in women aged 50–79 years. However, the confounding effect of age was not a very strong one, given the small magnitude of the differences between crude and adjusted ORs. The *negative* confounding effect of age (weakened relationship) occurred because:
1  Age is associated with exposure: 34% of cases and 23% of controls in the age group 50–60 years were current users, compared to 5% and 3% respectively, in the age group >60 years.
2  Age is associated with case–control status: 44.5% (4449/10000) of controls *vs.* 26% (76/292) of cases were in the younger age group.

Points 1 and 2 in Box C.2 describe two requirements for a factor to qualify as a potential confounder: it must be related to both outcome and exposure. In addition, it must not be a result or effect in the causal pathway between exposure and disease, such as an intermediary biochemical, physiological or structural change. However, as noted by HENNEKENS, BURING & MAYRENT (eds., 1987), the need to control for such a factor depends on the way the specific research question is posed. See also **propensity scores, residual confounding**.

## CONSORT statement

A collaborative statement published in 1996, the Consolidated Standards of Reporting Trials (CONSORT) statement sets out standards and checklists for reporting the rationale, methodology, results and conclusions of **clinical trials**, in order to facilitate the proper appraisal of the same. See BEGG *et al.* (1996), Sackett, in HAYNES *et al.* (eds., 2006), MOHER, SCHULZ & ALTMAN (2001), and www.consort-statement.org for further discussion and details, including various proposed revisions and extensions. See also **PRISMA statement**, **EQUATOR Network**, **critical appraisal**.

## Contingency coefficient

Also termed 'Pearson's contingency coefficient' (C). A measure of the **strength of association** between two variables that are cross-tabulated on a **contingency table**. It is calculated as follows:

$$C = \sqrt{[X^2/(X^2 + n)]}$$

where $n$ is the **sample size** and $X^2$ is the **chi-squared test statistic**. The latter is used to test the **null hypothesis** of no association or **independence** between the variables in question, but should not be interpreted as measuring the strength of their association: a large $X^2$ statistic simply indicates a small probability of having observed the association seen in the study sample (however weak) given that in reality there is no association. $C$ can take values between 0 (no association) and <1. See also **Cramér's V**.

## Contingency table

Tables 2.a and 2.b are examples of contingency tables, or, more specifically, **two-by-two** (**2 × 2**) **tables**. These are used to summarize the **association** between two **categorical variables**. The rows represent the different levels of one of the variables (usually, **exposure** or **treatment**), and the columns the different levels of the other variable (usually, disease status or **outcome**). The cells contain the observed frequencies resulting from the cross-tabulation of the two variables. These cells are **mutually exclusive**, where each observation can be in one and only one of the cells. Margin totals and row percentages should be presented whenever possible, though results from **case–control studies** may only show meaningful totals for the number of cases and the number of controls. The **chi-squared**

**Table 2** Contingency tables

**a. Observational study**

|  |  | Disease | | |
|---|---|---|---|---|
|  |  | Yes | No | Total |
| Exposure | Present | a | b | a + b |
|  | Absent | c | d | c + d |
|  | Total | a + c | b + d | a + b + c + d |

**b. Clinical trial/intervention study**

|  |  | Outcome | | |
|---|---|---|---|---|
|  |  | Occurred | Did not | Total |
| Treatment/intervention | Active | a | b | a + b |
|  | Placebo | c | d | c + d |
|  | Total | a + c | b + d | a + b + c + d |

test and related methods are often indicated for the analysis of contingency tables. For the chi-squared test, **degrees of freedom** are calculated as $(r - 1) \times (c - 1)$, where $r$ is the number of rows and $c$ is the number of columns. When one variable is **ordered categorical** and the other is **binary** (e.g. amount of smoking and occurrence of heart disease), or both are ordered categorical (as for example, cancer stage and level of pain), a **trend test** should be used. The **Kruskal–Wallis test** or **one-way ANOVA** are indicated when one variable is ordinal or interval/ratio and the other has three or more unordered categories. When variables are ordinal (i.e. given ranks or scores), **Kendall's correlation coefficient** may be calculated. Cross-tabulations involving more than two variables are summarized by **multidimensional tables** and analysed using **log-linear modelling**. See also **continuity correction**, **Fisher's exact test**, **McNemar's test** (paired data), **contingency coefficient**, **Cramér's V**, **risk** (proportion), **odds**, **measures of effect**, **stratification**; ARMITAGE, BERRY & MATHEWS (2002).

## Continuity correction

An adjustment made to the **test statistic** produced by a **significance test**, for the purpose of approximating a **continuous** distribution (usually, the **Normal** or the **chi-squared**) to its **sampling distribution**, if **discrete** (e.g. **binomial, Poisson, multinomial**). The correction consists of subtracting (and sometimes adding) a certain amount from the test statistic (usually 0.5 or 1, depending on the test), which results in a smaller test statistic, and therefore, a slightly more conservative **P-value**. **Yates' continuity correction** is one such example. Corrections are usually not necessary with large samples, but should be used when the **sample size** is small. Alternatively, exact tests such as **Fisher's exact test** could be used. Continuity corrections should also be used with **non-parametric tests**, to approximate the Normal distribution to the sampling distribution of the test statistic whenever sample sizes are small. With the **Mann–Whitney U test**, for example, the continuity correction usually consists of subtracting ½(interval between adjacent discrete values) from the observed value of $U$, so that if the test statistic goes up by increments of 1 unit, one needs to subtract ½, and if it goes up by increments of 2 units, 1 unit is subtracted. See BLAND (2015) for formulae, illustrative examples and discussion. See also **approximation**. Cf. **mid P-value**.

## Continuous sequential design

See **sequential designs**.

## Continuous variable

A **quantitative variable** that may, theoretically, take any real value within a given range. Examples are 'mass' (weight), 'height' and 'temperature'. This is in contrast to a **discrete variable**. When using statistical analysis software for **model selection**, continuous variables should usually be included as such, and not as the different classes or levels of a categorized continuous variable (i.e. not as **dummy variables**). The assessment of **confounding** should also usually be based on the uncategorized variable. See also **variable**, **categorized continuous variable**, **random variable**.

## Contrast

A term used in the context of **analysis of variance**, to refer to a function (usually, a linear function or combination) that is created to give a zero sum for its **coefficients**. This enables different comparisons to be made among the various treatment or exposure groups, as relevant, by using sets of coefficients (also commonly referred to as 'contrasts') as **weights**. For example, in an analysis of variance involving three comparison groups (for instance, two experimental treatment groups and one **control group**), a contrast or linear combination enabling the **mean** of the experimental groups to be compared to the mean of the control group is given by:

*Contrast = (mean of control group) – ½ (mean of first treatment group)*
*– ½ (mean of second treatment group)*

When a comparison is made between the means of just two groups, the implicit set of coefficients is {1 –1}, although not usually specified. In the example in Box O.3, p. 246 (**One-way ANOVA**), there are 4 different comparison groups under the 'type of household' categorical variable or factor. A set of coefficients to test for a difference in mean BMI between urban dwellers and displaced persons (both in private accommodation and in collective centres), on the one hand, and rural dwellers, on the other hand, could be specified as {1 1 1 –3}, and the estimated difference, linear combination, or contrast as follows:

*Contrast = 22.5 + 22.7 + 23.0 – 3 × 24.0*

where the three comparison groups whose means are being averaged are given each weight 1, and the fourth comparison group (rural dwellers) is given weight 3 with opposite sign. The comparison between urban and rural dwellers, on the one hand, and displaced persons, on the other hand, is given by the set of coefficients {1 –1 –1 1}, and the comparison between urban and rural residents (ignoring all displaced persons) is given by {1 0 0 –1}, i.e. any level or category not involved in the comparison is given weight zero. The test for a **linear trend** could be given by the set {–3 –1 1 3}. The **significance test** for a contrast effect involves the calculation of the **sum of squares** for the contrast ($SS_{contrast}$), which, with 1 **degree of freedom** ($df$), is equal to its **mean square** ($MS_{contrast}$). The ratio $MS_{contrast}$ to $MS_{residual}$ gives the $F$-statistic with 1 and $df_{residual}$ degrees of freedom (see **F-test**). See MITCHELL (2012b) and ARMITAGE, BERRY & MATHEWS (2002) for additional details.

## Control group

A group of individuals participating in a **comparative study** who act as the standard against which new treatments or interventions are to be tested (as in a **randomized controlled trial**), or against which the risks connected with a particular **exposure** are evaluated (as in a **case–control study**). Controls may be concurrent or historical, depending on whether they are contemporaneous with the treatment or exposure group(s) (or with the cases, in case–control studies), although rarely there is justification for use of historical controls (POCOCK, 1983). **Crossover trials** use a single group of patients who act as their own controls. Case–control studies are defined by the way in which the control series is selected (ROTHMAN, 2012), giving rise to three basic types: **cumulative case–control**

**studies** (the 'standard' type), **density case–control studies** and **case–cohort studies**. The **case–crossover design** combines features of case–control and crossover studies, such that the cases are also the controls. **Case–control studies** are usually conducted in one of two settings, as *population-based* case–control studies and *hospital-* or *facility-based* case–control studies. In the former, selection of controls is often through **random sampling** (requiring a register of the **source population**), and in the latter through **matching** with neighbourhood, member of household/family member or same health-facility controls, as the source population may not be easily enumerated. In **cohort studies**, and depending on the prevalence of the exposure under study, controls may be identified following an assessment of exposure status on the whole cohort (also termed *general population cohort*) that basically divides the main cohort into two or more subcohorts, or a suitable control group may be identified following the selection of the *special exposure cohort*. See also **active control group**, **blinding**, **placebo effect**, **matching**.

## Control group event rate

Or CER. Usually referring to the **risk** or **rate** of occurrence of the event of interest in a research study among the controls. Cf. **experimental group event rate** or EER. See **risk** or **rate difference**; **risk** or **rate ratio**.

## Cook's distance

In the context of **regression analysis**, where the resulting **model** estimates the value of the **regression coefficient** for each **independent variable** included, Cook's distance measures the **influence** a particular **observation** exerts on the model when included (cf. **DFBETA**, **DFFITS**). The higher the **leverage** and the larger the size of the observation's **standardized residual**, the greater the magnitude of Cook's $D$. Observations with values of $D$ greater than 1, or greater than $4/n$, where $n$ is the number of observations, are considered influential. See HAMILTON (1992) for further details. See also **regression diagnostics**.

## Correlation

A **linear association** between two **quantitative** or **ordinal variables**. The variables in question may vary concurrently toward higher values (positive correlation), or in opposite directions, with increasing values for one of the variables corresponding to decreasing values for the other (negative correlation). The **strength** and **direction** of the correlation is measured by the **correlation coefficient**. Correlation should only be assessed on **random samples**, and not when the values for one of the variables have been predetermined, as for example in a lab experiment gauging a **dose–response relationship**. See ALTMAN (1991) for a discussion of spurious correlations in the medical literature. See also **Pearson's** *r*, **rank correlation**, **Spearman's** ρ, **Kendall's** τ.

## Correlation coefficient

A measure of the **strength** and **direction** of the **linear association** between two **quantitative** or **ordinal variables**. The correlation coefficient may be calculated using **parametric** (**Pearson's** *r*) or **non-parametric** (**rank correlation**) methods (Figure P.1, p. 257).

The values taken by the correlation coefficient range from -1 (perfect negative association) to +1 (perfect positive association), with 0 representing absence of a *linear* association. (Note that for rank correlation, it is the linear association between the **ranks** given to the data values of each variable.) **Scatterplots** should be presented in addition to the correlation coefficient, to 'disclose' fully the shape of the relationship between the variables in question, since very different patterns can lead to the same value of the correlation coefficient. This is illustrated in Figure C.2 (from Bland, in EVERITT & PALMER (eds., 2011), p. 103), in which correlation coefficients are calculated for a number of different relationship shapes. In graph (e), a correlation of zero is obtained despite a very defined, albeit non-linear, U-shaped relationship; in graph (f), a strong positive correlation is obtained for a J-shaped relationship. The correlation between the observed values of a **dependent** (or $y$) **variable** and the values **predicted** (or fitted) by a **multivariable regression** model is measured by the **multiple correlation coefficient** (**R**). KIRKWOOD & STERNE (2003) give a useful interpretation of the correlation coefficient in reference to **simple linear regression**, as the number of standard deviations by which the $y$ variable changes for each standard deviation change in the independent or $x$ variable. See also **correlation**, **correlation matrix**, **r-squared** ($r^2$), **partial correlation coefficient**, **covariance**. Measures of correlation are also employed as **standardized measures of effect**.

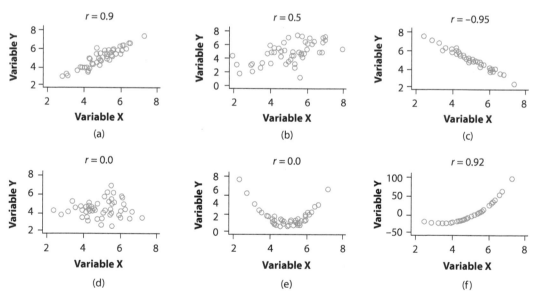

**Figure C.2** Correlation coefficients for linear and non-linear relationships: (a) $r = 0.9$ (close to perfect positive correlation); (b) $r = 0.5$ (weak to moderate positive correlation); (c) $r = -0.95$ (close to perfect negative correlation); (d) $r = 0$ (lack of correlation, although some heteroscedasticity is present); (e) $r = 0$ (lack of correlation, but strong non-linear relationship); (f) $r = 0.92$ (strong positive correlation, but relationship is non-linear). (Reproduced from Everitt BS, Palmer CR (eds., 2011). *Encyclopaedic Companion to Medical Statistics, 2nd edition.* Wiley (with permission).)

## Correlation matrix

A matrix that gives the **correlation coefficients** and/or the **scatterplots** for the **associations** between the variables in a data set, a useful tool when carrying out **exploratory data analyses** and assessing **collinearity**. The variables are each represented twice: once as rows and again as columns. Thus, the matrix is square. The entries in the **correlation** matrix give the corresponding correlation coefficients between the variables (that is, between a row variable and a column variable). Since each variable has perfect correlation with itself, each of the entries in the main diagonal of a correlation matrix (from the top left-hand cell to the bottom right-hand cell) has the value 1. Clearly, the matrix is symmetrical about the main diagonal, and so it is only necessary to report the upper half (or lower half) of the matrix. An example is given in Table 3, from the study by ARGOS *et al.* (2010) seeking to evaluate the effects of dietary B vitamin intakes on arsenic excretion, as measured by creatinine-adjusted urinary total arsenic concentration among individuals participating in the Health Effects of Arsenic Longitudinal Study (HEALS) cohort in Araihazar, Bangladesh. As the authors state, arsenic exposure is a major public health problem in Bangladesh due to consumption of naturally contaminated groundwater, and dietary factors may influence the metabolism of ingested arsenic (due to improved methylation), and may potentially be important modifiers of the health effects of arsenic in this population. High correlations between nutrients likely reflect their joint occurrence in certain food items. An adjusted analysis did not find significant associations for dietary riboflavin, cobalamin or folate, but found the other four nutrients to be significantly associated with the outcome variable.

**Table 3** A correlation matrix: Pearson correlation coefficients of weight-standardized nutrients ($n$ = 9,833), in the study by Argos *et al.* (2010) on dietary B vitamin intakes and total urinary arsenic concentration among members of the HEALS cohort, Bangladesh. (Reproduced from Argos *et al.* (2010). Dietary B vitamin intakes and urinary total arsenic concentration in the Health Effects of Arsenic Longitudinal Study (HEALS) cohort, Bangladesh. *Eur J Nutr* **49**: 473–81 (with permission).)

| Variable | Thiamin | Riboflavin | Niacin | Pantothenic acid | Pyridoxine | Cobalamin | Folate |
|---|---|---|---|---|---|---|---|
| Thiamin | 1.00 | 0.65 | 0.98 | 0.96 | 0.94 | 0.15 | 0.57 |
| Riboflavin | | 1.00 | 0.59 | 0.75 | 0.72 | 0.60 | 0.82 |
| Niacin | | | 1.00 | 0.94 | 0.92 | 0.19 | 0.46 |
| Pantothenic acid | | | | 1.00 | 0.96 | 0.31 | 0.63 |
| Pyridoxine | | | | | 1.00 | 0.25 | 0.62 |
| Cobalamin | | | | | | 1.00 | 0.37 |
| Folate | | | | | | | 1.00 |

## Correlation ratio

Synonym for **eta squared** ($\eta^2$).

## Correlation structure

A term used in the analysis of **longitudinal** and other **clustered data**, to refer to the pattern of association among **observations** or **residuals** pertaining to the same **study unit**.

For valid **inference**, data analyses must take account of this *within-cluster* correlation or **dependence**. This is often achieved in one of the following ways: by employing statistical models that assume cluster-specific or between-cluster effects to be **random effects** with a given **probability distribution** (which induces the correlation pattern among clustered or repeated observations given the predictors), by employing statistical models for continuous outcomes that induce an **autoregressive** or **moving average** autocorrelation structure among the residuals, by employing **transition models** that assume present responses to be dependent on past responses, or by introducing a 'working correlation matrix' into the analysis framework, which is used to approximate the correlation pattern of the residuals. For example, in random *intercept* models, the implicit pattern is *uniformity*, with the common **correlation coefficient** given by the **intraclass** or intracluster **correlation coefficient** (**ICC**), and a **covariance matrix** for within-unit observations characterized by *compound symmetry* (i.e. main diagonal elements are identical, off-diagonal elements are also identical). **Generalized estimating equations** (**GEEs**) are semi-parametric models that use the working correlation matrix approach. The values of the correlation coefficients are estimated from the data given the choice of correlation structure. The most commonly assumed correlation structure is termed *exchangeable*, with uniform within-unit correlations. The *autoregressive* structure allows for correlations to depend on the time-lag between observations. (Transition models are based on autoregressive outcomes or responses (not residuals), what is also termed lagged regression.) An *unstructured* correlation matrix is one that allows the correlation to be defined separately for each given pair of observations, often resulting in an excessive number of model parameters. For data that are uncorrelated, the correlation structure assumes *independence* of the residuals, i.e. the correlation coefficients are all equal to zero. For binary outcomes, the **odds ratio** may be used preferably as the measure of association (AGRESTI, 2007). These different correlation models and structures are discussed by DIGGLE *et al.* (2002), SINGER & WILLETT (2003), SKRONDAL & RABE-HESKETH (2004), AGRESTI (2007) and MITCHELL (2012b). See also **correlation matrix**.

## Correlogram

A graph that displays the **correlations** between two **time series**, i.e. two variables measured over time (**cross-correlation** – see Figures C.3a and C.3b, p. 85), or between the time series and itself (**autocorrelation** – see Figures A.3a and A.3b, p. 21), across various time lags. The **correlation coefficients** may be *positive* or *negative*, depending on whether positive departures from the mean tend to follow positive departures (and negative departures tend to follow negative departures), or, instead, positive departures tend to follow negative departures and vice-versa. Typically, the wider the time-lag, the weaker the correlation, but different patterns may be observed, especially where there is **cyclic variation**. Lags are ordered relative to any given present observation, so that, for example, if values are monthly observations, lag 1 corresponds to an observation made the previous month, lag 2 corresponds to an observation made 2 months prior, etc. The autocorrelation coefficient between any present month and the previous month is the first-order coefficient, and the one between present month and 2 months prior is the second-order coefficient. For **autoregressive models**, it is assumed the series is 'weakly stationary', i.e. the autocorrelation for any particular lag remains the same, regardless of the point in time at which it is measured. Autocorrelation (ACF) and partial autocorrelation (PACF) functions may aid in measuring the correlation between present observation and previous observations, and in identifying lags of response that may be useful predictors of present response. Correlograms may be used also to identify the appropriate error lags for **autocorrelation models**, i.e. regression models with autocorrelated *errors*. Lag 1 or first-order autocorrelation is given by $r_1$, lag 2 or second-order by $r_2$, etc. See also **Durbin–Watson statistic**. See HAMILTON (1992; 2012) for further details and illustrative examples.

## Cost-benefit analysis

A comparison of the costs and **outcomes** of different treatments/interventions when these interventions have either different effects, or similar multiple effects of different **magnitude**. In these situations, simple **cost-effectiveness** comparisons are difficult to make, and outcomes and costs are usually translated into their monetary value. A ratio of money spent (cost value) to money gained (outcome value) can be used to compare different interventions (e.g. a hypertension screening programme *vs.* an influenza immunization programme – DRUMMOND, 1994; DRUMMOND *et al.*, 2015; the outcomes are prevention of premature death and prevention of days with disability). Cf. **cost-utility analysis**. See also AJETUNMOBI (2002), THOMPSON & BARBER (2000).

## Cost-effectiveness analysis

A comparison of the costs and **outcomes** of alternative treatments/interventions, when these interventions are thought to have the same effect, but not the same **magnitude** of effect (e.g. kidney transplantation and inpatient dialysis for patients with renal failure – DRUMMOND, 1994; DRUMMOND *et al.*, 2015; the outcome is the same, survival, which could be longer with one treatment compared to the other). Cf. **cost-minimization analysis**. See also AJETUNMOBI (2002), THOMPSON & BARBER (2000).

## Cost-minimization analysis

A comparison of the costs and **outcomes** of alternative treatments/interventions, when these interventions can be shown to have comparable results or impact (e.g. day-surgery *vs.* inpatient surgery for patients with haemorrhoids – DRUMMOND, 1994; DRUMMOND *et al.*, 2015; the outcome is successful correction of the problem). Cf. **cost-effectiveness analysis**. See also AJETUNMOBI (2002), THOMPSON & BARBER (2000).

## Cost-utility analysis

A comparison of the costs and **outcomes** of different treatments/interventions, when these interventions have different effects, or similar single or multiple effects of different **magnitude**. Thus, simple **cost-effectiveness** comparisons are difficult to make, since their impact or importance may not be the same from patient to patient or from situation to situation. This type of analysis allows individual preferences, values and circumstances to be taken into account. Outcomes are translated into their utility value, usually 'quality-adjusted life-years' or **QALYs**, which may then be used to compare the costs of different interventions – DRUMMOND, 1994; DRUMMOND *et al.*, 2015. Cf. **cost-benefit analysis**. See also AJETUNMOBI (2002), THOMPSON & BARBER (2000).

## Count variable

A **quantitative discrete variable** that arises by counting the number of times a particular occurrence takes place over a given period of time or over a defined surface area or capacity volume (e.g. the number of new cases of a rare cancer in a given state or county and over a 5-year period). The number of occurrences of an event is the numerator in the calculation of **rates** and **risks**. The **sampling distribution** of the number of events – when these take place **randomly** and **independently** over time or space, and at a constant rate – is said to follow a **Poisson distribution** with parameter, mean, given by the number of observed events (or by the observed rate of occurrence per unit of time, area or volume). *Individual* count data (e.g. number of asthma attacks in a year, number of children, number of cigarettes smoked per day) may be also appropriately described by a Poisson distribution, as their **frequency distribution** is often positively **skewed** (due to the impossibility of negative counts, and/or high frequency of low counts), with variance proportional to the mean (likely resulting in lack of **homoscedasticity**), which violates **assumptions** for use of **ordinary least squares** as a method of regression analysis. However, the presence of **overdispersion** (variance larger than the mean) may also preclude **Poisson regression** as a method of analysis, with overdispersed Poisson and **negative binomial** models commonly used as alternatives. **Zero-inflated** models may be used when overdispersion is due (or due in part) to an excess of zero counts. The **square root transformation** is sometimes used as a **normalizing** and **variance-stabilizing** transformation for count variables, and **non-parametric methods** may also be employed. See also **geometric mean**. Cf. **proportion**, i.e. the number of times a specific occurrence takes place out of the total number of occurrences. Cf. **measurement**. See GARDNER *et al*. (1995), DWIVEDI *et al*. (2010), and ALEXANDER (2012) for illustrative examples of data analyses.

## Covariance

The joint **variance** of two variables (or **random variables**). It is estimated as the average cross-product between deviations from the **mean**, where for each observation, the difference between the observation value for variable $x$ and the mean of $x$ is calculated, and likewise for variable $y$. The covariances between pairs of variables may be displayed in a covariance or variance-covariance matrix, a symmetrical matrix in which the elements in the main diagonal represent the variances of the variables, and the off-diagonal elements represent the covariance between pairs of variables. With standardized variables (**z-scores**), the covariance matrix is given by the **correlation matrix**. **Correlation** is a standardized covariance (HAMILTON, 1992). The covariance matrix often holds the necessary and sufficient building blocks for statistical analysis.

## Covariance matrix

See **covariance, correlation matrix**.

## Covariate

A variable that is a **baseline measurement** for a **quantitative outcome variable**, and is included in an **analysis of covariance** (or **multivariable regression model**), in order to reduce random error **variability** in the outcome variable. A covariate may also be a quantitative **predictor variable** that is strongly associated with the outcome, although not a baseline measurement of the same. The purpose of adjusting for this type of predictor is as stated above: reduced variability in the outcome variable and greater **precision** of interval **estimates**. In a wider sense, the term covariate refers to any predictor variable, or to any quantitative predictor. **Categorical** predictors are usually termed **cofactors**. See also **time-varying covariate**.

## Cox–Mantel $\chi^2$ test

Synonymous with **logrank test**. See also **Mantel–Haenszel $\chi^2$ test** for survival curves.

## Cox regression

A **regression** method for the analysis of **survival times** (COX, 1972). Also known as proportional hazards **model** since it assumes the **hazard ratio** (**HR**) for the event in question (e.g. death) at any particular time and between any two groups being compared, is constant. Cox regression is a **semi-parametric method**, since no other **assumptions**, namely about the **distribution** of survival times, are made. The **outcome variable** is 'time to the event', if it has occurred, and if not (i.e. if **censored**), the duration of **follow-up**. The *predicted* outcome is the **logarithm** to base $e$ of the **hazard** or instantaneous rate at any given time $t$. **Predictor variables** are various prognostic factors. The model estimates a **regression coefficient** for each predictor variable. **Exponentiating** (or anti-logging) these regression coefficients gives the hazard ratio, i.e. the factor by which the hazard increases for each unit increase in the corresponding predictor variable. As mentioned above, the model is specified to predict the logarithm (to base $e$, i.e. **ln**) of the hazard, $h(t)$, at any given time, as a linear function (**multiplicative** on the original scale) of $\ln[h_0(t)]$ (i.e. the log *baseline* hazard, which is the value of the hazard when the value for all predictors is zero), and of the linear predictive function:

$$\ln[h(t)] = \ln[h_0(t)] + b_1x_1 + b_2x_2 + b_3x_3 + \dots$$

or equivalently,

$$h(t) = h_0(t) \times \exp(b_1x_1 + b_2x_2 + b_3x_3 + \dots)$$

where the linear predictive function, $b_1x_1 + b_2x_2 + b_3x_3 + \dots$, is sometimes designated by $\eta$ (lower case Greek letter eta), and the $b$s represent the regression coefficients associated with each predictor variable $x$. The Cox regression model may *not* in fact predict $h(t)$, as the baseline hazard function is not given directly (CLEVES, GOULD & MARCHENKO, 2016). However, it may predict the **cumulative hazard function**, $H(t)$, and the **survival function**, $S(t)$. Furthermore, the model's linear predictive function ($\eta$) may be used as a **prognostic index**, and a prognostic score may be derived for each individual in the data set. Box C.3 gives an example of Cox regression, from the study by CHATURVEDI *et al.* (1996). The Cox regression model can also incorporate predictor variables whose values change over time (**time-varying covariates**). As an alternative to the Cox model,

## BOX C.3

Based on data from Chaturvedi N *et al.* (1996). Differences in mortality and morbidity in African Caribbean and European people with non-insulin dependent diabetes mellitus: results of a 20-year follow-up of a London cohort of a multinational study. *Br Med J* **313**: 848–52.

The results presented are for a 20-year follow-up study of all cause and cardiovascular mortality among a London cohort of 77 African Caribbeans and 150 Europeans with non-insulin dependent diabetes mellitus. Patients (aged 35–55 years) were recruited into the study over a 2-year period from 1975 to 1977. Median duration of follow-up was 18 years, and time to death is measured in years. Some observations are censored (patient alive at the end of the study period or lost to follow-up). Fifty-nine and 16 deaths were observed in the European and African Caribbean cohorts, respectively, over 3498 person-years of follow-up (see **person-time at risk**). An adjusted hazard ratio for the comparison between the two groups was obtained by fitting a Cox regression model that included sex, smoking habits, proteinuria and body mass index, in addition to the binary variable 'ethnicity'.

The Cox regression analysis yielded the following results for all-cause mortality (see also Figure K.1 and Box L.2, pp. 181 and 201):

| | HR | 95% CI | P-value |
|---|---|---|---|
| **Unadjusted analysis:** 'ethgrpAFRCRB' (coded 1) *vs.* 'ethgrpEUR' (coded 0): | | | |
| | 0.41 | 0.23–0.73 | 0.002 |
| **Adjusted** for the effects of sex, smoking, proteinuria, and BMI: | | | |
| | 0.59 | 0.32–1.10 | 0.1 |

*Interpretation:*
1   The unadjusted analysis gives a death hazard in the African Caribbean group that is 0.41 that in the European group, i.e. $h(t) = h_0(t)*\exp(-0.892*\text{ethgrpAFRCRB})$, and therefore the hazard ratio = $\exp(-0.892) = 0.41$.
2   After adjusting for additional prognostic factors, the effect of 'ethnicity' was reduced (hazard ratio changed from 0.41 to 0.59), still a clinically significantly result, albeit no longer statistically significant. The 95% CI was compatible with an *HR* as low as 0.32, and also with an *HR* of 1.10. The latter would suggest a death hazard in the African Caribbean group that could be 10% higher than in the European group.
3   The authors concluded "...African Caribbeans with diabetes maintain their protection from heart disease and [...] this protection may be due to a low degree of central obesity, resulting in a reduced atherogenic lipid profile. Further investigations are required to disentangle these complex relations."

**parametric survival models** are usually more **efficient**, provided a functional form can be chosen for the **baseline hazard function** and a **probability distribution** can be specified for the distribution of **survival times**. See ALTMAN (1991), BLAND (2015), POCOCK (1983) and KIRKWOOD & STERNE (2003) for further discussion. See also **proportional hazards assumption, Kaplan–Meier method, logrank test, generalized linear model, conditional model, intercept**. See **hazard rate** for the baseline and cumulative baseline hazard functions.

## Cramér's V

A measure of the **strength of association** between two variables, which are cross-tabulated on a **contingency table**. Cramér's $V$ is calculated as follows:

$$V = \sqrt{[X^2/n(k-1)]}$$

where $n$ is the **sample size**, $X^2$ is the **chi-squared test statistic** and $k$ is the lesser of the number of rows or the number of columns in the contingency table. The $X^2$ statistic is used to test the **null hypothesis** of no association between the variables in question, but should not be interpreted as measuring the strength of their association: a large $X^2$ statistic simply indicates a small probability of having observed the association seen in the **study sample** (however weak) given that, in reality, there is no association. $V$ can take values between 0 and 1, with values closer to 1 indicating stronger association. See also **contingency coefficient**.

## Credible interval

In the context of **Bayesian inference**, a credible interval is a range of likely values for a parameter that is being estimated, which is given by its **posterior distribution**, i.e. by the conditional probability distribution for the parameter *given* the sample data. For a 95% credible interval (95% CrI), for example, it may be stated that there is a 95% chance that the population parameter lies within its limits. Cf. **confidence interval (CI)** in **frequentist inference**, where a similar statement of belief cannot, strictly speaking, be made. See also **supported range, Bayes' factor**; GREENLAND (2008).

## CrI

Abbreviation for **credible interval (Bayesian inference)**.

## Critical appraisal

The evaluation of the methods, results and conclusions of a research study, based on an understanding of research methodology and accepted standards of quality and validity, in the context of the particular clinical or public health issue being investigated. See also **hierarchy of evidence, evidence-based medicine, clinical epidemiology, epidemiology, Cochrane Collaboration**. For a comprehensive guide, see GUYATT *et al.* (2014). See also GREENHALGH (1997; 2014), AJETUNMOBI (2002) and HENEGHAN & BADENOCH (2006). See the UK-based Critical Appraisal Skills Programme (CASP, www.casp-uk.net) for critical appraisal checklists. HIGGINS *et al.* (2011) report on the Cochrane Collaboration's tool for assessing risk of bias in randomized trials. For reporting guidelines, see **CONSORT statement, PRISMA statement, STROBE statement, STARD statement, TRIPOD statement**. For additional reporting guidelines see SIMERA *et al.* (2010) and **EQUATOR Network** (www.equator-network.org). See also **GRADE approach** (www.gradeworkinggroup.org).

## Critical value

In the context of **significance testing**, the critical value of a **test statistic** is the threshold value in its **sampling distribution** under the null hypothesis that corresponds to a given cumulative probability or **significance level** (one- or two-sided). The critical value is also referred to for **confidence interval** estimation: in the formulae used to calculate the limits of a confidence interval, it is the value that is multiplied by the **standard error** of the **estimate**. From Tables 1 (p. 53), 6 (p. 234), and 7 (p. 358), each displaying select **percentage points** of the chi-squared, Normal, and $t$ distributions, respectively, the critical value of $X^2$ with 2 **degrees of freedom** (as in the case of a 3 × 2 contingency table, for example) is 5.99 (for a 0.05 or 5% level of significance); the critical value of $z$ at the 0.01 or 1% level of significance is 2.58 (two-sided); and the two-sided critical value of $t$ with 30 degrees of freedom (as would be the case with a one-sample test with $n = 31$, or a two-sample test with $n_1 + n_2 = 32$) is 3.65, for a 0.001 (0.1%) significance level.

## Cronbach's alpha

A measure of the **reliability** of a **composite rating scale** made up of several items or sub-scales. Psychological and mental health tests are common examples of this type of scale. Alpha ranges in value from zero to one, with $\alpha = 1$ reflecting perfect **correlation** between the subscales and a high degree of internal consistency. It is also an indication that the scale could be simplified (in terms of number of items) without significant loss of information, in the same way that regression models with collinear or highly correlated predictors may be simplified. See BLAND (2015) for additional details and interpretation. See also **factor analysis**.

## Cross-correlation

The **correlation** between the values of two variables (e.g. two **time series**), as measured across various time (or space) lags. The purpose of the analysis may be to determine which variable 'leads' and which variable 'lags', or it may be to determine by how much the 'output' variable lags the 'input'. Lags may be positive or negative, depending on which variable is assumed to lead. A **correlogram** helps in evaluating the pattern of cross-correlation, and in particular the presence of delayed effects, i.e. which lags of 'input' might be predictors of 'output' in a **lagged regression**. An example is given in Figures C.3a and C.3b (HUANG *et al.*, 2011), in which cross-correlations of monthly time series of malaria incidence and meteorological data help uncover the time-lag(s) of preceding meteorological factors at which there is strongest correlation. The **correlation coefficient** will be positive or negative, depending on whether positive departures from mean 'output' tend to follow positive departures from mean 'input' (or negative departures tend to follow negative departures), or, instead, positive departures from mean 'output' follow negative departures from mean 'input' and vice-versa. When evaluating the relationship between the variables, a **confounding** effect of 'time' may be present as the variables are each measured over the same time-period. It is important to control for this effect, by including time-varying factors that are associated with both series as predictor variables, and also by filtering seasonal variation. Detrending techniques, such as inclusion of time as a predictor, may also be employed (Hertz-Picciotto, in ROTHMAN, GREENLAND & LASH [eds., 2012]). Special techniques are also used to address the issue of **autocorrelation** within each series, if present. These techniques are often referred to as 'prewhitening', a reference to producing 'white noise' errors in the series (see **Normal i.i.d.**). In the illustrative example, Figure C.3b, a seasonal **ARIMA model** was fitted to the monthly malaria incidence series, and to each of the series of monthly meteorological data, which was able to remove both seasonality and autocorrelation from each series. **Autocorrelation models** are sometimes necessary when

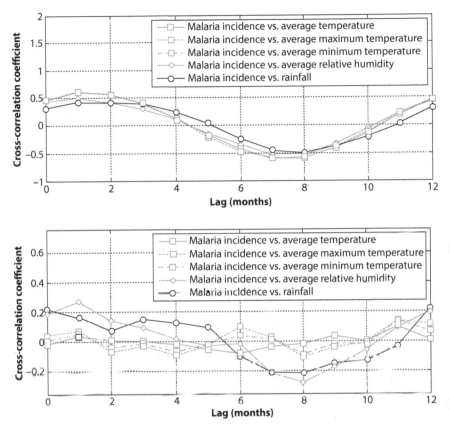

**Figures C.3a and C.3b** Cross-correlation functions (CCF): cross-correlation coefficients between monthly time series of meteorological variables and malaria incidence at 1-, 2-, ..., and 12-month lags. Data are from the Motuo County in Tibet, for the period 1986 through 2009. The analysis in Figure C.3b is after 'prewhitening' each series and removing seasonality, which has generally weakened or reversed the cross-correlations previously observed. See also Figures T.1a and T.1b, p. 362. (Reproduced from Huang F *et al.* (2011). Temporal correlation analysis between malaria and meteorological factors in Motuo County, Tibet. *Malar J* **10**: 54.)

exogenous predictors are included in the analysis of a time series, if standard regression methods produce autocorrelated errors. See HAMILTON (2012) for further details.

## Cross-overs

Participants in a **clinical trial**, who, despite having been assigned through **randomization** to a given treatment or intervention, end up receiving an alternative treatment. In studies of treatment **effectiveness**, **intention-to-treat analysis** is recommended to minimize the **bias** that results from these **protocol breaches**. However, this also leads to **misclassification** of 'exposure', i.e. treatment, with the resulting underestimation of treatment effects itself a bias. In studies looking at safety issues, **perprotocol analysis** may be a preferable approach in order to prevent underestimation of effect with regard to the occurrence of adverse reactions and side-effects (ROTHMAN, 2012). See also **pragmatic trial**, **sensitivity analyses**, **selection bias**.

## Cross-sectional study

An **observational study** in which all pertinent data is collected at a single point in time (cf. **follow-up** or **longitudinal study**). **Descriptive** cross-sectional studies are often referred to as **surveys**, and are usually concerned with estimating different parameters in reference to a given **source population**. Often, source and **target population** are one and the same. Non-**random** selection of the **study sample** and non-response or **volunteer bias**, can all lead to lack of representativeness, and therefore, **sampling bias**. A cross-sectional study gives estimates of disease **prevalence** (how many cases of a given disease there are at a certain point in time) rather than **incidence** (how many *new* cases develop over a certain period of time). **Analytical** cross-sectional studies, on the other hand, tend to investigate the **association** between any two or more factors, commonly disease and **exposure**. Since disease and exposure status are ascertained simultaneously in a cross-sectional study, it becomes more difficult to infer **cause–effect relationships** from this **study design** (see Box C.4 – MORIOKA *et al.*, 2015). Still, such a study can provide useful information, provided prevalence of disease is not low, as this would require very large sample sizes (BLAND, 2015). ROTHMAN (2012) discusses a few instances in which the cross-sectional design might be as informative as a longitudinal study, as, for example, where current exposure status is a good proxy for, or more reliable than, the recollection of past exposure. Cross-sectional studies are sometimes carried out to assess **baseline characteristics** and follow-up results in large **intervention trials** (KIRKWOOD & STERNE, 2003). See also MACHIN & CAMPBELL (2005). Cf. **cohort study**, **case–control study**.

### BOX C.4

Adapted from Morioka TY *et al.* (2015). Vitamin D status modifies the association between statin use and musculoskeletal pain: A population based study. *Atherosclerosis* **238**: 77–82.

The distribution of comorbidities according to serum 25-hydroxyvitamin D (25(OH)D) concentrations (in ng/ml) among 5907 participants (age ≥40 years) in the US National Health and Nutrition Examination Survey (NHANES, 2001–2004) shows an **association** between serum vitamin D levels and coronary heart disease, stroke, congestive heart failure and diabetes. There appears to be a weak to no association with lung disease, arthritis and osteoporosis. Though suggestive of a real effect with regard to cardiovascular diseases and diabetes, **causality** may not however, be inferred from this cross-sectional study.

| Characteristics (results are shown as percentages) | Overall % (SE), n = 5907 | 25(OH)D ≥15 ng/ml % (SE), n = 4626 | 25(OH)D <15 ng/ml % (SE), n = 1281 |
|---|---|---|---|
| Comorbidities | | | |
| Coronary heart disease | 10.5 (0.7) | 9.9 (0.7) | 13.8 (1.5) |
| Stroke | 3.4 (0.4) | 3.1 (0.4) | 5.2 (1.0) |
| Congestive heart failure | 3.7 (0.4) | 3.3 (0.4) | 5.5 (0.8) |
| Diabetes | 11.4 (0.6) | 10.2 (0.6) | 18.2 (1.6) |
| Lung disease | 11.4 (0.7) | 11.3 (0.7) | 11.9 (1.5) |
| Arthritis | 34.2 (1.1) | 34.9 (1.2) | 35.6 (1.7) |
| Osteoporosis | 8.8 (0.6) | 8.9 (0.6) | 8.0 (1.1) |

## Cross-tabulation

See **contingency table**.

## Cross-validation

See **validation**.

## Crossover design

A **study design** for a **clinical trial** in which all patients are given the two or more treatments under investigation, such that each patient acts as his own **control**. As a result, required **sample sizes** are smaller than with the **parallel design** (where different groups are given different treatments), given the lesser degree of **variability** of within-patient responses compared to between-patient responses. SENN (2002; 2008) points out, however, that evaluation of **safety** in later clinical trials usually requires larger numbers than even in a parallel design trial, for which reason crossover trials may be a less appropriate design for **Phase III trials**, and most useful in studies of pharmacokinetics and pharmacodynamics (**bioequivalence studies**, **Phase I** and **Phase II trials**). **Randomization** is used to assign the order in which the treatments are to be administered (Box C.5 – two-period crossover trial), mainly to avoid **period effects**. The crossover design has limitations in that it cannot be used to study acute conditions, or illnesses that could be cured after the first treatment is administered. It is more suitable to investigate immediate/short-term treatment effects for chronic conditions, where symptoms are expected to return upon cessation of treatment. In addition, long treatment periods pose a problem as patients may be prone to **dropping out**. There is also the potential for **carry-over** of **treatment effects** from one period into the next, resulting in **treatment–period interaction**. The latter should be given careful consideration in the planning stages of a trial so that it may be avoided by inserting appropriate **wash-out periods** between treatments. Appropriate methods for statistical analysis are those discussed under **paired data**. See POCOCK (1983), ALTMAN (1991), FLEISS (1999) and MACHIN & CAMPBELL (2005) for further details and illustrative examples, and SENN (2002; 2008) for a comprehensive presentation. See also **multiperiod crossover design**.

---

### BOX C.5

Based on data from Weinshenker B *et al.* (1992). A double-blind, randomized crossover trial of pemoline in fatigue associated with multiple sclerosis. *Neurology* **42**: 1468–71.

**Total number of patients = 46**

Five patients dropped out due to exacerbation of their condition

23 randomized to receive pemoline first (pemoline has since been withdrawn from the market due to adverse effects)

18 randomized to receive placebo first

**Wash-out period: 2 weeks**

| First period (4 weeks) | | Second period (4 weeks) |
|---|---|---|
| N = 23 pemoline | → | placebo |
| N = 18 placebo | → | pemoline |

## CRT

Abbreviation for **cluster randomized trial**.

## Crude estimate

As opposed to **adjusted estimate**. In the context of **comparative studies**, it refers to an estimate of **exposure** (or treatment) **effect** that is computed without controlling for potential **confounding factors** (or for baseline imbalances). In the presence of confounding, crude estimates are said to be **biased**. See Box C.2 (Confounding, p. 70) for an illustrative example.

## Crude rate

The **rate** or frequency of occurrence of an event among an entire group or population, without reference to specific age- or sex/age groups. Cf. **age-specific rate, standardized event rate**. See also **overall rate, cause-specific rate**.

## Cubic power transformation

See **transformations, polynomial regression**.

## Cubic spline

See **spline regression**.

## Cumulative baseline hazard function

Or $H_0(t)$. This function and the baseline hazard function $[h_0(t)]$ are discussed under **hazard rate**/hazard function $[h(t)]$ and under **cumulative hazard function** $[H(t)]$. Cf. **baseline survival function** $[S_0(t)]$.

## Cumulative case–control study

A **case–control study** in which **controls** are sampled or selected from the non-diseased in the **source population** at the end of the 'at-risk' period. This is the standard case–control design. As with the **case–cohort design**, the **odds ratio** (calculated as a measure of association between exposure and disease) gives an estimate of the **incidence risk ratio** between the two exposure groups. How good an estimate depends on whether the disease in question is more or less common, the approximation being closer for rare diseases. For common diseases, the odds ratio likely overestimates the risk ratio, as the distribution of exposure among controls does not reflect the distribution in the source population. This case–control design lends itself to the study of epidemics, and to situations where the 'at-risk' period is well defined and somewhat limited (ROTHMAN, 2012). Cf. **density case–control study**.

## Cumulative distribution function

Often referred to as CDF or $F(x)$. The theoretical equivalent of a **cumulative frequency distribution (CFD)**. See also **probability density function**, also denoted by pdf or $f(x)$.

## Cumulative frequency distribution

Or its abbreviation, CFD. A **frequency distribution** for a **quantitative** or **ordered categorical variable** in which, for each **class interval** or **category**, the cumulative or added frequency – up to and including the frequency of the class in question – is given. For example, consider the following hypothetical frequency distribution (or frequency table) of the IQ scores of a class of 120 first-year medical students:

| IQ score | n |
|---|---|
| 100–109 | 42 |
| 110–119 | 34 |
| 120–129 | 26 |
| 130–139 | 12 |
| 140–149 | 6 |
| **Total** | **120** |

The corresponding cumulative frequency distribution is as follows:

| IQ score | n |
|---|---|
| <100 | 0 |
| <110 | 42 |
| <120 | 76 |
| <130 | 102 |
| <140 | 114 |
| <150 | 120 |

The cumulative frequency in the final row should be equal to the total frequency, which in this case is 120. To calculate the *relative* cumulative frequency at any interval, the corresponding cumulative frequency is divided by the total frequency, and multiplied by 100 to be expressed as a percentage. For example, for the data above, the *percentage relative cumulative frequency* of IQs under 120 is given by $(76/120) \times 100\% = 63\%$ (to two **significant figures**). See also **cumulative frequency polygon, cumulative distribution function** or F(x), **quantiles**.

## Cumulative frequency polygon

The graphical representation of a **cumulative frequency distribution**. Figure C.4 shows a graphical representation of the relative cumulative frequency use of paracetamol in children under 2 years, in the study by LOWE *et al.* (2010). It can be seen that by age 2, or more exactly, 100 weeks, nearly all children in the sample have been administered this antipyretic drug. By approximately age 12 weeks, over 50% of infants will have been administered paracetamol. See also **frequency polygon, cumulative distribution function**.

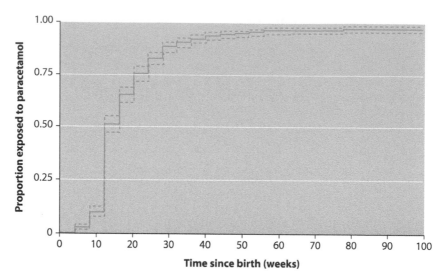

Figure C.4 Cumulative frequency distribution: paracetamol use in infants and toddlers under 2 years of age according to time since birth (in weeks) (with 95% CI). (Reproduced from Lowe A *et al.* (2010). Paracetamol use in early life and asthma: prospective birth cohort study. *Br Med J* **341**: c4616 (with permission).)

## Cumulative hazard function

In the context of **survival analysis**, the cumulative hazard function, $H(t)$, is the set of estimates of total hazard that is experienced up to and including any given time $t$. Cumulative hazards may be calculated by integration, from time zero to $t$, of the **hazard function**. They may also be estimated by a **non-parametric method** (the Nelson–Aalen estimator) that parallels the **Kaplan–Meier estimator** of the survival function, $S(t)$, in the following way: for each time $t$ at which an event has occurred, the cumulative hazard is estimated as the running sum of the 'probabilities of failure', up to and including the probability of failure at time $t$. These probabilities are calculated at the exact times (and based on the same **risk sets**) at which 'probability of survival' is calculated (see **survival function** or [$S(t)$]). Alternatively, cumulative hazards may be calculated from the Kaplan–Meier estimates of survival probability up to and including any given time $t$ at which an event of interest has occurred, by using the following equivalence:

$$H(t) = -\log[S(t)] \text{ and, conversely,}$$

$$S(t) = e^{-H(t)}$$

where *log* is the natural logarithmic function, and *e* is the mathematical constant 2.718.... The cumulative hazard function may be illustrated graphically as a cumulative hazard curve, which, in similar fashion to the **Kaplan–Meier survival curve**, is also expressed as a step function (albeit one that increases over time). When **hazard rates** ($\lambda$) are constant over time, the survival function decreases exponentially over time, in what is termed an **exponential** decay curve. The cumulative hazard and survivor functions are now given by:

$$H(t) = \lambda t \text{ and, conversely,}$$

$$S(t) = e^{-\lambda t}$$

The cumulative hazard, or accumulated risk up to and including time $t$, may be interpreted as the number of times we would expect an event to be repeated (if that were possible) over the period up to and including time $t$. This is the count-data interpretation of cumulative hazard (CLEVES, GOULD & MARCHENKO, 2016). The risk itself, or cumulative probability of failure at each time $t$, is calculated as 1 *minus* the cumulative probability of survival, i.e. $1 - S(t)$. (See **rate** for the relationship between rates and risks.) See also **Cox regression**.

## Cumulative incidence

An alternative term for **risk** or **incidence risk**. The cumulative incidence is the **proportion** of individuals who have developed the outcome of interest by the end of the **follow-up period** for a research study, in reference to the number at risk at the start of the study. This is in contrast with the **incidence rate**, which also measures incidence, but in reference to the total **person-time at risk**. The cumulative incidence tends to increase in magnitude the longer the follow-up period, as more cases are likely to occur in reference to the same initial number at risk. On the other hand, the higher the rate of occurrence of the outcome in question (assuming it remains constant over time), the fewer cases are produced as time goes on, as the pool of individuals at risk will decrease concomitantly. See also **attack rate**.

## Cumulative meta-analysis

A **meta-analysis** technique that combines the results from individual studies, as these studies are carried out and results become available. The **graphical display** of a cumulative meta-analysis shows the **pooled** estimates of effect for all studies carried out up to a particular point in time, going from the first study (at the top) to the last (at the bottom), which includes all previous studies. As new data are included at each additional step, the **sample size** increases and the **confidence interval** for the pooled estimate of treatment (or exposure) effect becomes narrower, reflecting increasing certainty. Figure C.5 shows the results of one of the early meta-analyses (DAVEY SMITH, SONG & SHELDON, 1993) of the effects of cholesterol lowering on total mortality (with a further distinction between deaths due to coronary heart disease (CHD) and deaths from all other causes). According to the authors, "The present analysis [...] examines the manner in which the outcome of cholesterol lowering is related to initial risk of coronary heart disease and the implications of this for current practice with regard to pharmacological treatments to lower cholesterol.". Results are stratified by risk of CHD in the control group. The interested reader is

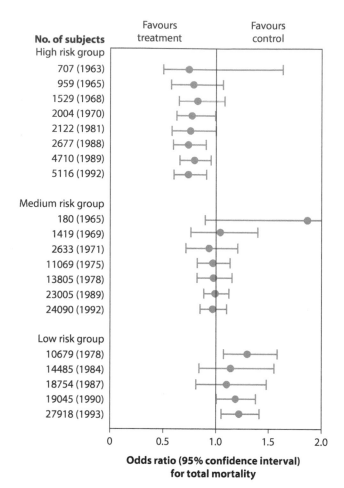

**Figure C.5** Cumulative meta-analysis of the effect of cholesterol lowering treatment on total mortality stratified by risk, as measured by number of deaths from coronary heart disease per 1000 PYAR among controls (high risk >50, medium risk 10–50, low risk <10). (Reproduced from Davey Smith G *et al.* (1993). Cholesterol lowering and mortality: the importance of considering initial level of risk. *Br Med J* **306**:1367–73 (with permission).)

referred to THOMPSON, SMITH & SHARP (1997), and Sharp, in EGGER, DAVEY SMITH & ALTMAN (eds., 2001), for discussion of the relationship between treatment benefit and underlying risk. See also **forest plot**.

## Cumulative sampling

See **cumulative case–control study**. Cf. case–cohort sampling, **density sampling**.

## Cumulative survival function

Synonym for **survival function** or $S(t)$. See also **cumulative hazard function** or $H(t)$.

## Curvilinear regression

A method of **regression analysis** in which a **non-linear relationship** may be summarized by means of a linear model, following a suitable **transformation** of the continuous outcome, continuous predictor, or both. Plotting the **predicted outcome** thus obtained (or its **back-transformed** values) against the continuous predictor, gives the predicted *curve*. HAMILTON (1992) gives examples of **monotonic** and **non-monotonic** **curves** resulting from curvilinear models, which include semi-log and log-log **exponential** curves (see Figure E.2, p. 125, for an example of the latter), and **polynomial** curves (obtained by inclusion of **quadratic** and higher order terms – see Figure Q.1, p. 292). MOSTELLER & TUKEY (1977) and KIRKWOOD & STERNE (2003) give a general guide for choosing a transformation for outcome and/or predictor variable, for simple monotonic curves (see **Tukey and Mosteller's bulging rule**). See also **fractional polynomials**. Cf. **non-linear regression**.

## Cusum

Or cumulative sum, in reference to **serial measurements** where at each time point the cusum chart stays flat or shows level changes with regard to a reference value.

## Cut-off point

In the context of **screening** and **diagnostic testing** using biochemical markers, clinical measurements and other tests measured on a **ratio** or **ordinal scale**, the cut-off point or **diagnostic threshold** for a given test is the test result above (or sometimes, below) which a decision is made to **classify** an individual as being diseased or at high risk for a particular disease (see Figure R.1, **ROC curve**, p. 319). It is often preferable to have several test result categories, as opposed to a dichotomized test result, in order to make better use of the entire range of results (see **likelihood ratios**). See also **classification table**, **categorized continuous variable**.

## Cuzick's test

A **non-parametric** test for **trend**. The test is carried out to evaluate the presence of a trend in some measurement or quantity across the levels of an **ordinal variable**. Cf. **chisquared test for trend**, in which the possible trend involves an increase or decrease in the **proportion** with a given binary outcome across the levels of an **ordered categorical variable**.

## Cyclic variation

A **non-linear** pattern of change over time, characterized by the repetition of cycles with a given periodicity. Cycles may span relatively shorter or longer lengths of time, with regard to morbidity and mortality measures, or any given measurements or characteristics. For example, daily (circadian) variation is characteristic of blood pressure measurements and cortisol levels, whereas the cycle of female reproductive hormones tends to be repeated on an approximate monthly basis. Seasonal variation is seen where a cycle or sequence spans an entire year, and is typical of the incidence of certain infectious diseases such as influenza and malaria. Secular cycles may have decennial or greater periodicity, as illustrated by many socioeconomic indicators. Cyclic variation may be modelled by fitting sinusoidal curves, which necessitates the inclusion of special functions in **regression models** that estimate the amplitude, lag and periodicity of the cycles. An example is given in Figure C.6, from the study by MAEDA *et al.* (2013) on

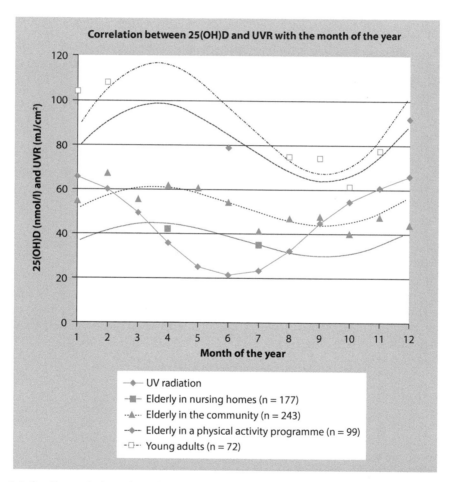

**Figure C.6** Cyclic variation: distribution of mean ultraviolet radiation (UVR, in mJ/cm²) and serum 25-hydroxyvitamin D (25(OH)D, in nmol/l) levels over the course of a calendar year, in four different age/level of physical activity groups in São Paulo, Brazil. For the 'nursing' group, the graph also shows the time delay (early June to mid-September) between lowest levels of UVR and lowest levels of vitamin D3. (Reproduced from Maeda SS *et al.* (2013). Seasonal variation in the serum 25-hydroxyvitamin D levels of young and elderly active and inactive adults in São Paulo, Brazil – The São PAulo Vitamin D Evaluation Study (SPADES). *Dermatoendocrinol* **5**: 211–17 (with permission).)

the seasonal variation in serum 25-hydroxyvitamin D levels of young and elderly active and inactive adults in São Paulo, Brazil. **Smoothing** techniques may be employed to uncover cyclic patterns where there is excessive fluctuation, and also to better perceive longer-term trends. See ALTMAN (1991) and BLAND (2015) for additional details and illustrative examples. See also **time series**, **serial measurements**.

# D

*d*

The **Durbin–Watson** (D–W) **test statistic**.

*D*

See **deviance statistic**.

## Data

Measurements, counts or observations; the term is plural, with the singular form being datum. See also **independent data, paired data, clustered data, longitudinal data, aggregate data, individual participant data, censored data, missing data, variable**.

## Data set

A collection of **data** that usually includes information pertaining to a number of different **variables**, of which one or more give information on responses or **outcomes**, and one or more on factors and measurements thought to affect those responses, such as age, gender, treatment or exposure status, and other risk and prognostic factors. Commonly presented in tabular form, each row representing a separate **observation**, and each column representing a different variable. An additional column will record an identifier for each of the different observations. Observations are assumed to be **independent**, except in the case of multilevel or **clustered data**.

## Data summaries

See **summary measures, aggregate data, descriptive statistics**.

## Death rate

See **mortality rate**.

## Deciles

The 10th, 20th, 30th... **quantiles**. Deciles divide the total number of observations in a given variable into ten equal-sized groups. The 10th decile, for example, is the observation value below which we find 10% of all observations, when these are sorted in ascending order. See also **tertiles, quartiles, quintiles, centiles**.

## Decision analysis

A systematic approach to reaching medical decisions, based on evidence extracted from research studies. Information stemming from these studies is translated into **probabilities**, and incorporated in diagrams or decision trees that direct the clinician through a succession of possible scenarios, courses of action and **outcomes**. An important concept in decision analysis is that of patient's utilities, i.e. the relative value of each possible outcome for an individual patient. Decision trees are also used in **diagnostic testing**. Figure D.1 shows an example of a decision tree (van CREVEL, HABBEMA & BRAAKMAN, 1986), for the management of incidental intracranial saccular aneurysms (i.e. unruptured, asymptomatic and discovered in the course of an angiography or high-resolution CT scan for unrelated symptoms; the analysis did not consider patients with multiple aneurysms and subarachnoid haemorrhage). The starting point of the decision tree is a specific medical problem. The different possible *courses of action* branch out of the *decision node*, represented by a square. They are, in this case, surgery, or not, and the possible *outcomes* branch out of the *chance nodes* (represented by the circles). An *utility* (ranging from 0: no value, to 100: ideal outcome) is attached to each of these outcomes. The *probabilities* of the different outcomes, shown on the branches of the tree, are extracted from the results of previous research. The tree is analysed starting from the outcomes (their probabilities and utilities), and working 'back' to obtain the *expected utilities* or EU (see van CREVEL *et al.* for details on methodology) for the different courses of action. In this example (a 45-year old woman with migraines and no other symptoms), and given the probability and the value or utility attached to each outcome, the authors concluded surgery was the preferred course of action (EU = 96.5 for 'preventive surgery' *vs.* EU = 93.3 for 'do not operate'). See also STRAUS *et al.* (2010); **cost-utility analysis**.

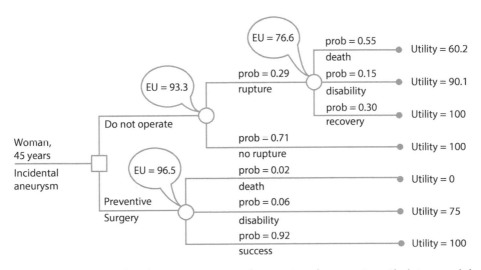

**Figure D.1** Decision tree for the management of unruptured, asymptomatic intracranial saccular aneurysms, with probabilities, utilities, and expected utilities included. (Adapted from van Crevel H *et al.* (1986). Decision analysis of the management of incidental intracranial saccular aneurysms. *Neurology* **36**: 1335–9 (with permission).)

## Degrees of freedom

In the context of **significance testing** and **estimation** of **means**, the number of degrees of freedom (*df* or v) is a measure that reflects the **sample size(s)** of the study group(s), and plays a role in determining the **significance level** of **test statistics** and the width of **confidence intervals**. The number of degrees of freedom is usually calculated as the total sample size *minus* the number of parameters to be estimated, which gives a measure of how many unconstrained or independent observations contribute to the calculation of the estimate of variability (i.e. the **variance**, or its square root, the standard deviation), and the estimate of sampling error (i.e. the **standard error**). For the one-sample *t*-test, for example, the number of degrees of freedom is $n - 1$ (where $n$ is the sample size), as the standard deviation of the differences between paired variables must be estimated. When a two-sample *t*-test is carried out, the number of degrees of freedom becomes $n_1 + n_2 - 2$, as two separate standard deviations must now be estimated from the data, one for each group. The larger the sample size(s), the greater the number of degrees of freedom. The large sample **z-test** does not depend on degrees of freedom, as in this case sample variances are considered reliable estimates of population variances. For **contingency tables** summarizing the association between two categorical variables, each cell of the table contributes $(O - E)^2/E$ to the chi-squared test statistic (*E* stands for expected frequency). However, only a given number of observed frequencies (*O*) can vary independently in a cross-tabulation, the others being constrained by the **marginal totals**. Thus, $(r - 1)$ rows are unconstrained, and $(c - 1)$ columns are unconstrained, giving a total of $(r - 1) \times (c - 1)$ unconstrained *cells*, i.e. the number of degrees of freedom for the **chi-squared ($\chi^2$) test**. This represents the number of cell frequencies in the cross-tabulation that can vary freely before the remaining frequencies are fixed due to the constraint imposed by the marginal totals, i.e. the number of independent contributions to the test statistic (HAMILTON, 1990). In addition to the *t* and **chi-squared distributions**, another distribution that depends on degrees of freedom is the *F* **distribution**, which is referred to in the context of **analysis of variance** (see also *F*-**test**). Here, two sets of degrees of freedom are calculated as $(m - 1)$ and $(n - 1)$, where $m$ is the number of groups and $n$ is the total number of observations. See also **critical value**; ALTMAN (1991), BLAND (2015). See also **residual degrees of freedom**.

## Delta method

A technique that is used to calculate the **standard error (SE)** of a **transformed** variable, based on the mean and standard error of the *untransformed* variable (KIRKWOOD & STERNE, 2003). A common application of the delta method is in calculating the standard error of the **logarithm** of various measures of **relative risk** (risk ratio, rate ratio, and odds ratio). The SE of log-transformed ratio measures may then be used to calculate **confidence intervals** for those measures. **Back-transforming** the limits of confidence intervals thus obtained gives a confidence interval in the original, untransformed scale. Alternatively, the standard error of the log ratio measure may be used to compute an **error factor (EF)** for the untransformed ratio measure, so that dividing and multiplying the untransformed risk, rate or odds ratio by the error factor gives the limits of the relevant confidence interval (90% or 95% CI, for example), on the untransformed scale. CIs for ratio measures are asymmetrical around the point estimate. See also **Woolf's formula**.

## Demographic indicators

Summary measures for human populations, regarding, in particular, their magnitude, characteristics and dynamics, and how these interplay with different socioeconomic and health-related factors. The subset of indicators that relates to births and deaths (and also marriages and divorces) and reflects the rate of growth and health of a population is termed vital statistics. Examples of the latter include the **birth rate, fertility rate, mortality rate, stillbirth rate, infant mortality rate, neonatal mortality rate, perinatal mortality rate, child mortality rate** and **maternal mortality rate**. See also **standardization**, which covers methodology often used to compare **populations**.

## Density

See **frequency density, probability density function, incidence density, density sampling**.

## Density case–control study

A **case–control study** in which the selection of **controls** is based on **density sampling**, and, as such, the **odds ratio** (the measure of association between exposure and disease) can provide a good estimate of the **incidence rate ratio**, as would be obtained in a **follow-up cohort study** based on the same **source population**. This estimate of the incidence rate ratio will not, however, have the same **precision** as the estimate obtained from the cohort study. Selection of multiple controls per **case** is a strategy that is often utilized to address this shortcoming. See ROTHMAN (2012) for further discussion and an illustrative example. Cf. **cumulative case–control study** and **case–cohort study**, in which the odds ratio gives an estimate of the **incidence risk ratio**.

## Density sampling

A method for choosing a **control series** in **density case–control studies**. Here, and in contrast to the manner in which controls are selected in **cumulative case–control studies** and in **case–cohort studies**, controls are selected by sampling from the **risk set** for each newly occurring or incident **case**, i.e. the set of people in the **source population** who are at risk of becoming a case at that same time (ROTHMAN, 2012). With density sampling, the distribution of **exposure** in the control series reflects the distribution of **person-time** in the source population, and the ratio 'exposed/unexposed' in the control series approximates the ratio 'person-time among exposed/person-time among unexposed' in the source population, provided selection of controls was independent from exposure status. The **odds ratio** now gives an estimate of the **incidence rate ratio**. Density sampling is a form of **matching**, and can account for changes in the pattern of exposure over the 'at-risk' period. This matching with respect to time is often disregarded in the data analysis (CLAYTON & HILLS, 1993). See ROTHMAN (2012) for further details and discussion.

## Dependence

As opposed to **independence** of observations. This term is used with reference to a degree of correlation or lack of independence among observations pertaining to a **study unit** (commonly, an individual or a cluster), which often results from between-subject or between-cluster **heterogeneity**. Allowances for **overdispersion** and/or **random cluster effects** are usually necessary when analysing correlated data. Where time dependence is a feature of serial observations, **autoregressive (time series)** and **transition (longitudinal data)** regression models may be used, where a previous value of the observation is used as a predictor of present value. Dependence, or in other words, heterogeneity, may sometimes be 'explained away' by including a previously omitted **predictor variable**(s) in the regression model. Likewise, for **autocorrelation** in a time series. See also **paired data**.

## Dependent variable

Synonym for **outcome variable**.

## DerSimonian and Laird random effects model

A **pooling** method (DerSIMONIAN & LAIRD, 1986) that combines **estimates** of absolute or relative effect, for both binary and continuous outcomes, to produce a single summary, which is a **weighted average** across the different **primary studies** in a **meta-analysis**. This method differs from the **inverse variance method** in that the weights incorporate an additional variance component, $\tau^2$ (**Kendall's correlation coefficient**, tau, squared), the estimated variance of the **sampling distribution** of treatment effects of which the primary studies in the meta-analysis are assumed to be a **random sample**. In other words, the underlying 'true' exposure or treatment effect is assumed to vary from study to study. As KIRKWOOD & STERNE (2003) point out, a random effects model gives an estimate of 'average effect', whereas a fixed effect model gives an estimate of 'true effect'. The calculation of $\tau^2$ is based on $Q$, the test statistic for the test of **heterogeneity**, the number of **degrees of freedom** ($df$) for the test and the inverse variance weights. This between-study variability adds uncertainty, so confidence intervals for the pooled estimate are wider and significance tests more conservative than with a **fixed effect** approach. On the other hand, if heterogeneity is not accounted for when present, it leads to spurious **precision**. The closer $\tau^2$ is to zero, the closer the results of random effects and fixed effect approaches. The **random effects** approach gives less weight to larger studies than does the fixed effect approach (thus affecting also the value of the pooled estimate), as weights for small and large studies are less dissimilar (BLAND, 2015). Relative effect measures for binary outcomes (including hazard ratios for 'time to event' data) are combined on the **log scale**. See also **index of heterogeneity** ($I^2$), **meta-regression**. See Deeks, Altman & Bradburn, in EGGER, DAVEY SMITH & ALTMAN (eds., 2001), for formulae and illustrative examples, and RILEY, HIGGINS & DEEKS (2011) for additional details on interpretation.

## Descriptive statistics

Data summaries that describe the **distribution** of a given variable or characteristic in a population or study group. Examples include the **mean**, **standard deviation**, **minimum** and **maximum** values, **reference interval**, **proportion** with a given trait or condition, etc. The presentation of descriptive statistics does not involve **hypothesis testing** or **estimation**, i.e. **statistical inference**. See also **exploratory data analysis**, **descriptive study**.

## Descriptive study

A study that aims to provide **descriptive statistics** for a given group or population, and which may also explore the relationships and associations between measurements and characteristics pertaining to the same, through **graphical displays** and **cross-tabulations**. A common example is a **cross-sectional survey**. Cf. **analytical study**.

## Design effect

The effect of **study design** features such as clustering on the **power** of a statistical test, i.e. on its ability to detect real effects as statistically significant. The design effect may be defined as the factor by which a **sample size** must be multiplied in order for a statistical test to retain a given level of power. Design effects are often applied to sample size calculations for **clustered designs**, as the **effective sample size** will be reduced. Larger sample sizes are usually required to make up for the fact that clusters, not individuals, are the **study units**. The magnitude of a design effect depends on the extent of clustering, as measured by the **intraclass correlation coefficient** (**ICC**), and on the intended average cluster size. The larger the ICC and average cluster size, the larger the magnitude of the design effect. See BLAND (2015), KIRKWOOD & STERNE (2003), MACHIN & CAMPBELL (2005) and ELDRIDGE & KERRY (2012) for further discussion and formulae.

## Design variable

A variable the value of which is determined by the investigator. This term may also be used as a synonym for **dummy** or indicator **variable**.

## Detection bias

See **selection bias**.

## Detection rate

Synonym for **sensitivity**.

## Deterministic model

A **model** that does not contain probabilistic or **random** elements, in contrast to a **probabilistic** (i.e. random or stochastic) model. For example, Einstein's equation for mass–energy equivalence does not contain any aleatory factors whose effects have to be **estimated**: $E = mc^2$. For this reason, **coefficients** are not estimated in a deterministic model.

## Deviance statistic

A **test statistic** that is used to assess the overall **goodness-of-fit** (**GoF**) of **regression models** fitted by the method of **maximum likelihood**. The deviance statistic ($D$) is based on deviance residuals (see **standardized residual**), and reflects the difference in **log likelihood** between a given model and the corresponding **saturated model** (see AGRESTI, 2007).

This statistic plays a similar role to the **residual sum of squares** in least squares regression, in that the latter decreases as predictor variables are added to a model and the sum of squares due to regression increases, in the same way that the deviance decreases as variables are added to a model and the likelihood (or log likelihood) of the data given the model parameters increases. A related statistic is **G**, which is the difference between the deviances of any two **nested models**. *D* and *G* are the test statistics for the residual deviance test (the GoF test) and the **likelihood ratio test** (a **significance test**). The equation for their calculation may be simplified as follows:

$$D \text{ or } G = -2\log_e \left[ \frac{likelihood\ of\ simpler\ model}{likelihood\ of\ fuller\ model} \right]$$

$$= -2\left[ \log_e likelihood\ of\ simpler\ model - \log_e likelihood\ of\ fuller\ model \right]$$

where the fuller model is either the saturated model or a model on which a simpler model is nested. The likelihood of the fuller model is always higher than that of the simpler model (i.e. the *log* likelihood of the fuller model is always less negative than that of the simpler model). It is the trade-off between a decrease in likelihood and a simplified model that must be evaluated as reasonable or not (see **parsimony**). Under the **null hypothesis** of a similar fit, *D* follows a **chi-squared ($\chi^2$) distribution** with **degrees of freedom** equal to the difference in number of **parameters** between the saturated model and the current model. With binary outcomes and data that are individual-level records (i.e. ungrouped), the validity of these assessments depends on the number of unique covariate patterns. When the model contains **continuous variables**, the number of unique covariate patterns (and therefore the number of parameters in the saturated model) may be approximately equal to the total sample size, which invalidates the test. The **Hosmer and Lemeshow $\chi^2$ test** may be used in these situations. See CLAYTON & HILLS (1993), HOSMER, LEMESHOW & STURDIVANT (2013), and Greenland, in ROTHMAN, GREENLAND & LASH (eds., 2012), for further details. A related statistic is the **Pearson chi-squared** goodness-of-fit statistic. See also **overdispersion**.

## df

Sometimes also denoted by ν (lower case Greek letter nu). See **degrees of freedom**.

## DFBETA

In the context of **regression analysis**, where the resulting **model** estimates the value of the **regression coefficient** for each **independent variable** included, DFBETA is a statistic that measures the amount of change in a given regression coefficient when a particular **observation** is excluded from the analysis, i.e. how much **influence** the observation exerts on the magnitude of the coefficient when included. DFBETA is expressed in units of the **standard error** of the estimated coefficient (calculated from a model that excludes the observation in question). For any given observation, the larger the value of this standard error, the smaller the **absolute value** of its DFBETA. Observations with absolute value of DFBETA greater than 2 or greater than $2/\sqrt{n}$, where *n* is the number of observations, are considered influential. See HAMILTON (1992) and AGRESTI (2007) for further details. See also **regression diagnostics**, **DFFITS**, **Cook's D**.

## DFFITS

In the context of **regression analysis**, DFFITS is a statistic that measures the amount of change in the **predicted value** of a particular **observation** when this same observation is excluded from the analysis, i.e. how much **influence** the observation exerts on the magnitude of its predicted outcome when included. DFFITS is calculated with reference to the **residual standard deviation** (of a model that excludes the observation in question) and the square root of the observation's **leverage** statistic, $h$. For any given observation, the larger this residual variance and the lower the leverage, the smaller the **absolute value** of its DFFITS. Observations with absolute value of DFFITS greater than $2\sqrt{(k/n)}$, where $n$ is the sample size and $k$ is the number of estimated coefficients in a model, are considered influential. See HAMILTON (1992) for further details. See also **regression diagnostics**, **DFBETA**, **Cook's D**.

## Diagnostic odds ratio

A measure of overall **accuracy** for a dichotomous (or dichotomized) **diagnostic test**. It is the ratio between the **odds** of a positive test result among the diseased and among the non-diseased. It is calculated as follows:

$$DOR = \frac{LR+}{LR-} = \frac{a \times d}{b \times c}$$

where, from Table 4, p. 191, LR+ is the likelihood ratio of a positive test result and LR− is the likelihood ratio of a negative test result (see **likelihood ratios**). The DOR may be calculated also from the **sensitivity** and **specificity** of a test. However, once calculated, it no longer discriminates between, for example, high sensitivity/low specificity and vice-versa. Deeks, in EGGER, DAVEY SMITH & ALTMAN (eds., 2001), discusses the calculation of summary diagnostic odds ratios across primary studies, in **meta-analyses** evaluating diagnostic and screening tests, when varying **diagnostic thresholds** preclude the calculation of pooled estimates of sensitivity, specificity and likelihood ratios (LRs). A summary **ROC curve** may be plotted using estimates of sensitivity and specificity calculated on the basis of the **pooled** DOR, which is assumed to be constant for different diagnostic thresholds. Alternatively, methods that allow for varying DORs may be employed (see Deeks for methodology and interpretation).

## Diagnostic test

A clinical, laboratory, radiological or other type of test, which is carried out for the purpose of establishing an actual diagnosis as to the presence or absence of disease. Unlike **screening**, diagnostic testing is usually prompted by the presence of signs and/or symptoms of disease. Test results are often dichotomized according to the categories of a **binary variable** as, for example, positive/negative, above threshold/below threshold. For this type of test, diagnostic accuracy is measured by its **sensitivity** and **specificity**, but its usefulness in practice is given by its **predictive** ability, given the actual **prevalence** of disease. A measure of *overall* accuracy is the **diagnostic odds ratio**. For test results on an **ordinal** or **quantitative scale**, the choice of **diagnostic threshold** may be made by plotting sensitivity (detection rate) *vs.* false-positive rate for different **cut-off points** – what is known as a **ROC curve**. However, a different utilization of these test results is also possible, given by the likelihood of different test results *conditional* on the presence (or absence) of disease, that results in the calculation of **post-test odds** and **post-test probabilities** of disease for different test results. Errors or **misclassification** with respect to disease status may lead to underestimation of exposure and treatment effects. See also **classification table**, **false-positive rate**, **false-negative rate**, **predictive values**, **likelihood ratios**. MACHIN & CAMPBELL (2005) give details of the design of studies to establish diagnostic accuracy. See Guyatt, Sackett & Haynes, in HAYNES *et al.* (eds., 2006), for further details and discussion, with a focus on the evaluation of diagnostic tests. Deeks, in EGGER, DAVEY SMITH & ALTMAN (eds., 2001), discusses the undertaking of systematic reviews of studies evaluating diagnostic and screening tests, to which special quality and bias assessment criteria apply, and which require specific methodology. A comprehensive overview of statistical methods for the evaluation of diagnostic and screening tests is also given. See **STARD statement** for reporting guidelines for studies of diagnostic accuracy.

## Diagnostic threshold

The **cut-off** test result for a quantitative or semi-quantitative **diagnostic** (or **screening**) **test** above, or sometimes, below which a diagnosis of disease (or a determination of high risk) is made. Deeks, in EGGER, DAVEY SMITH & ALTMAN (eds., 2001), discusses varying diagnostic thresholds as a source of **heterogeneity** in **systematic reviews** of studies evaluating diagnostic and screening tests. See also **diagnostic odds ratio**, **ROC curve**, **net benefit**.

## Dichotomous variable

Synonym for **binary variable**.

## Difference *vs.* average plots

See **Bland–Altman plot** (Figures B.5a and B.5b, pp. 36, 37), and **Oldham plot** (Figures O.1a and O.1b, p. 244). These plots are useful when conducting **method comparison studies** and also in the study of **change**, and are used preferentially to plots of 'difference' *vs.* 'baseline measurement'. In the study of change, the latter often show a characteristic downward slope indicative of a negative association, which could be simply due to **regression to the mean**, leading one to believe the amount of change correlates with the magnitude of the measurements when this may not be the case (the downward slope is present when the 'change' variable is calculated as 'post measurement' *minus* 'baseline measurement'). A plot of 'difference' *vs.* 'average' circumvents this problem. Similarly, when comparing methods, the average of the two measurements gives a better estimate of the underlying 'true value' of the measurement.

## Differential censoring

See **censoring**, **selection bias**. See also **informative censoring**.

## Differential loss to follow-up

See **loss to follow-up, selection bias**. See also **informative loss to follow-up**.

## Differential misclassification

See **misclassification, information bias**.

## Digit preference

A systematic error in recording measurements and other assessments, due to a tendency to round off numbers either to the nearest unit, to multiples of 5 or 10, or to the nearest even number. Digit preference may contribute to **misclassification** of disease and exposure status. See also **significant figures**.

## Direct standardization

See **standardization**.

## Direction of effect

The positive or negative association between **exposure** and disease, or between **treatment** and **outcome**. For absolute measures of effect such as the **absolute risk difference** (for example, control *minus* treatment), the direction of effect is given by the sign of the measure: a positive-sign difference indicating a beneficial or risk reduction effect on the part of the treatment and a negative-sign risk difference indicating the opposite. For relative effect measures, the direction of effect is given by a ratio that is greater or lesser than 1. For example, taking the **risk ratio** as the measure of association (exposed *over* unexposed), a risk ratio greater than 1 indicates a detrimental exposure effect, whereas a risk ratio lower than 1 indicates a protective effect. Where relative effect is given by **relative differences** (such as the excess relative risk, the attributable fraction, or the relative risk reduction), the null value is 0 (or 0%), not 1. Different signs or directions across different strata of a confounding variable (or the different primary studies in a meta-analysis) could be evidence of significant **heterogeneity**. Direction of effect is also given by the sign of **correlation** and **regression coefficients**. See also **measures of effect, magnitude of effect, strength of association**.

## Discrete variable

A **quantitative variable** which, unlike **continuous variables**, may only take certain discrete values, usually non-negative integers (e.g. number of children, number of patients on a practice list, number of asthma episodes in a year, total score in a quality-of-life or other questionnaire). Discrete variables may be analysed with methods for quantitative or ordinal variables, depending on the range of values and shape of distribution of the variable, among other considerations. Additional details are given under **count variable**. Cf. discrete **categorical variable** (binary and nominal data). See also **variable, random variable**.

## Discriminant analysis

A **multivariate method** for **classifying** individuals into known groups, on the basis of their profile of measurements (e.g. physiological function and laboratory test results). This is a form of computerized diagnosis, also known as supervised pattern recognition in artificial intelligence language. Linear discriminant analysis (see **MANOVA**) is sometimes employed, but simple regression methods (for example, various types of **logistic regression**) are also commonly used for this purpose, with the profile variables included as **predictors**. The search for the subset of predictor or explanatory variables that maximizes **discrimination** may be carried out through a **stepwise** procedure. In addition to finding a discriminant rule or **model**, it is important to assess its performance, i.e. its **misclassification rate** or proportion of individuals incorrectly classified. Ideally, a **training set** is used to build the discriminant model, and a separate **validation sample** to evaluate its performance. See ALTMAN (1991) and ARMITAGE, BERRY & MATHEWS (2002) for further details, and AFIFI, MAY & CLARK (2011) for a comprehensive presentation. Cf. **cluster analysis**, which classifies into *unknown* (not yet defined) groups.

## Discrimination

The ability of a classifying tool (for example, the range of **predicted probabilities** computed from a logistic regression model, or the range of values of a **prognostic index**) to differentiate between individuals in distinct categories, as, for example, diseased and non-diseased, or favourable and unfavourable prognosis. This may be assessed by drawing a **classification table** or by plotting a **ROC curve** for different cut-off points of the relevant range of values, to check whether sufficient discrimination may be achieved, and is sometimes carried out as part of a **goodness-of-fit** assessment for a **regression model**. It is however possible to have good discrimination and poor fit, and vice-versa. HAMILTON (1992) discusses the problem of too high discrimination in **logistic regression**, which often leads to inefficient and invalid estimation. See also **classification, discriminant analysis**. Cf. **calibration**.

## Disease cluster

See **clustering**.

## Disease surveillance

See **surveillance**.

## Dispersion

The degree of spread or **variability** around a **measure of central tendency** (such as the **mean**) that is displayed by the values of a **quantitative** (or ordinal) **variable**. Measures that express **absolute dispersion** include the **standard deviation, variance, range, interquartile range** and other **central ranges** (including **reference intervals**), and **limits of agreement**. The **coefficient of variation** is a measure of **relative dispersion**. See also **dispersion parameter**.

## Dispersion parameter

A measure that accounts for extra-binomial and extra-Poisson variation in the **distribution** of a **discrete variable**. The dispersion parameter is a component of the **variance** estimate for the variable. In the presence of **overdispersion**, this parameter is usually greater than zero, and the data may be said to conform to a **beta-binomial** or a **negative binomial distribution**. Where the dispersion parameter is equal to zero, the observed variability is as expected under the **binomial** and **Poisson distributions**, and **beta-binomial** and **negative binomial regression** yield the same results as **logistic** and **Poisson regression**, respectively. Negative binomial regression fits **generalized linear models** with an additional parameter, the dispersion parameter. See AGRESTI (2007; 2013), DIGGLE *et al.* (2002). See also **underdispersion**. Cf. **scale parameter** (under overdispersion), **index of dispersion**.

## Distribution-free method

See **non-parametric method**.

## Distributions

The count or frequency of occurrence of the different values in a set of observations, as determined by a set of **probabilities** for each of the **mutually exclusive** values, characteristics or events, such that the sum of these probabilities is equal to 1 or 100%. The set of probabilities may be given by an observed **relative frequency** distribution, or it may be given by a theoretical **probability distribution**, on the basis of its **parameters**. The description above fits **discrete** numerical or categorical data. For **continuous** data, reference is made to the probability that the value of an observation is less than or greater than some value (as, for example, the probability or area under a Normal curve below a certain value), or between any two given values. **Empirical** and **theoretical distributions**, which result from the application of relative frequencies or of probability distributions, may take different shapes: they may be symmetrical or skewed, unimodal or bimodal, bell-shaped, J-shaped or uniform, peaked or U-shaped, etc. In addition, empirical distributions may be said to follow one of a number of theoretical distributions, as, for example, a Normal, binomial, Poisson, exponential, lognormal, or uniform distribution. This has implications for the choice of methods of statistical analysis. Statistical methods that do not rely on distributional **assumptions** for the data are termed distribution-free or **non-parametric**. See also **marginal distribution**, **sampling distribution**, **approximation**.

## DOR

Abbreviation for **diagnostic odds ratio**.

## Dose–response relationship

The relationship between a response variable and the corresponding values of a drug dose or exposure level. This is often plotted as a two-dimensional dose–response curve or plot, with response as the **ordinate** and dose or exposure as the **abscissa**, as illustrated in Figure D.2 (HACKSHAW, LAW & WALD, 1997) with the relationship between exposure to cigarette smoke (second-hand exposure, expressed as number of cigarettes smoked by spouse and years lived with spouse who is a smoker) and relative risk of lung cancer. The graph strongly suggests increased risk of lung cancer with greater second-hand exposure. WALD (2004) discusses the interpretation of a graphed dose–response relationship, depending on the **measurement scale**(s) (*arithmetic* or *logarithmic*) on which dose and response have a linear relationship (with dose measured on a **continuous** scale). This allows for the estimation of a *constant* absolute or proportional change in outcome for specified absolute or proportional changes in level of exposure. Also of interest is whether those with *zero exposure* experience the outcome to any degree, and if not, at which dose does response occur (*threshold dose*). For those exposed, it might be possible to estimate the average length of the **induction** and **latency periods**. Also of importance is the degree of individual **variability** of response within each exposure level (PORTA (ed.), 2014). See also **trend** (test for), **linear relationship**, **non-linear relationship**, **cause–effect relationship**; CLAYTON & HILLS (1993).

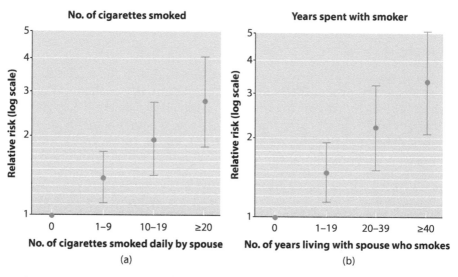

Figure D.2 Dose–response relationship: linear trend between second-hand cigarette smoke exposure (measured as (a) number of cigarettes smoked daily by spouse; and (b) number of years living with cigarette smoking spouse) and log of relative risk (RR) of lung cancer; 95% confidence intervals (CIs) for RR estimates are also shown. (Reproduced from Hackshaw A *et al.* (1997). The accumulated evidence on lung cancer and environmental tobacco smoke. *Br Med J* **315**: 980 (with permission).)

## Dot plot

A **graphical display** that is similar to a **scatterplot**, but with one of the two variables plotted being a **categorical** or grouped variable. A dot plot may be preferable to a **bar chart** to display this type of data, as the latter can conceal important aspects of the data. For example, in the upper panel of Figure D.3 (DRUMMOND & VOWLER, 2011), although the two variables have the same value for the **mean**, one has a **symmetrical** distribution, while the other has a positively **skewed** distribution. This difference is not evident on the corresponding error bar charts (also termed 'plunger plots'). Despite the presentation of the 'error bars', which express degree of uncertainty as given by the **standard error** (some authors use them to represent the standard deviation, a measure of variability), the reader might erroneously assume dispersion to have similar range above and below the mean.

Bar charts are best used to display the *univariate* **frequency** and **relative frequency** of the various categories that comprise a categorical variable. However, in the study by MUSCATELLO *et al.* (2006), lay persons found it easier to interpret bar charts than dot plots. Cf. scatterplot, which displays the *bivariate* relationship between two **quantitative variables**.

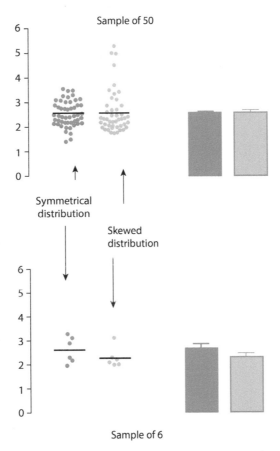

**Figure D.3** Comparison of dot plots with corresponding error bar charts: the horizontal lines on the dot plots are mean values, while the error bars on the bar charts denote the standard errors of the means. The comparison illustrates how dot plots are more informative than bar charts in what concerns the distribution of the data. (Reproduced from Drummond GB, Vowler SL (2011). Show the data, don't conceal them. *Br J Pharmacol* **163**: 208–10 (with permission).)

## Double blind

See **blinding**.

## Drop-outs

See **withdrawals**.

## Drop-the-losers design

A type of **adaptive design** that is used in a **clinical trial** in which the **treatment group** (or groups) with the poorest responses to a treatment regimen can be dropped, following an **interim analysis**. This study design could be used, for instance, in a **Phase II trial**, to help determine the optimum dose for a given pharmaceutical drug. The treatment arms with the poorest responses could then be dropped before the end of the trial. Once a group has been dropped, a new treatment arm may be included, in accordance with a preset **protocol**. This adaptive design is sometimes termed 'pick-the-winners' design. See CHOW & CHANG (2008; 2011) for further discussion.

## Dummy variable

A **binary variable** whose two levels are usually coded 0 and 1. In the context of **regression analysis**, dummy or indicator variables are created to allow the inclusion of **categorical variables** into **models**. If this step is not taken, categorical variables such as blood group, whose levels are coded with labels, for example, from 1 to 4 (O, A, B, AB), will be interpreted as **quantitative**, since the labels will be given numerical meaning. In the example above, three new dummy variables are created (for blood groups A, B, and AB). Blood group O is taken as the reference level or category, and is coded '0' for all three dummy variables, BGA, BGB and BGAB:

|  |  | Dummy variables | | |
| --- | --- | --- | --- | --- |
| Patient | Blood group | BGA | BGB | BGAB |
| 1 | 1 (O) | 0 | 0 | 0 |
| 2 | 3 (B) | 0 | 1 | 0 |
| 3 | 4 (AB) | 0 | 0 | 1 |
| 4 | 1 (O) | 0 | 0 | 0 |
| 5 | 2 (A) | 1 | 0 | 0 |

When these three new dummy variables are included in a regression model, their **coefficients** each express the comparison between the category they represent and the baseline category, group O. See **model** (Box M.1, p. 219) for an example of the use and interpretation of dummy variables in regression models. See also **analysis of covariance**, **Dunnett's correction**.

## Duncan's multiple range test

See **multiple-comparison procedures**.

## Dunnett's correction

A procedure that applies a correction or adjustment to **P-values** produced by **multiple significance testing**. This particular correction is employed when the non-independent tests or comparisons are between the different levels of a **categorical variable** and the level that is taken as the baseline or **control** level. See **Bonferroni correction** for further details. See also **dummy variable**.

## Durbin–Watson statistic

A statistic that tests the significance of first-order **autocorrelation** among the **residuals** from a **linear regression** model. It is calculated as being approximately equal to $2(1 - r_1)$, where $r_1$ is the first-order autocorrelation coefficient for the residuals. A D–W ($d$) statistic of 2 indicates absence of autocorrelation. Positive autocorrelation is given by $d < 2$ and negative autocorrelation by $d > 2$. $d$ (with **degrees of freedom** equal to the sample size, $n$, and the number of variables in the regression model) is referred to tables of its **critical values** for an assessment of **statistical significance**. For positive autocorrelation, the test is inconclusive if $d$ is between $d_L$ and $d_U$, the critical values for $d$ according to sample size and desired level of significance. Evidence to reject the **null hypothesis** of no first-order autocorrelation is given by $d < d_L$; $d > d_U$ means lack of evidence to reject NH. For negative autocorrelation, the statistic is $(4 - d)$. The D–W statistic may not be used with **autoregressive models**, in which a previous value of the **outcome variable** becomes a **predictor** of the present value. SKRONDAL & RABE-HESKETH (2004) point out the need to distinguish between the latter (models with lagged responses) and models for autocorrelated errors (**autocorrelation models**), and to rule out the former before applying the D–W test. See also **correlogram**, **time series**. See HAMILTON (1992; 2012) and HUITEMA (2011) for additional details and an alternative test.

*e*

The mathematical constant 2.7182818… See **logarithmic scale, ln, log$_{10}$, exponentiation**.

*E*

See **expected frequency, expected value**.

## EBM

Abbreviation for **evidence-based medicine**.

## Ecological bias

An error that arises when measuring an **association** in an **ecological study**. This error or distortion can be in the form of a *spurious* association (due to difficulties in adequately controlling for the presence of **confounding**), or it can be in the form of *dilution* of association (due to the use of 'averaged' measurements at the population level, and proxy measures for exposure and disease). See ALTMAN (1991), ROTHMAN (1986). See also **regression dilution bias**.

## Ecological study

A **descriptive study** that measures the **association** between any two factors or characteristics (commonly, **exposure** and disease, or their proxies) in the broadest way possible, by using *population* summaries as opposed to *individual* measurements or observations. An illustrative example is given in Figure E.1 (OWEN, WHINCUP & COOK, 2005), which shows a negative association between early life factors (as measured by infant mortality rates approximately 25 years earlier, in 1963) and standardized mean systolic blood pressure (SBP) in adulthood among 20- to 29-year-olds, for a number of countries participating in the INTERSALT study (an international study of electrolyte excretion and blood pressure, 1988/1989). **Correlation** is often used to measure association in ecological studies. **Causal inferences** cannot be drawn from this type of study, and, sometimes, associations that are observed at the population level cannot be similarly found in studies that measure the same characteristics at the individual level, as proper control of **confounding** is often not feasible (ALTMAN, 1991). The opposite may also occur, as measurements at the group or population level represent 'averaged values', which may result in the dilution or attenuation of associations. A similar effect may result from the use of proxy measures for exposure and disease (ROTHMAN, 1986). OWEN, WHINCUP & COOK concluded that

"The directions of these associations suggest that [low mean birthweight and] high infant mortality are not important determinants of high population mean adult blood pressure levels." See Morgenstern, in ROTHMAN, GREENLAND & LASH (eds., 2012), for a fuller discussion, and also ELLIOTT & WARTENBERG (2004). See also **ecological bias**, **regression dilution bias**, **spatial epidemiology**.

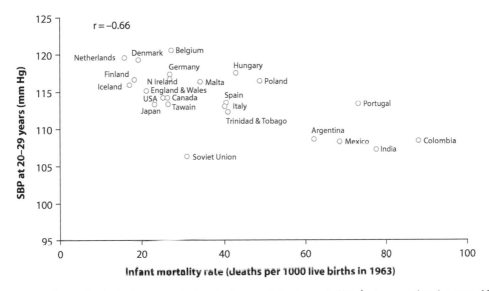

Figure E.1 Ecological study: correlation between infant mortality (rates as deaths per 1000 live births, measured 25 years earlier) and standardized mean systolic blood pressure (SBP, in mmHg) in adulthood, for different countries included in the INTERSALT study. (Reproduced from Owen CG et al. (2005). Are early life factors responsible for international differences in adult blood pressure? An ecological study. *Int J Epidemiol* **34**: 649–54 (with permission).)

## EDA

Abbreviation for **exploratory data analysis**.

## EER

Abbreviation for **experimental group event rate**.

## EF

Abbreviation for **error factor**.

## EFA

Abbreviation for exploratory factor analysis. See **factor analysis**.

## Effect measure

See **measures of effect**.

## Effect-measure modification

Or statistical **interaction**. With regard to two (or more) factors that may affect a given outcome, statistical interaction is said to be present when the effect of one factor changes across the range of values for the other factor. It is important to note that a statistical interaction will be present (or not), depending on the choice of **measure of effect** or **measurement scale**: if there is no interaction when an *absolute* measure is used (e.g. the **risk difference**), there will be an interaction when a *relative* measure (e.g. the **risk ratio**) is used to analyse the same data, and vice-versa (HILLS, 1974). Statistical interaction is represented in **linear** and **generalized linear regression models** by **product terms** that may involve two or more **predictor variables**. Use of these product terms may be helpful when fitting **predictive models**, where greater **saturation** leads to greater predictive ability. For **causal models**, a proper evaluation of **biological interaction** is needed. See ROTHMAN (2012) for further discussion.

## Effect size

The magnitude of a **measure of effect**, which may be *standardized* or *unstandardized*. Unstandardized effect measures are often used in the analysis of **primary studies**, and give an estimate of **treatment** or **exposure effect** through measures such as differences between means and risk and rate differences. Standardized measures, on the other hand, are particularly useful in the context of **meta-analysis**, when the individual studies included have different, albeit related, **outcomes** (e.g. degree of flexibility and level of pain in patients with arthritis). More details are given under **standardized measures of effect**, for both **binary** and **continuous** outcomes. As a rough guide, and for *standardized differences,* 0.2 might be considered a small effect, 0.5 a medium effect, and 0.8 a large effect. Standardized measures relate to the concept of *practical significance,* i.e. **clinical significance**, which is expressed in a manner that facilitates comparison between different studies. Methodological complexities and difficulties with correct interpretation should be kept in mind when evaluating standardized effects. See MACHIN & CAMPBELL (2005), ELLIS (2010) and BORENSTEIN *et al.* (2009) for further details and discussion.

## Effective sample size

The **sample size** available to detect real effects as significant at the desired **level of significance**, after taking into account factors such as **attrition**, **protocol breaches**, invalid **assumptions** or **design effects**, which reduce the initial or total sample size, thus decreasing the **power** of a given statistical test. Examples of instances leading to a reduced effective sample size are the **exclusion** of ineligible individuals from the data analysis, **losses to follow-up**, incorrect **assumptions** about the variability of a measurement, revised hypotheses regarding the magnitude of treatment effects in **adaptive designs, treatment–period interaction** in a crossover trial (that then becomes a parallel design trial – see **carry-over**), the presence of synergistic effects in a trial that employs a **factorial design** and **clustered designs** in which the study unit is the group or cluster, not the individual. KIRKWOOD & STERNE (2003) give formulae for adjustments to standard sample size calculations, which may be used when **losses to follow-up, confounding** and **subgroup analyses** are anticipated, and also when employing clustered designs. See ELDRIDGE & KERRY (2012) for a comprehensive discussion in the context of cluster randomized trials.

## Effectiveness

The extent to which a treatment or intervention works in real life settings and benefits its intended **target population**. Treatments of proven **efficacy** may show little or no benefit when adopted in every day practice. Patient **compliance**, side-effects and **adverse reactions**, and **concomitant treatments** are some of the factors affecting efficacy to determine effectiveness. See also **pragmatic trial**, **Phase III trial**, **intention-to-treat analysis**; Sackett, in HAYNES *et al*. (eds., 2006).

## Efficacy

The extent to which a treatment or intervention has a beneficial effect under controlled, **experimental** conditions. Efficacy may be evaluated against a **placebo** treatment where no effective treatments exist for a given target disease, or by comparing the effect of the new or experimental treatment against an established treatment of known efficacy, which is tantamount to an indirect comparison with a placebo treatment. Sackett, in HAYNES *et al*. (eds., 2006), provides further discussion around these evaluations. Efficacy alone may not be sufficient in determining that a given drug or treatment will have a significant impact when adopted in every day practice, as many other factors (such as compliance and unexpected adverse reactions) interact to determine **effectiveness**. It should always be balanced against **safety** considerations. See also **explanatory trial**, **Phase III trial**, **perprotocol analysis**. The **relative risk reduction** (**RRR**), a measure of the impact of treatments and interventions, is also referred to as 'efficacy' or 'preventable fraction', especially when evaluating vaccine efficacy.

## Efficiency

The extent to which a given statistical method is able to produce **precise** results or **estimates** from the **sample size** at hand, i.e. its ability to extract the maximum amount of information from the data available. Greater efficiency does not, however, exclude the possibility of **bias**. An example is the greater efficiency of **multiple regression** as compared to **stratification** methods, at the possible expense of **validity**. Some **study designs** are also more efficient than others: a much smaller **case–control study** can estimate an exposure effect with the same level of precision as a larger **cohort study**, and a **crossover trial** is more efficient than a **parallel trial** of the same size. **Stratified sampling** is also more efficient than **simple random sampling**. FLEISS (1999) and MACHIN & CAMPBELL (2005) illustrate the relative efficiency of various experimental (and observational) designs and **analysis of covariance**. Rothman & Greenland, in ROTHMAN, GREENLAND & LASH (eds., 2012), discuss strategies to increase cost efficiency (in case–control studies, in particular), and how **matching** and **stratification** affect efficiency. See also **effective sample size**.

## Egger's regression asymmetry plot

See **Egger's test**, **Galbraith plot**.

## Egger's regression intercept

See **Egger's test**.

## Egger's test

A test that is commonly used in conjunction with a variation of the **Galbraith plot** (Egger's regression asymmetry plot), and which provides a formal assessment as to the presence of **publication bias** in the results of a **meta-analysis** (EGGER *et al.*, 1997). As with the **Begg and Mazumdar test**, the aim is to evaluate whether the **magnitude** of estimates of effect is related to **study size**, as results from smaller, poorer quality studies are often overestimated. Egger's test is based on the **linear regression** of the standardized **estimate** (i.e. estimate/SE) on the inverse of the standard error (1/SE or **precision**), and tests the extent to which the regression line is removed from the origin, i.e. it is a test of the **null hypothesis** that the **intercept** equals zero. A regression line going through the origin gives the best indication of no evidence of publication bias, or more generally, of small study effects. On the other hand, a deviation of the intercept from zero indicates that smaller studies (with less precise results) have produced large estimates of effect. See Sterne, Egger & Davey Smith, in EGGER, DAVEY SMITH & ALTMAN (eds., 2001), STERNE *et al.* (2011) and BLAND (2015) for further discussion on the evaluation of publication bias/funnel plot asymmetry. See also **funnel plot**, **meta-regression**, **regression through the origin**.

## $e_i$

In the context of **regression analysis**, the **residual** of the *i*th observation.

## Eigenvalue

See **principal components analysis**, **scree plot**.

## Eligibility criteria

In the context of **clinical trials**, it refers to the criteria used by researchers for selecting patients for possible inclusion in a trial. The criteria should include detailed and objective **diagnostic** criteria for the disease or condition for which treatments are being tested, and any patient characteristics deemed relevant, such as age group, gender and ethnicity. **Exclusion criteria** are also commonly used, to further refine the criteria for inclusion. Eligibility criteria are also pertinent in **case–control studies**, to help determine which patients qualify as **cases**, and, by extension, who constitutes the **source population** from which **controls** will be selected. An important consideration when setting out inclusion criteria for a case–control study is that selection of cases and controls should be *independent* from **exposure** status. See also **restriction**.

## Empirical distribution

An actual or observed **frequency distribution**. Cf. **theoretical distribution**.

## Endpoint

Synonym for **outcome**. See also **surrogate endpoint**, **multiple outcomes**.

## Enrolment

See **accrual period**, **eligibility criteria**, **exclusion criteria**. Cf. **attrition**.

## Epidemics (Study of)

The application of epidemiological and statistical principles and methodology to the study of the occurrence of disease (either communicable or non-communicable) in a given population and over a given time-period, such that the **incidence** of the disease in question is considerably greater than would be expected, or than has been detected during the preceding time-period by disease **surveillance** systems. The **case–control design** is often used in the study of epidemics and disease outbreaks. Special statistical methods may be employed to analyze **clustering** patterns. See ROTHMAN (2012) for an overview.

## Epidemiological study

A study that aims to evaluate the relationship between one or more **exposures** and occurrence of disease. This is in contrast with **clinical trials**, which are mainly concerned with the evaluation of treatments and interventions that prevent adverse disease outcomes. Epidemiological studies tend to be **observational** in nature, especially where the exposure in question is believed to be detrimental. **Intervention studies** may also be carried out to answer epidemiological questions involving protective or preventive exposures. Examples of the latter are **field** and **community intervention trials**. **Cohort** and **case–control studies** are study designs often used when conducting observational studies, though pertinent questions may sometimes be adequately answered using the **cross-sectional design**. In community intervention trials, **cluster randomization** is used to assign the **study units** to the different interventions under study. See WALD (2004), ROTHMAN (2012) and HENNEKENS, BURING & MAYRENT (eds., 1987) for a comprehensive overview, and ROTHMAN, GREENLAND & LASH (eds., 2012) for in-depth discussion. ARMITAGE, BERRY & MATHEWS (2002) give an overview of statistical methods in epidemiology. See also **epidemiology, study design, prospective study, retrospective study, ecological study, exposure effect, measures of effect, bias, confounding**.

## Epidemiology

The branch of medical science that studies disease **distribution** in populations, i.e. *who* gets diseased, *where* and *when*. Epidemiology is also concerned with the study of disease determinants, i.e. the reasons *why* people are affected by disease. Other health-related outcomes such as causes of death, disease outcomes, behaviours and provision and use of health services are also the focus of epidemiology (PORTA (ed.), 2014). The main areas of epidemiological study are disease **surveillance** and **analytical research**, the latter entailing observational and intervention studies. An important goal of epidemiological research is to identify the **causative factors** for different diseases, which can lead to the development and implementation of appropriate disease control and disease prevention measures. See also **spatial epidemiology, clinical epidemiology, epidemiological study**.

## EQUATOR Network

From the website (www.equator-network.org; accessed 12/2016): "The EQUATOR (Enhancing the QUAlity and Transparency Of health Research) Network is an international initiative that seeks to improve the reliability and value of published health research literature by promoting transparent and accurate reporting and wider use of robust reporting guidelines. [...]" The organization's website serves as a hub for well over 300 reporting guidelines, including **CONSORT**, **PRISMA**, **STROBE**, **STARD**, and **TRIPOD**.

## Equipoise

Or more specifically, clinical equipoise. In the context of medical research, the lack of certainty regarding the comparative merits of alternative therapies for a given target disease among certain patient groups or populations (FREEDMAN, 1987). Sackett, in HAYNES *et al.* (eds., 2006), discusses equipoise and uncertainty, and points out the need to take the individual clinician's and individual patient's uncertainty into account, in addition to the more general uncertainty of the professional community. Clinical equipoise provides ethical justification (among other factors) for **randomization** in the conduct of **clinical trials**, and individual-level uncertainty provides justification for the enrollment of a particular patient into a clinical trial. SENN (2008) provides additional discussion. See also **eligibility**, **exclusion criteria**.

## Equivalence studies

See **active control equivalence study**, **bioequivalence study**.

## Equivalence trial

Equivalence and non-inferiority trials are discussed under **active control equivalent study** (**ACES**).

## ERR

Abbreviation for **excess relative risk**.

## Error

This term has different meaning depending on usage and context. As in ordinary, non-statistical usage, it refers to a mistake – usually one that is made when making or recording an observation, or when taking or recording a measurement. For example, a subject may be recorded as being male when they are female; this would usually be a recording error but might sometimes be an observing error. In contrast, a subject may be recorded as weighing 70.1 kg when, in fact, they weigh 70.2 kg; this may be because the scales are not very accurate, or perhaps the person has stood rather awkwardly on the scales and they have not recorded the weight properly. The term is also used in the context of **regression analysis**, where errors, also known as **residuals**, provide a means of evaluating the extent to which a model has been correctly specified and provides a good fit for the data. Error also comes into play when establishing disease and exposure status, and here it is evaluated by studying the **accuracy** of diagnostic tests and the **reliability** of measurements, methods and tools. Attention to study design, trial protocol, correct classification and minimization of measurement error, avoidance of systematic errors (**selection biases**, **information biases** and **confounding**; also, **misspecification**) and use of appropriate methods of statistical analysis are all steps that can and should be taken to eliminate as much error as possible from the results and conclusions of an investigation. See additional details under non-differential **misclassification** and **measurement error** (random errors), **bias** and **measurement bias** (systematic errors), and **sampling error, standard error, type I error** and **type II error** (inferential errors).

## Error bar chart

See **dot plot**, where these two graphical displays are compared and contrasted. Error bar charts are also termed 'plunger plots'.

## Error factor

A quantity that is used to compute the limits of a **confidence interval** (**CI**) for a *ratio* **measure of effect**. This quantity or factor is based on the **standard error** (**SE**) of the **log** of the ratio, which prevents negative values from being obtained for the *lower limit* of the confidence interval, especially in cases where the ratio measure is close to zero and imprecise. The ratio measure is divided by the error factor (EF) thus calculated to give the lower limit of the confidence interval, and multiplied to give the upper limit. This is equivalent to calculating the limits of a confidence interval on the log scale and then **back-transforming** the lower and upper limit, as, for example, when calculating confidence intervals for the regression coefficients estimated by a **generalized linear model**. For a 95% CI, the error factor is given by:

$$EF = \exp[1.96 \times SE\,(\log_e \text{ of ratio measure})]$$

where 'exp' is the **exponentiation** or antilog function, 1.96 is the 2.5% **critical value** of the standard Normal distribution, and 'ratio measure' refers to the **risk ratio**, the **odds ratio** or the **rate ratio**. CIs will be asymmetrical. KIRKWOOD & STERNE (2003) give formulae for calculating the standard error of the log of these ratio measures using the **delta method**.

## Error rate

Synonym for misclassification rate. See **classification table**.

## Estimate

A **summary measure** (e.g. a **mean, proportion, regression coefficient, relative risk**, etc.) that is calculated from **sample** data. A single-value estimate may be more precisely termed a *point* estimate. Estimates are used to draw **inferences** about the true values or **parameters** of **populations**, and about **treatment** and **exposure effects**. Estimates should be reported with the corresponding **standard errors** (**SE**), usually translated into **confidence intervals** (*interval* estimates) for ease of interpretation. See also **precision, bias, crude estimate, adjusted estimate, measures of effect**.

## Estimation

The process of deriving point and interval **estimates** from **sample** data. See also **confidence interval**. Cf. **significance testing**.

## Estimator

A formula or equation that is used to estimate the value of a given **parameter** (e.g. a **mean**, an **incidence rate** or a **risk ratio**). The term is also used to refer to the **estimate** itself. Ideally, an estimator will be **efficient** (or **precise**) and **unbiased**. An estimator is said to be unbiased if the mean of its **sampling distribution** (i.e. its **expected value** or long-run expectation) equals the true value of the parameter that is being estimated. Precision is given by the variance of the estimator, i.e. the **mean squared error** or its square root, the **standard error**: the lower the variance or the standard error, the greater the precision of the estimator. A biased estimator may nonetheless be efficient. See also **bootstrapping, jackknifing**.

## Eta squared

A **standardized measure of effect** that is equivalent to $R^2$, the square of the **multiple correlation coefficient, $R$**, and which is calculated in the context of **analysis of variance** (**ANOVA**) as the ratio of the between-groups **sum of squares** to the total sum of squares. Eta squared ($\eta^2$) is considered a more **biased** measure than **omega squared ($\omega^2$)**, especially with small **sample sizes**. Similarly to the latter, it gives the proportion of total variance that is accounted for by an effect or factor under study. A *partial* measure may also be calculated for an effect where additional factors and/or covariates add to, rather than reduce, the variability in the **outcome variable** (see **partial correlation coefficient**). A *generalized* eta squared has been proposed for comparing results from different experimental designs (e.g. including just the **factor** of interest, a **covariate** and/or additional factors, **blocking** factors, and mixed fixed and random effects – see **linear mixed effects model**) (OLEJNIK & ALGINA, 2003). See also **effect size**.

## Etiological fraction

See **aetiological fraction, attributable fraction**.

## Evidence-based medicine

Often referred to by its abbreviation, EBM. Defined by STRAUS *et al.* (2010) to be the integration of best clinically relevant research evidence with clinical expertise and patient values and circumstances (the unique preferences, concerns and expectations each patient brings to a clinical encounter, in the context of their clinical state and setting). The *Evidence-Based Medicine Working Group* at McMaster University, Canada, and the *Centre for Evidence-Based Medicine*, Oxford University, UK, are among the institutions that have played a significant role in the development, promotion, and implementation of this approach. Dr. Gordon Guyatt of the EBM Working Group is credited with having coined the term in a 1991 editorial of the ACP Journal Club (Annals of Internal Medicine). See also **clinical epidemiology, hierarchy of evidence, critical appraisal, Cochrane Collaboration, science-based medicine**; EVIDENCE-BASED MEDICINE WORKING GROUP (1992), HENEGHAN & BADENOCH (2006).

## Exact method

A method for interval **estimation** or, more commonly, for evaluating **statistical significance**, which is based on the discrete **probability distribution** (for example, the **binomial, hypergeometric** or **Poisson distribution**) that best describes the **sampling distribution** of the outcome of interest (usually, a count or observed frequency). This is in contrast with methods based on **approximations** by continuous probability distributions (usually, the

**Normal** or the **chi-squared distribution**). Exact methods give the **exact probability** (under the **null hypothesis**, and assuming relevant totals are fixed) of each and all possible outcomes that are equal to, or more extreme than, the outcome observed in a study. (More extreme outcomes are those still farther from the null hypothesis. In a 2 × 2 table, for example, the observed frequencies – given margin totals that remain unchanged – that would suggest even stronger association between, for instance, exposure and disease.) These probabilities are then added up to give the exact significance level or **P-value** for the test. Exact methods do away with the **assumption** of a large enough **sample size** and with the need for **continuity corrections**. However, modified P-values may need to be calculated as exact P-values are usually too conservative (see **mid P-value**). See **Fisher's exact test**. Cf. **asymptotic method, large sample method, z-test, chi-squared test**.

## Exact probability

The **probability** of each distinct value of a **discrete random variable**. It is calculated from the equation or **probability mass function** for the relevant **probability distribution**. When carrying out an exact test of significance, the resulting **P-value** is a cumulative sum of exact probabilities. Exact probabilities cannot be calculated for the values of a **continuous** random variable (see **Normal distribution curve**, p. 235). See also **exact method**.

## Excess relative risk

An alternative way of expressing **relative risk**, the **excess relative risk** (ERR) or **relative risk increase** (RRI) is a measure of **relative effect** that relates the **absolute risk increase** (ARI) or attributable risk to the risk in the *unexposed*. It is calculated as follows:

$$ERR = \frac{absolute\ risk\ increase}{risk\ in\ unexposed} = \frac{risk_1 - risk_0}{risk_0}$$

where, from Table 2.a (**Contingency table**, p. 72), $risk_1$ is the risk among the exposed, and $risk_0$ among the unexposed. The ERR may be multiplied by 100 to be expressed as a percentage. Alternatively, it may be calculated from the **risk ratio** (**RR**):

$$ERR = (RR - 1) \times 100\%$$

The excess relative risk or relative risk increase is interpreted as the percentage increase in risk in the exposed group relative to the risk in the unexposed (see Box E.1).

### BOX E.1

Based on data from Sodemann M *et al.* (2008). Hypothermia of newborns is associated with excess mortality in the first 2 months of life in Guinea-Bissau, West Africa. *Trop Med Int Health* **13**: 980–6.

In the study by SODEMANN *et al.* (2008) on the long-term effects of neonatal hypothermia (HT) on survival in the west African country of Guinea-Bissau, 2926 live births were identified that took place in a maternity ward between 1997 and 2002. Axillary temperature was measured within 12 h of birth, and 238 newborns were diagnosed with HT. Based on

*continued...*

*continued...*

mortality risk, HT was defined as body temperature below 34.5°C. Infants were followed up for 6 months through regular home visits, using a community- and hospital-based surveillance system. 177 deaths before 6 months of age were registered. Controlled for birthweight, HT was associated with a nearly fivefold increase in mortality during the first 7 days: mortality ratio = 4.81 (infants with HT as newborns *vs.* infants with normal temperatures), with 95% CI = 2.90–8.00. The ERR is therefore (4.81 – 1) × 100% = 381%. Increased risk of death associated with hypothermia as a newborn was seen up to at least 2 months of age.

*Interpretation:* The mortality risk at 7 days (within the perinatal period) increased by 381% in infants with HT as newborns, as compared to those with normal axillary temperatures, with 95% CI from 190% to 700%.

See also **attributable fraction (AF$_{exposed}$)**, which relates the absolute risk increase to the risk in the *exposed*; **relative risk reduction (RRR)**, also termed efficacy or preventable fraction.

## Exchangeable correlation matrix

See **correlation structure, generalized estimating equations (GEEs)**.

## Exclusion criteria

In the context of **clinical trials**, it refers to the criteria used by researchers to determine which patients, among those eligible for inclusion in a particular trial, should nonetheless be excluded due to either ethical, safety or practical considerations. In other words, exclusion criteria are further refinements to the **eligibility criteria**. A reason for excluding eligible patients from trial participation is the possibility that their **prognoses** will be worse with the trial treatment(s) than without. Another reason is the fact that too much **heterogeneity** in terms of patient characteristics may result in excessive **variability** of response, which can lead to inconclusive results. **Restriction** offers a possible solution to the latter. Checklists are often used to ensure that eligibility and exclusion criteria are applied objectively, not only in experimental studies, but also in observational studies, as for example in **case–control studies**, to define who qualifies as a **case**.

## Expected frequency

As opposed to **observed frequency (O)**. In a **contingency table**, the frequency expected in each cell, under the **assumption** of **independence** or lack of association between **exposure** (or treatment) and **outcome**, or between any two categorical variables of interest. For each cell, it is calculated as follows:

$$E = \frac{row\ total \times column\ total}{grand\ total}$$

where the row and column totals are also known as **marginal totals**. In Table 2 (p. 72), for example, the expected frequency in the first cell (*a*) is: $(a + c)(a + b)/(a + b + c + d)$. The formal comparison of *O vs. E* is given by the **chi-squared test**. These comparisons form the basis of **goodness-of-fit** (**GoF**) tests such as the **Hosmer and Lemeshow test** used in the context of logistic regression, and GoF tests that compare the frequency in each category, value, or class interval of a categorical or quantitative (discrete or continuous) variable (i.e. the observed **frequency distribution**) to the frequency that is expected based on the parameters of a **theoretical distribution**.

## Expected outcome

The **outcome** or response that is **predicted** on the basis of a **model**, as opposed to the actual outcome that is measured or **observed** to have occurred.

## Expected value

The expected value of each observation of a **continuous variable**, under the **assumption** the variable in question follows a given **theoretical distribution** with **parameters** given by the sample statistics. The meaning here is equivalent to 'fitted' or 'predicted' value in the context of **regression analysis**. A common application of this concept is the **Normal plot**, which is used to assess the extent to which the distribution of a given variable may be said to follow an approximately **Normal distribution**. Reference is also made to the expected value of a continuous or discrete **random variable** $X$, $E(X)$, as being either the mean of a **population distribution** or the mean of a **sampling distribution**. Likewise, the expected value of an **estimator** is the mean of its sampling distribution.

## Experimental group event rate

Or EER. Usually referring to the **risk** or **rate** of occurrence of the event of interest in a research study among the treated. Cf. **control group event rate** or CER. See **risk** or **rate** **difference**; **risk** or **rate ratio**.

## Experimental study

A study in which investigators attempt to isolate a **treatment effect** by comparing groups of individuals thought to be similar overall in every respect except for the factor or factors under study, which are usually under experimental control. **Comparability** between study groups is crucial for an **unbiased** assessment, and is normally achieved through **random allocation** of individuals or **study units** to the treatments being compared. **Simple randomization** may be employed, which does not always result in study groups with similar distribution of important **baseline characteristics** (i.e. with similar overall **prognosis**). Prognostic balance through randomization limits the number of competing explanations for an effect that is observed. Greater control of prognostic factors may be achieved through two additional strategies, **blocking** (see block or **restricted randomization/randomized block design**) and **stratified randomization**. This greater control of factors that account for between-subject variability further reduces **response variability**, which increases the **precision** of estimates of treatment effect. **Analysis of covariance** (**ANCOVA**) is an approach to data analysis that is used to the same aim.

Simple randomization and block randomization result in **parallel group** comparisons (unmatched and matched). Blocking can be made more **efficient** still by treating each patient as a 'treatment block', i.e. by administering all treatments under study to each and all study participants, as in a **repeated measurements** randomized block design, or in a two-period or multiperiod **crossover trial**. These are examples of one-factor designs in which there is a single treatment factor, which is the factor of interest, and one or two blocking factors. In clinical experiments, there is often interest in the joint effect or **interaction** between two (or more) factors. **Factorial** and **split-plot designs** may be used to this aim, the former corresponding to a comparison between independent groups, and the latter to independent-group comparisons between levels of factor A, and within-subject comparisons between levels of factor B (i.e. it also involves repeated measurements). See FLEISS (1999), ARMITAGE, BERRY & MATHEWS (2002), MACHIN & CAMPBELL (2005) and HUITEMA (2011) for further details and illustrative examples. See also **clinical trial**, **intervention study**.

## Explanatory trial

A **clinical trial** such as a **Phase III drug trial**, in which researchers are mainly concerned with assessing the **efficacy** of a treatment regimen. For this reason, explanatory trials usually employ stricter **eligibility criteria** and a number of **exclusion criteria**. Data analysis is typically carried out **perprotocol**, as opposed to by **intention-to-treat**. Cf. **pragmatic trial**.

## Explanatory variable

See **predictor variable**.

## Exploratory data analysis

Sometimes denoted by the abbreviation EDA, it refers to data analysis to check for errors and inconsistencies (also referred to as 'initial data analysis' or IDA), and to develop an understanding of the **distribution** of, and **relationships** between, variables. **Cross-tabulations** and **graphical displays** play an important role in these initial assessments, and inform how subsequent **inferential analysis** (or **confirmatory data analysis**) should best be performed. See TUKEY (1977) for methods and application.

## Exploratory factor analysis

Or its abbreviation, EFA. See **factor analysis**. Cf. confirmatory factor analysis (CFA).

## Exponential curve

A depiction of a **non-linear relationship** between two **continuous variables**, where a unit increase in the $x$-variable is associated with an increase in the value of the $y$-variable by a fixed multiple (HILLS, 1974). For example, in the relationships $y = e^x$ and $y = 10^x$ (depending on whether base $e$ or base 10 is used – see **ln, log$_{10}$, exponentiation**) $y$ increases by a factor of $e$ (the mathematical constant 2.718…) or by a factor of 10, for each unit increase in *x*. This curve is characteristic of a rapid *growth* process, such as that of population growth over time in the absence of environmental resistance or constraints (constrained population growth may be better described by a *negative exponential* curve, a curve displaying accelerated initial growth that decelerates at a particular point in time). The reverse curve is characteristic of a rapid *decay* process, such as loss of radioactivity over time. Exponential curves may be fitted through **curvilinear** and **non-linear regression** (HAMILTON, 1992). The specific curve obtained depends on the magnitude and direction of the parameters of a given model, and the values of the *x*-variable. An example is the log-log curve or log-log plot in Figure E.2 (SHROFF *et al.*, 2008). Such a relationship is modelled by taking logs of both the *y* and the *x* variable (see also semi-log plot). Cf. **sigmoid curve, J-shaped curve, U-shaped** (quadratic) **curve,** two-term exponential curve **(non-monotonic).** See also **exponential distribution.** Exponential curves are also referred to as J-shaped growth curves (not to be confused with non-monotonic J-shaped curves).

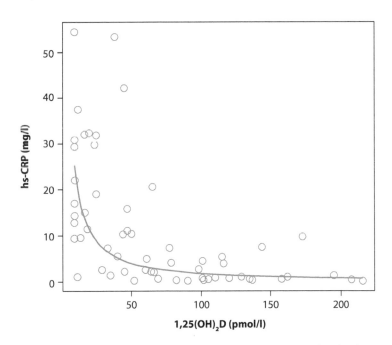

**Figure E.2** Decay exponential curve for the relationship between 1,25(OH)$_2$D (active vitamin D3, in pmol/l) and hs-CRP (high sensitivity C-reactive protein, in mg/l) levels, in children on dialysis; the regression line was fitted on the log-log scale and is shown back-transformed. (Reproduced from Shroff R *et al.* (2008). A bimodal association of vitamin D levels and vascular disease in children on dialysis. *J Am Soc Nephrol* **19**: 1239–46 (with permission).)

## Exponential distribution

A continuous **probability distribution** that describes the distribution of a 'time to event' variable, where the rate of occurrence of the event in question is constant over time.

This is the distribution of **survival times** when the **hazard rate** remains constant over time. It is also the distribution of a 'waiting time' or 'time between consecutive events' variable, when the event in question occurs as a **Poisson** process, i.e. independently, at random, and at constant rate $\lambda$. This establishes a relationship between these two distributions (Poisson and exponential), whereby if the sampling distribution of the 'number of events per unit of time' follows a Poisson distribution, the frequency distribution of 'time to event' or 'time between events' follows an exponential distribution. The exponential distribution is said to be 'memoryless', as the probability of the event per unit of time is not conditional on time already waited. The rate **parameter**, $\lambda$ (lambda), defines the exponential distribution. The **mean** and **variance** are given by $1/\lambda$ and $1/\lambda^2$, where the mean represents the average number of time units 'until the event'. The higher the rate, $\lambda$, the lower the mean of the distribution. The **probability density function (pdf)** is given by $f(x) = \lambda e^{-\lambda x}$ and the **cumulative distribution function (CDF)** is given by $F(x) = 1 - e^{-\lambda x}$, where $\lambda$ is the rate of occurrence of the event (always positive), $x$ is the value of the time variable at which these functions are to be evaluated (always non-negative), and $e$ is the mathematical constant 2.718... The exponential distribution is sometimes referred to as negative exponential distribution (see Figure E.3). Continuous variables that display an approximate exponential distribution are often referred to as having a reverse **J-shaped distribution** (not to be confused with J-shaped curves). These are distributions with an extreme positive **skew**. See also **exponential curve** (a plot of the relationship between two variables, mathematically defined as exponential).

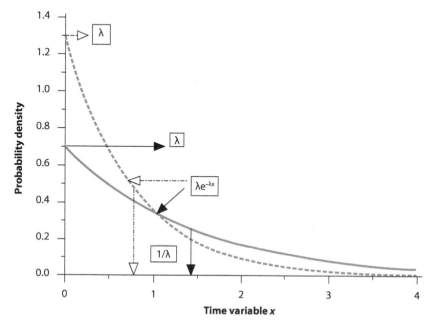

**Figure E.3** Probability density function for two negative exponential distributions (rate parameter is $\lambda$, and mean or expected value is $1/\lambda$): rate and mean are, for the solid line, 0.7 and 1.43, respectively; for the dashed line, 1.3 and 0.77 (drawn using MedCalc Statistical Software).

## Exponential model

In the context of **generalized linear models**, an *exponential risk model* of the form:

$$Predicted\ risk = \exp(\alpha + \beta x)$$

may be specified as a **log-linear risk model**, by taking logs of both sides of the equation:

$$Log(predicted\ risk) = \alpha + \beta x$$

where $\beta$ is the estimated log risk ratio and $\exp(\beta)$ is the estimated **risk ratio** (Greenland, in ROTHMAN, GREENLAND & LASH [eds., 2012]). See also **accelerated failure time models**, **proportional hazards models** (parametric survival models).

## Exponentiation

Exponentiation of $y$ to the power $x$ is the process of calculating $y^x$. It is the inverse of the process of calculating a **logarithm**. If using the base 10, application of exponentiation to the values 2 and 3 gives 100 and 1000, respectively (i.e. $10^2 = 100$ and $10^3 = 1000$). Often, the base $e$, the base of natural logarithms, is chosen (see **ln**). Note that $y^0$ is taken to be equal to 1, regardless of the value of $y$. Exponentiation or 'anti-logging' is often carried out when analysing results from medical research, as many biological measurements follow a **lognormal distribution**. In addition, a number of frequently used regression models are specified on a logarithmic or logit **transformation** of the **predicted outcome** variable, and therefore **regression coefficients** must be **back-transformed** to the original scale by taking antilogs. The following arithmetic equivalences involving exponentiation have frequent practical application:

$$\exp(a + b) = \exp(a) \times \exp(b)$$

$$\exp(a - b) = \exp(a) \div \exp(b)$$

For example, and in the simplest case, the combined effect of two or more binary variables in a **multiplicative model** is calculated by anti-logging the sum of their regression coefficients, or by multiplying the antilogs of each coefficient. Also, the antilog of the coefficient for each of the binary variables is really a ratio of $\exp(a)$, where $a$ is the regression coefficient, to $\exp(b)$, where $b$ is the implicit coefficient for the reference or unexposed group and taken to be 0, with $\exp(b)$ taken to be 1. See also **geometric mean**, **logistic regression**, **Cox regression**, **Poisson regression**, **delta method**.

## Exposure

In its widest sense, any biological characteristic, genetic predisposition, behaviour, environmental or occupational hazard, treatment or intervention that is thought to be associated with the development (**risk factor**) or prevention (protective or **preventive factor**) of a given disease or **outcome**. Often, a distinction is made between 'exposures', whose effects are evaluated in **observational studies**, and 'treatments' or 'interventions', the focus of **experimental studies**. Uncovering the role of exposures in disease **causation** is one of the main objectives of **epidemiological research**. See **exposure effect**, **measures of effect**. See also **propensity scores**.

## Exposure effect

The **comparative** effect of an **exposure** on a response or **outcome variable**, which is obtained by comparing groups with different levels of exposure, or with and without exposure (as in a **cohort study**, for example). Commonly used measures of exposure effect are the **absolute risk increase**, the **attributable fraction** and the **risk ratio**. See **measures of effect**.

## Extra-binomial variation

See **overdispersion**, **beta-binomial distribution**.

## Extra-Poisson variation

See **overdispersion**, **negative binomial distribution**.

## Extrapolation

In regression analysis, the **prediction** of the value of the **outcome variable** for a given value of a **predictor variable**(s) that is outside of the **range** of the **sample** data. Extrapolation may result in incorrect predictions as the pattern of relationship outside of the stated range may deviate markedly from what is specified by the **model**. For instance, in **simple linear regression**, the relationship between outcome and predictor variable may no longer be assumed to be linear. See also **generalizability**.

## Extreme observation

See **outlier**.

# F

## *F* distribution

The **probability distribution** that is followed by the ratio of two independent **chi-squared** random variables, each divided by the corresponding degrees of freedom. The **parameters** of the *F* distribution are given by the numerator and denominator **degrees of freedom** ($v$ or $df$). See **distributions, F-test**.

## *F*-test

Also known as variance-ratio test. A **significance test** that is carried out to compare the **variances** of two independent groups with respect to a Normally distributed variable, i.e. to test the assumption of **homoscedasticity**. The **test statistic**, with **degrees of freedom** equal to each respective sample size, is calculated as the ratio of the larger to the smaller variance (see below). Another common application of the *F*-test is in comparing between-groups to within-groups **variability** when an **analysis of variance** is carried out to compare the **means** of several groups (Box O.3, p. 246). Under the **null hypothesis** of no difference between the groups, these two components of variability are the same and their ratio (*F*-statistic) is equal to one. The *F* distribution (which is followed by the *F*-statistic when the null hypothesis is true) has two different degrees of freedom: the number of groups *minus* 1 (between-groups), and the total number of observations *minus* the number of groups (within-groups). When comparing two **independent** groups, the *F*-test yields the same **P-value** as the unpaired **t-test**. An overall *F*-test is used in **least squares regression** to test the joint significance of all variables in a **model**. **Nested models**, where one model is an extension of the other, may be compared using a partial *F*-test. See also **Bartlett's test, likelihood ratio test, stepwise regression, residual F-test**.

## Factor

Synonym for **categorical variable**. In a general sense, any condition, event or characteristic that may affect disease occurrence or its outcome. See **exposure, treatment, risk factor, preventive factor, prognostic factor, confounding factor**, causative factor (**component cause**), blocking factor (**block**).

## Factor analysis

A **multivariate method** that analyses the **correlations** between sets of observed measurements, with the view to estimate the number of different factors that explain these correlations. For example, correlations between the components of a composite intelligence rating scale are inferred to arise from the fact that they (the subscales or sets of measurements) are all measures of intelligence (the factor, or latent variable). An *exploratory* factor analysis (EFA) looks at these correlations, assesses the number of factors that might need to be postulated to provide an explanation for the correlations, and decides which variables might be indicative of which factors. A *confirmatory* factor analysis (CFA) evaluates whether a set of correlations can be adequately explained by a factor **model** specified *a priori*. Factor models are regression-like models that estimate standardized regression coefficients (termed 'factor loadings') for the postulated factors. This helps to determine which unobserved or unmeasurable factors explain the observed variation in each of the measured variables, and in turn which observed variables are indicative of which factors. A **composite factor score** (weighted or unweighted) may then be computed for each observation. A procedure known as 'rotation' is often used, and factors derived in this way are more easily interpreted. Rotation produces either *orthogonal* (uncorrelated) or *oblique* (correlated) factors. See also **correlation matrix**, **latent variable**, **Cronbach's alpha**, **principal components analysis**. See HAMILTON (1992; 2012) and BLAND (2015) for further details and illustrative examples.

## Factorial

For a positive **integer** $x$, factorial $x$ (or $x$ factorial) is conventionally denoted by $x!$ and is given by:

$$x! = x \times (x-1) \times (x-2) \times \ldots \times 2 \times 1$$

For example, $5! = 5 \times 4 \times 3 \times 2 \times 1 = 120$. Note that $0!$ is defined as being equal to 1. Factorials appear in the formulae for calculating **exact probabilities** under the **binomial** and **Poisson distributions**.

## Factorial design

A **study design** for a **clinical trial** that allows two or more different treatments to be evaluated simultaneously, such that both **treatment effects** and **interactions** between treatments can be estimated. In a $2 \times 2$ factorial design, patients are randomly allocated to one of the treatment groups or to a placebo control group, following which they are independently randomized to the other treatment group or, again, to a placebo control group. Four **treatment groups** result from this double **randomization**, each receiving either: the control (or **placebo**) treatment, treatment A, treatment B, or both treatments A and B. This design allows the testing of several **hypotheses** simultaneously, including that of synergism or **biological interaction** between the two treatments (Box F.1). **Sample size** calculations should take the possibility of interaction into account, as testing for the presence of an interaction usually requires larger sample sizes. See POCOCK (1983), FLEISS (1999), SENN (2002), MACHIN & CAMPBELL (2005) and HUITEMA (2011) for illustrative examples and further details. POCOCK also describes a three-treatment factorial design in which the eight different treatment regimens (A, B, C, AB, AC, BC, ABC, and no treatment) are assigned as **random permutations** within **blocks** of eight patients. Cf. **parallel design**, **crossover design**. See also **two-way ANOVA**, **split-plot design**.

## BOX F.1

From **Box A.1**, p. 3.

In the ISIS-2 trial, patient randomization was first to streptokinase *vs.* placebo, and then to aspirin *vs.* placebo, resulting in four treatment groups. Since the authors concluded the effects of aspirin and streptokinase are **additive*** (for vascular mortality at 5 weeks), it is appropriate to evaluate the effect of each treatment 'at the margins' (Sackett, in HAYNES *et al.* [eds., 2006]), i.e. by comparing all patients receiving aspirin *vs.* all not receiving aspirin (and all receiving streptokinase *vs.* all not receiving streptokinase), also referred to as **main effects**. In the presence of **biological interaction** (or departure from additivity of absolute effects) between the two treatments, the synergism or antagonism between them would make it necessary to compute separate estimates of effect (for example, effect of aspirin with streptokinase and effect of aspirin without streptokinase). The arrows represent the different comparisons made possible by the study design:

|  |  | Streptokinase | | |
|---|---|---|---|---|
|  |  | Yes $\rightarrow$ | No | Total |
| Aspirin | Yes | 4292 | 4295 | 8587 |
|  | No | 4300 | 4300 | 8600 |
|  | Total | 8592 | 8595 | 17,187 |

***Additivity of risk differences:**
Effect of aspirin (*vs.* placebo): 1016/8600 – 804/8587 = 11.8% – 9.4% – 2.4%
Effect of streptokinase (*vs.* placebo): 1029/8595 – 791/8592 = 12% – 9.2% = 2.8%
Effect of both (*vs.* neither): 568/4300 – 343/4292 = 13.2% – 8% = 5.2%, i.e. 2.4% + 2.8%

## Failure

The occurrence of the event of interest in studies of **survival**. Failure, in this context, refers to the occurrence of any event, not just adverse outcomes, and is usually measured as 'time to failure', 'survival time' or 'time to event'. Individuals whose **outcomes** are not known, or have not yet occurred by the end of the **follow-up period**, are said to have **censored** outcomes. See also **survival time**.

## False-negative rate

The complement of **sensitivity**, i.e. FNR = 100 – sensitivity%. See also **diagnostic test**.

## False-positive rate

The complement of **specificity**, i.e. FPR = 100 – specificity%. See also **diagnostic test, ROC curve, screening**.

## Familywise error rate

See **multiple-comparison procedures**.

## Fertility rate

The number of live births during a given period of time and in a given population, divided by the number of women in the population who were potentially fertile during the same time-period (alternatively stated as aged 15–44 years or 15–49). See also **demographic indicators, population pyramid, maternal mortality rate**.

## Field trial

A type of **epidemiological study** in which **interventions** such as treatments for actual diseases, preventive treatments and vaccines, vector and environmental control and behaviour-changing and educational interventions are tested. Field trials are often conducted to evaluate measures and policies that might bring about control and prevention of endemic diseases, and thus focus on the overall health of a community as opposed to individual patients. Thus, researchers conducting a field trial may have to visit study participants in their homes, places of work (or equivalent, e.g. at school or university) or at purpose-made centres, which usually involves significant logistical planning. Further details on the planning and conduct of field trials, including discussion of community participation, ethical considerations, censuses and mapping and development of questionnaires, among other topics, are given by SMITH & MORROW (eds., 1991). A distinction is usually made between different types of intervention studies at the community level on the basis of the **randomization** scheme that is employed. See also **community intervention trial**.

## Fieller's theorem

Application of this theorem allows **confidence intervals** to be constructed for the *ratio* of two **random variables** when the variables each follow (or nearly follow) a **Normal distribution** (EVERITT & SKRONDAL, 2010). See also ARMITAGE, BERRY & MATTHEWS (2002).

## Finite population correction

For a given **sample** of size $n$ which is drawn from a **population**, the **standard error** of the sample **mean** is given by:

$$\text{Standard error of the mean} = s/\sqrt{n}$$

where $s$ is the sample **standard deviation**. If, however, the population is finite in size, then its size will diminish as each sample value is drawn from it, if the sample values are not immediately replaced. If a finite population is of size $N$ to begin with, then the corrected standard error of the mean when a sample of size $n$ is taken *without replacement* is given by:

$$\text{Corrected standard error of the mean} = s\sqrt{[(1/n)(N-n)/(N-1)]}$$

where a correction factor of $\sqrt{[(N-n)/(N-1)]}$ is now applied (HAMILTON, 1990; COCHRAN, 1977; LEVY & LEMESHOW, 2009).

## Fisher's exact test

A **significance test** that is carried out to compare two or more groups with respect to the **proportion** in each group with a given outcome or characteristic. Unlike the **chi-squared**

**test**, Fisher's exact test is not based on an **approximation** by a continuous probability distribution. Its validity does not rely on **assumptions** being met or the application of **continuity corrections**. The test gives **exact probabilities** (under the **hypergeometric distribution**) for the observed cross-tabulation, and for each and all cross-tabulations that are more extreme (i.e. farther away from the **null hypothesis** of independence), given the table's **marginal totals**. These probabilities are then added up to give the test's **P-value**, which is a *cumulative* hypergeometric probability (see also **mid P-value**). An important reminder is that the test produces **one-sided** P-values, which may need to be doubled if the **alternative hypothesis** is better stated as a **two-sided test**. Commonly used with **two-by-two (2 × 2) tables**, the test may also be used with larger tables. ALTMAN (1991), BLAND (2015) and AGRESTI (2007) give additional details and illustrative examples.

## Fisher's Least Significant Differences test

See **multiple-comparison procedures**.

## Fisher's transformation

A **transformation** that is applied to **Pearson's correlation coefficient** (*r*), which allows **confidence intervals** to be calculated for *r* when the **sample size** is roughly less than 100 (BLAND, 2015; KIRKWOOD & STERNE, 2003). This prevents values outside of the range −1 to +1 from being obtained for the limits of the confidence interval.

## Fit

See **goodness-of-fit (GoF)**.

## Fitted value

In the context of **regression analysis**, the predicted value of the **outcome variable**, based on the estimated **coefficients** for a given regression **model** and the specific values of the **predictor variables** included in the model. For each observation, the difference between **observed** and fitted value is the **residual**. These may be analysed to evaluate the **goodness-of-fit** and adequacy of regression models. **Prognostic indices** and **risk scoring** tools derived from **predictive regression models** rely on the ability of fitted values to **discriminate** between competing outcomes and diagnoses.

## Fixed effect model

As opposed to **random effects model**. In the context of **meta-analysis**, where results from several studies are combined into a single **estimate** by taking a **weighted average** of individual study results, a fixed effect model is one that assumes an underlying 'true' effect exists that is the same for all **primary studies** included, differences between the various studies being the result of **sampling error**. The **Q test**, the **index of heterogeneity** ($I^2$) and graphical methods may all be employed to decide on the choice of model. See BLAND (2015), KIRKWOOD & STERNE (2003), EGGER, DAVEY SMITH & ALTMAN (eds. 2001) and BORENSTEIN *et al.* (2009) for additional details.

## Fixed effects

As opposed to **random effects**. A term that is used in the context of **analysis of variance** (**ANOVA**) and **multilevel modelling** to describe **factors** (e.g. gender, ethnicity, treatment group) all of whose categories will remain the same if a different study sample is chosen, in contrast to random effects factors (e.g. the different patients in a clinical trial in which serial measurements are taken, or the different schools selected for a community intervention trial). Usually, there is interest in the effect and significance of factors considered to be fixed, whereas random factors are usually of interest only to the extent that they account for a particular design feature (e.g. **repeated measurements** and other **clustered designs**), and to the extent that predictor variables measured at these levels may affect the outcome. See BLAND (2015) and KIRKWOOD & STERNE (2003) for additional details.

## Fleming–A'Hern design

A one-stage **Phase II trial** design in which the number of patients recruited into the trial is calculated in advance based on the proportion of responses deemed necessary to warrant further investigation, and based on the proportion of responses below which no further investigation is warranted. MACHIN & CAMPBELL (2005) give details.

## Follow-up period

The length of time subjects are kept under observation in a follow-up or **longitudinal study**. A distinction is sometimes made between the actual follow-up period, and the **accrual period** during which patients or healthy individuals are recruited to the study. In a clinical trial where the aim is to compare **survival times**, length of follow-up should be measured from **randomization**, and not from the actual time treatments are given (PETO *et al.*, 1977). For example, if patients are randomized to receive either medical (e.g. a pharmaceutical drug) or surgical treatment for the management of unstable angina, patients having surgery may have to wait longer for their treatment. Thus, were follow-up time to be measured from beginning of treatment, patients receiving the medical treatment would be given a clear advantage. See also **person-time at risk** or PTAR.

## Follow-up study

A **clinical trial** or **epidemiological study** in which information is collected by following study participants over a period of time, thus allowing temporal relationships to be investigated. The terms **prospective** and **longitudinal** are sometimes used as synonymous with follow-up study, but the former simply indicates that a study is conducted looking forward in terms of data collection and occurrence of events, even when there is no follow-up in the usual sense of the expression (e.g. prospective **nested case–control study**). On the other hand, a **retrospective cohort study** is a longitudinal study, although study participants are not actually followed up as all exposures and events of interest have already taken place. Follow-up studies are often concerned with estimating the **incidence** over time of some occurrence or disease, or the average 'time to event' and/or probability of **survival**.

## Force of morbidity

Also, force of mortality. See **hazard rate**.

## Forecast

For a given individual or **study unit**, the projection of the value of an **outcome variable** at a given time *t*, based on a **model** that includes as **predictor variables** past values of the outcome variable, or past regression errors. See also **autoregressive model**, moving average model **(time series), transition model (longitudinal data)**, autocorrelation model. Cf. **prediction**.

## Forest plot

A graphical technique for presenting the results of a **meta-analysis**, which enables a visual assessment of statistical **heterogeneity** to be made (see also **L'Abbé plot, Galbraith plot**). The point **estimate** for each individual study is displayed on either side of a solid vertical line (representing absence of **treatment** or **exposure effect** – zero if a difference is being estimated, or 1 for a relative risk measure), and represented by a solid box, the area of which is directly proportional to the study's **sample size**. This allows the magnitude and

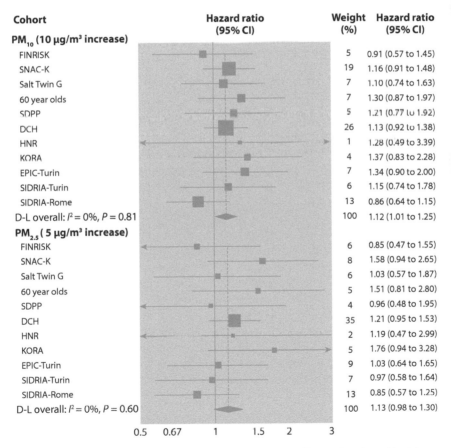

Figure F.1 A forest plot displaying estimates of exposure effect (hazard ratios of incident coronary events) for 11 cohorts (primary studies), by pollutant particulate diameter; pooled estimates of effect (diamond shapes) are also presented. (Reproduced from Cesaroni G *et al.* (2014). Long term exposure to ambient air pollution and incidence of acute coronary events: prospective cohort study and meta-analysis in 11 European cohorts from the ESCAPE Project. *Br Med J* **348**: f7412 (with permission).)

direction of effect in each **primary study** to be assessed. In addition, **confidence intervals** are also presented, which readily give information on the **statistical significance** and **precision** of individual estimates. The **pooled estimate** of effect is given by a diamond shape (often superimposed on a broken, vertical line), and its confidence interval is represented by the width of the same. An example of a forest plot is shown in Figure F.1, which displays the results from 11 cohorts participating in the European Study of Cohorts for Air Pollution Effects (ESCAPE Project – Cesaroni *et al.*, 2014). The aim of this study was to look for evidence of an association between long-term exposure to particulate air pollution and increased risk of acute coronary events. Exposure effect is given as **hazard ratios**. The relative weights attributed to each primary study are also shown (see **weighted average**).

## Forward variable selection

See **stepwise regression** (stepwise model selection).

## Fourfold table

Synonymous with **two-by-two (2 × 2) table**.

## Fractional polynomials

An extended family of curves with **power transformation** terms from the restricted set of powers {−2, −1, −0.5, 0, 0.5, 1, 2, 3}, which may be used to improve the fit of the relationship between a **continuous covariate** and a continuous outcome variable, as in **linear regression** (ROYSTON & ALTMAN, 1994), or, for models predicting risk, between the covariate and a suitable transformation of the predicted outcome such as the **logit** (see **logistic regression**) (ROYSTON, AMBLER & SAUERBREI, 1999). The powers in the restricted set include some standard transformations: **reciprocal** (−1), **square root** (0.5), **logarithmic** (0), **square** (2), and **cubic** (3). The power 1 transformation (identity) is equivalent to no transformation, and the assumption of a linear relationship with the predicted outcome. Use of fractional polynomials provides an alternative approach to analysing **non-linear relationships** with continuous risk factors or exposures, as opposed to the assumption of linearity, to **categorization** (and subsequent inclusion in a regression model as **dummy variables**), and to less flexible approaches such as fitting a **quadratic curve**. First-degree fractional polynomials may provide a good fit for modelling simple **monotonic curves** (Figure F.2; ROYSTON, AMBLER & SAUERBREI, 1999), whereas greater complexity (such as a J-shaped curve) may be better accommodated by a second or higher degree fractional polynomial. For example, a fractional polynomial of order 4 with powers chosen from the set {0, 0.5, 1, 2} is as follows:

$$\beta_0 + \beta_1 \ln x + \beta_2 \sqrt{x} + \beta_3 x + \beta_4 x^2$$

where $x$ is a continuous covariate, $\beta_0$ is the **intercept**, and $\beta_1$, $\beta_2$, … are the **regression coefficients** for each of the power terms. The quadratic curve (a lower order **polynomial**) corresponds to a fractional polynomial with powers from the set {1, 2}. See also **non-monotonic curve**, **curvilinear regression**; MITCHELL (2012b).

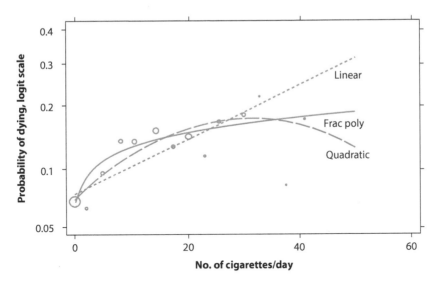

**Figure F.2** Fractional polynomials: comparing the fit of a first-degree fractional polynomial (Frac. poly.), a linear term and a quadratic curve in the relationship between all-cause mortality (log odds of dying) and cigarette consumption (number of cigarettes per day) (data from the Whitehall I study of British civil servants analysed by Royston *et al.*, 1999). Size of symbols indicates precision of estimates. (Reproduced from Royston P *et al.* (1999). The use of fractional polynomials to model continuous risk variables in epidemiology. *Int J Epidemiol* **28**· 964–74 (with permission).)

## Frailty model

A statistical **model** for **survival times** that does not assume the probability of a **censored outcome** to be the same for all individuals being followed up, due to the possible presence of **overdispersion** or random **heterogeneity** among study participants (for example, due to variability in genetic or congenital susceptibility to disease, or due to differences in lifestyle risk factors; these various factors are also termed 'frailties'). These unknown or unmeasurable factors cause individuals who are otherwise similar in their measurable risk or prognostic profile to have different probabilities of experiencing a given outcome. This is in contrast to the common assumption in standard **Cox regression** and other models for survival times of homogeneity with respect to factors other than those being analysed. Frailties may be modelled assuming variations at the individual level (overdispersion/heterogeneity model or *unshared* frailty), or at the group or cluster level (random effects model or *shared* frailty) (CLEVES, GOULD & MARCHENKO, 2016).

## Framingham risk score

See **risk score**.

## Frequency

The number of times a given category (i.e. an outcome or characteristic) occurs in the **raw data**, for any given **categorical variable**, or the number of times an observation value falls in a given **class interval**, for any given **quantitative variable**, continuous or discrete.

The frequencies for all the classes or categories of the variable in question form the **frequency distribution** for that variable. The *absolute* frequency for a category or class is the actual count or frequency in that group, whereas its *relative* frequency is the absolute frequency divided by the total frequency across all categories or classes. Multiplication of a relative frequency by 100 allows it to be expressed as a **percentage**. Box F.2 shows the frequency of various types of anaemia in non-institutionalized persons 65 years and older (data from the US Third National Health and Nutrition Examination Survey, NHANES III, Phase II, 1991 to 1994 – PATEL, 2008). Relative frequencies for each type of anaemia within two main classifications ('With nutrient deficiency' and 'Without nutrient deficiencies') and in reference to all anaemia are also shown.

## BOX F.2

Reproduced from Patel KV (2008). Epidemiology of anemia in older adults. *Semin hematol* **45**: 210–17 (with permission).

Frequency and relative frequency of various types of anaemia in non-institutionalized persons 65 years and older (data from the US Third National Health and Nutrition Examination Survey, NHANES III, Phase II, 1991 to 1994 – see also Figure F.3, p. 140). For example, the absolute frequency of '$B_{12}$ only' was 165,701, while its relative frequency within the 'With nutrient deficiency' group was 165,701/965,544, or (165,701/965,544) × 100%, which is approximately equal to 17.2% (to three **significant figures**). The overall relative frequency of $B_{12}$ deficiency anaemia was 165,701/2,814,875 × 100% or 5.9% (to two significant figures). ACI*: anaemia of chronic inflammation.

| Anemia | Number in the United States | Type, % | All anemia, % |
|---|---|---|---|
| **With nutrient deficiency** | | | |
| Iron only | 466,715 | 48.3 | 16.6 |
| Folate only | 181,471 | 18.8 | 6.4 |
| $B_{12}$ only | 165,701 | 17.2 | 5.9 |
| Folate and $B_{12}$ | 56,436 | 5.8 | 2.0 |
| Iron with folate or $B_{12}$ or both | 95,221 | 9.9 | 3.4 |
| **Total** | **965,544** | **100.0** | **34.3** |
| **Without nutrient deficiencies** | | | |
| Renal insufficiency only | 229,686 | 12.4 | 8.2 |
| ACI*, no renal insufficiency | 554,281 | 30.0 | 19.7 |
| Renal insufficiency and ACI* | 120,169 | 6.5 | 4.3 |
| Unexplained anemia | 945,195 | 51.1 | 33.6 |
| **Total** | **1,849,331** | **100.0** | **65.7** |
| **Total, all anemia** | **2,814,875** | N.A. | |

See also **bar chart, pie chart, histogram, frequency density**.

## Frequency density

An alternative way of expressing **frequency** on the vertical or **y-axis** of a **histogram**. Frequency must be expressed as density rather than a count whenever the **class intervals** of the **quantitative variable** in question are not of equal width. When this is the case, the frequency of the wider interval(s) will not take into account the fact that it is spread over a wider range of values. This problem is solved by dividing the frequency in each class interval by the width of the same, to give (within each class interval) the *frequency per unit* of the quantitative variable (BLAND, 2015). Frequency density may also be expressed as *relative frequency density*, by dividing the frequency density in each class interval by the total frequency across all class intervals, or equivalently, by dividing the *relative* frequency by the width of the class interval. When the y-axis of a histogram shows frequency densities, the frequency in each class interval is given by the *area* (not the height) of the bar for the same class interval. See also **probability density function**.

## Frequency distribution

The representation, graphical or tabular, of data in the form of **classes** or **categories** with their corresponding frequencies. An example, for a **categorical variable**, is the table given under the item **Frequency**. For a **continuous variable** such as height or body mass, or a variable that although not truly continuous, may be analysed as such, **class intervals** are formed. An example of the latter type of variable is the intelligence quotient (IQ) score, which is usually measured to the nearest integer (whole number). Suppose the IQs of all 120 first-year students at a particular medical school are measured. The following table shows the frequency distribution (also known as a 'frequency table') of these IQ scores:

| IQ score | $n$ |
| --- | --- |
| 100–109 | 42 |
| 110–119 | 34 |
| 120–129 | 26 |
| 130–139 | 12 |
| 140–149 | 6 |
| **Total** | **120** |

In this case, the range of scores was partitioned into five equal-sized class intervals (10 IQ points each). Choosing too few classes (for example, fewer than five) is likely to give too coarse a distribution. Choosing too many classes (for instance, with intervals of just one IQ point per class) does not provide a useful summary. The table above might have presented also the **cumulative frequency distribution**, alongside the column with the frequencies for each class interval. Frequency distribution and cumulative frequency distribution may also be expressed in *relative* terms. See also **bar chart**, **pie chart**, **histogram**. Cf. *empirical* or observed frequency distribution *vs. theoretical distribution*.

## Frequency matching

See **matching**.

## Frequency polygon

A line graph in which the **frequencies** (on the vertical axis) are plotted against the mid-points of the corresponding **class intervals** (on the horizontal axis). This line graph may be superimposed on the corresponding **histogram**, by simply joining together the middle points of the upper lines of the individual bars or rectangles that depict the **frequency density**. Figure F.3 (PATEL, 2008) shows the relative frequency distribution (%) of hae-moglobin measurements (in g/dl) in non-institutionalized persons 65 years and older, according to sex (data from the US Third National Health and Nutrition Examination Survey, NHANES III, 1988 to 1994). Frequency polygons allow several **distributions** to be plotted on the same graph, as is the case here with separate frequency polygons for men and women. This shows men to have higher haemoglobin levels, on average, with a range coinciding with that among women. See also **cumulative frequency polygon** (Figure C.4, p. 90).

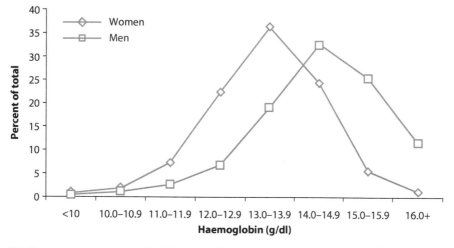

**Figure F.3** Frequency polygon: distribution of haemoglobin concentrations (in g/dl) in persons 65 years and older, according to sex (US NHANES III, 1988 to 1994). (Reproduced from Patel KV (2008). Epidemiology of anemia in older adults. *Semin hematol* **45**: 210–17 (with permission).)

## Frequentist inference

In contrast to **Bayesian inference**, frequentist inference is an approach to making statistical inferences that considers **probability** to be such that it may only be stated on the basis of repetition of observation. For example, the probability of the occurrence of a given event is the proportion of times the event occurs in a large number of observations. Thus, no statements of belief are made that would be taken into account and weighed against the actual data to arrive at an estimate of probability that goes beyond the information contained in the data. Error (as in **standard error**) and **likelihood** are key concepts in frequentist inference, as they provide a means to account for **sampling error** or variation while basing inferences on a single sample. In this way, hypotheses may be tested (**significance testing**), and confidence intervals may be calculated (**estimation**). Interpretation of **P-values** resulting from significance testing, and of confidence intervals, goes back to the idea of repetition: the $P$-value is the probability (or the *proportion of times* out of many repetitions of the study) one would come to a result of the same or greater magnitude as seen in the study sample if in fact the 'true' result were that of the **null hypothesis**. Likewise, for a 95% (for instance) **confidence interval**, we may state that 95% of the confidence intervals obtained from a large number of samples of the same size as our study sample *will contain* the 'true' value that is being estimated. See GREENLAND *et al.* (2016) for a discussion on misinterpretations of key concepts in statistical inference.

## Funnel plot

A graphical assessment of bias in **meta-analysis**, including **publication bias**. **Estimates** of **treatment** or **exposure effect** (on the **x-axis**) are plotted against the corresponding **sample size**, or, more often, the corresponding measure of **precision** (i.e. the *inverse* of the **standard error**, on the **y-axis**), for each of the individual studies (often clinical trials) included in a meta-analysis. Trials with smaller sample sizes (represented at the bottom of the graph) are subject to greater **sampling variation**, and therefore are more likely to contribute to greater scatter around the **pooled estimate** of treatment effect, and *vice versa*, with the larger trials (*smaller* standard errors, and therefore, *larger* inverse standard errors) at the top, and closer to the pooled value. A funnel-shaped (inverted V) plot that is symmetrical around the pooled estimate of treatment effect indicates absence of publication bias. On the other hand, publication bias is suspected if trials on the lower *right*-hand corner of the graph appear to be missing, as these would be trials showing absence of treatment benefit or a detrimental treatment effect. In addition, a seeming preponderance of trials on the lower left-hand corner may indicate yet another source of bias, in that when small trials display **clinically significant** results, this may be indicative of lower methodological standards, a situation often conducive to overestimation of treatment effects and consequent statistical significance. Another 'small study effect' that may explain funnel plot asymmetry are issues around *clinical* heterogeneity, where small trials are sometimes conducted in special settings, where patients, clinicians and the disease may all have unusual characteristics. In the example in Figure F.4, which looks at an association with a presumable harmful exposure, evidence of publication bias is suggested by the missing studies on the lower *left*-hand corner of the plot (and not the lower *right*-hand corner, in this instance) that would indicate a protective effect of Epstein–Barr infection with regard to multiple sclerosis. **Sensitivity analyses** ('trim and fill') may help evaluate the likely impact of missing studies, as well as the impact of excluding studies of possibly lower quality. See Sterne, Egger & Davey Smith, in EGGER, DAVEY SMITH & ALTMAN (eds., 2001), KIRKWOOD & STERNE (2003) and BLAND (2015) for a discussion of causes of funnel plot asymmetry (*small study effects*) that includes methodological approaches to its assessment. See also **Begg and Mazumdar test**, **Galbraith plot**, **Egger's test**, **meta-regression**. See **CONSORT**

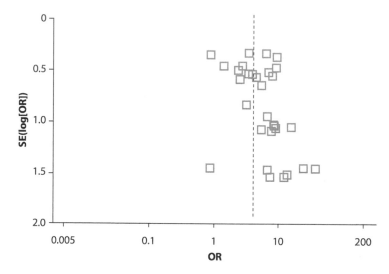

**Figure F.4** Funnel plot: meta-analysis of the sero-epidemiological association between Epstein–Barr virus and multiple sclerosis (studies testing for anti-EBNA IgG sero-positivity); missing studies on lower *left*-hand corner of the plot with regard to a presumable harmful exposure is suggestive of publication bias (the *y*-axis scale is inverted as standard errors, not inverse standard errors, are shown). (Reproduced from Almohmeed Y *et al.* (2013). Systematic review and meta-analysis of the sero-epidemiological association between Epstein–Barr virus and multiple sclerosis. *PLoS One* **8**: e61110.)

**Statement** (www.consort-statement.org) on the issue of quality standards. LAU *et al.* (2006) give a critique of the use and interpretation of the funnel plot. STERNE *et al.* (2011) give guidance on interpreting funnel plot asymmetry, make recommendations on testing, and explain implications for deciding on a **fixed effect** *vs.* a **random effects model** for summarizing the results of a meta-analysis.

## f(x)

**Probability density function** or pdf.

## F(x)

**Cumulative distribution function** or CDF.

# G

G

Or $G^2$. The **test statistic** for the **likelihood ratio test**. See also **deviance statistic**.

## Galbraith plot

Also known as Galbraith's radial plot, a graphical technique that is used to evaluate **heterogeneity** of effect among the different **primary studies** in a **meta-analysis** (GALBRAITH, 1988). For each individual study, the ratio of the **estimate of effect** (on the log scale, if ratio measures) to its **standard error** (i.e. the **test statistic**) is plotted against the reciprocal of the standard error. The latter, 1/SE, gives a measure of the **precision** of each estimate. A **regression line** is fitted through the plotted points, the **slope** of which gives the overall estimate of effect (here, unlike for **Egger's test**, the line is constrained to pass through origin, though it is also unweighted). An interval around the regression line is also plotted, which gives the limits within which most individual studies (approximately 95%, as the

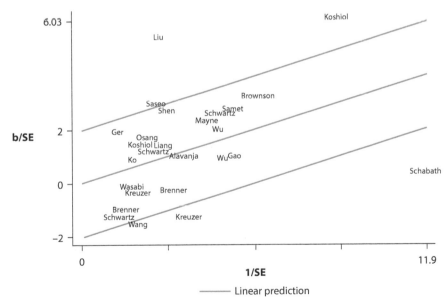

Figure G.1 Galbraith plot: assessment of heterogeneity of effect of chronic bronchitis across studies in a meta-analysis of the epidemiological evidence concerning previous lung diseases as risk factors for lung cancer. (Reproduced from Brenner DR *et al.* (2011). Previous lung diseases and lung cancer risk: a systematic review and meta-analysis. *PLoS One* **6**: e17479.)

interval is ±2) are expected to fall if there is no significant heterogeneity. Since small studies have large standard errors (and small *inverse* standard errors) they will be found on the left-hand side of the graph, with the larger studies on the right-hand side (farther away from origin), as shown in Figure G.1, from the meta-analysis by BRENNER, McLAUGHLIN & HUNG (2011) on the epidemiological evidence concerning previous lung diseases as risk factors for lung cancer. Studies falling outside the ±2 interval may be further investigated in order to evaluate what specific characteristics they display that could explain the statistical heterogeneity vis-à-vis other studies. Notice the studies by Koshiol, Schabath, Liu and Kreuzer fall outside the 95% interval. On a **forest plot**, studies falling outside the stated interval on the Galbraith plot are those whose interval estimates do not overlap the overall or **pooled** estimate of effect (BLAND, University of York MSc course materials – accessed August 2016). See also **L'Abbé plot**, **index of heterogeneity ($I^2$)**, **meta-regression**, **regression through the origin**.

## Gamma model

See **accelerated failure time models** (parametric survival models).

## Gaussian distribution

See **Normal distribution**.

## GCS

Abbreviation for Glasgow Coma Scale. See **severity of illness index**.

## GEEs

Abbreviation for **generalized estimating equations**.

## Gehan design

A two-stage **Phase II trial** design in which the trial is designed to end if there are no responses indicative of activity in the first stage, while the **sample size** calculation for the second stage is dependent on the number of responses in the first stage. MACHIN & CAMPBELL (2005) give details.

## General population cohort

See **cohort study**, **control group**. Cf. special exposure cohort.

## Generalizability

The ability to **extrapolate** study results beyond the **study sample**. Most research studies carried out in the medical/public health field are concerned with **estimating** the average value or the **prevalence** of some characteristic among specific populations, and with estimating and **testing hypotheses** regarding the effects of different **exposures** and the

**efficacy** or **effectiveness** of treatments and interventions. Representativeness of the study sample with regard to the **source population** is essential in **survey**-type studies seeking to estimate population **parameters**, where clearly one is using a sample to extrapolate to the source population. In studies testing hypotheses concerning the effects of exposures and interventions, the *internal* **validity** of the results is usually considered of greatest importance. However, the ability to extrapolate beyond the study sample (*external* validity) to groups and **target populations** that may differ from those who were studied (in terms of geographical location, age, gender, disease severity or any other characteristic that might be a **risk** or **prognostic factor**) will depend on an understanding of the underlying biological processes and how these might be affected by differing patient or population characteristics, rather than on statistical **sampling** (Rothman, Greenland & Lash, in ROTHMAN, GREENLAND & LASH (eds., 2012); ROTHMAN, 2012).

## Generalized estimating equations

Or its abbreviation, GEEs. A **semi-parametric method** (quasi-likelihood estimation) for the analysis of **longitudinal** and other types of **clustered data**, which may be extended to the analysis of non-**Normal** outcomes, **binary** responses in particular (LIANG & ZEGER, 1986). GEE regression models are specified around a 'working correlation matrix' that approximates the **correlation structure** between clustered observations (i.e. the residual correlation given the predictors) and thus takes data **dependence** into account. The values of the **correlation coefficients** are estimated from the data, given the choice of correlation structure. For binary outcomes, the **odds ratio** may be used preferably as the measure of association (AGRESTI, 2007). In contrast to **random effects** models in which the within-cluster **covariance** structure is specified and modelled, GEEs model only the mean response and variance (as in **cross-sectional studies**), for which reason they are also termed 'marginal' or 'population-averaged' models. Cluster effects are treated as **nuisance parameters**. The structure of the working correlation matrix determines the **efficiency** of parameter **estimation**. To take account of the clustering and ensure the validity of **inferences, robust standard errors** are estimated by the Huber–White or sandwich variance estimator, on the basis of an assumed covariance *and* the actual observed variability (see also **Wald test**, score test). **Missing data**, a common occurrence in longitudinal studies, are assumed to be missing 'completely at random' (or MCAR). Limitations of the method are that it allows for only two hierarchical levels (e.g. 'patients' within 'general practices' or 'observations' within 'individuals'), and it requires a relatively large number of **clusters** (BLAND, 2015). See KIRKWOOD & STERNE (2003), HOSMER, LEMESHOW & STURDIVANT (2013), and DIGGLE *et al.* (2002) for additional details. See also **generalized linear model** (in particular, **logistic regression**), **marginal model**.

## Generalized linear mixed model

Or GLMM. See **multilevel generalized linear model, multilevel model**.

## Generalized linear model

Or its abbreviation, GLM. A general extension of the **linear regression model** in which the predicted value of the **outcome variable** is a *linear function* of the independent or **predictor variables** in the model and their **coefficients**. The standard linear regression model is fitted to **interval/ratio** outcome variables that are **normally distributed** (their errors or **residuals** are expected to follow a Normal distribution). With outcome variables measured on other **measurement scales** (and following **probability distributions** other than the Normal) the simple linear model is usually unsuitable. GLMs make it possible for proportions, counts and other non-interval/ratio outcomes to be modelled by means of a linear model, provided an adequate **transformation** (link function) for the predicted outcome can be found. **Logistic regression** is an example of a GLM, where a **binary** outcome is modelled by a linear model that predicts not the probability of the binary outcome, but a transformation of this probability – the **logit** or log odds. **Poisson regression** is often used when the outcome variable is in the form of **count** data, or when analysing **rates**. Special methods are employed to deal with **overdispersion**, i.e. extra-binomial or extra-Poisson variation (see also **dispersion parameter**). **Cox regression** and **conditional logistic regression** are special types of generalized linear model in which exposure effects are estimated by carrying out comparisons within **risk sets** and **strata** (see **conditional model**). The logistic, Cox and Poisson models are examples of regression models that are specified as linear functions (additive on the transformed scales), with exposure or treatment effects having a **multiplicative effect** when regression coefficients are **back-transformed** to the original scales. The **link function** in ordinary linear regression is the identity function if the quantitative outcome variable remains untransformed. In the case of lognormal variables where the model is fitted to the logs of the original values, the link function is the logarithmic function. Although binary outcomes are often modelled through logistic regression, it is also possible to specify a generalized linear model that will predict the log of the risk, as opposed to the log of the odds (or logit). Here, the link function is the log or logarithmic transformation, and back-transforming the regression coefficients gives the **risk ratio** (rather than the **odds ratio**), i.e. the estimate of exposure or treatment effect for any given exposure or predictor variable in the model. KIRKWOOD & STERNE (2003) discuss the limitations of models predicting risks (and estimating risk ratios), which derive from the need for the predicted outcome to be constrained within a given range of values, and the fact that results are not interchangeable if the outcome variable is expressed in an alternative way (e.g. 'survived', as opposed to 'died'). See also AGRESTI (2007), HAMILTON (2012), MITCHELL (2012b); **maximum likelihood estimation**.

## Geometric distribution

A **discrete probability distribution** for the number of trials required before the first success (or event of interest) occurs, where the probability of a success in any given **independent** trial is $p$. It is therefore a special case of the **negative binomial distribution**, the probability distribution of the number of trials required until a fixed number of successes is observed. The **parameter** of the distribution is $p$, with **mean** $1/p$ and **variance** $(1 - p)/p^2$. As the continuous **exponential distribution**, it is characterized by a positive **skew**, and may sometimes be **approximated** by the latter with parameter $p$. See also **binomial distribution**, **hypergeometric distribution**.

## Geometric mean

The antilog of an arithmetic **mean** that was calculated from the log-transformed values of a quantitative variable, i.e. from a variable whose values have been **transformed** to a **logarithmic scale**. The geometric mean is thus obtained by **anti-logging** or **back-transforming** the arithmetic mean of the log values. Figure G.2 (JOSEPH *et al.*, 2007) shows the distribution of urinary cotinine levels in infants from non-smoking (a, $n = 33$) and smoking (b, $n = 71$) households. Cotinine levels were measured at around 12 weeks of age. Both distributions have a positive **skew**, with arithmetic means of 5 µg/mmol creatinine and 39 µg/mmol creatinine, respectively. The geometric means were lower in both cases, 3.47 µg/mmol creatinine and 19.05 µg/mmol creatinine, respectively (3.47 = exp[0.54] and 19.05 = exp[1.28], where 0.54 and 1.28 are the arithmetic means of the log-transformed cotinine levels). In general, the value of the geometric mean is lower than the value of the arithmetic mean of the original values, since it is less affected by high value **outliers**. See BLAND (2015) for an illustrative example of how to interpret the back-transformed **confidence interval** for the difference between two means. ALEXANDER (2012) draws a distinction between the geometric mean and 'Williams mean'. The latter is often calculated when one or more observations in a positively skewed **count variable** has a zero count, as the log of zero may not be calculated (see **ln**). The calculation of Williams mean is similar to the calculation of the geometric mean, but a quantity (usually 1) must be added to all observation values before log transforming the variable, and the same quantity must be subtracted from the geometric mean. See also **lognormal distribution**, reverse **J-shaped distribution**.

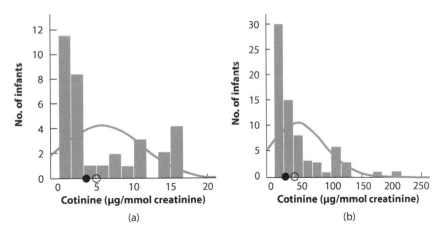

**Figure G.2** Arithmetic (○) and geometric mean (●) for a positively skewed distribution: urinary cotinine levels (in µg/mmol creatinine) in infants from non-smoking (a) and smoking (b) households. (Reproduced from Joseph DV *et al.* (2007). Effect of parental smoking on cotinine levels in newborns. *Arch Dis Child Fetal Neonatal Ed* **92**: F484–8 (with permission).)

## Glasgow Coma Scale

Or its abbreviation, GCS. See **severity of illness index**.

## Glass's Delta (Δ)

A standardized measure of the difference between two **means**, often calculated in the context of **meta-analysis**. The **standard deviation (SD)** in the **control group** is used as the scaling factor. Delta is indicated when treatment or exposure effect impacts both mean response and variability of response. See **standardized difference, standardized measures of effect, effect size, weighted average**. See also **Cohen's $d$** and **Hedges' adjusted $g$**.

## GLM

Abbreviation for **generalized linear model**.

## GLMM

Abbreviation for **generalized linear mixed model**.

## GoF

Abbreviation for **goodness-of-fit**.

## Gold standard

In the context of **diagnostic testing**, a gold standard is a **valid** diagnostic tool or method that consistently gives the correct diagnosis (i.e. it is **reliable** and **accurate**). In practice, gold standards are rarely 100% accurate. They are simply the best method of diagnosis according to current dogma. Gold standard tests can be invasive and expensive, and thus may be used in studies that evaluate the accuracy (**sensitivity, specificity**) of simpler and/or less costly methods. Sackett, in HAYNES *et al.* (eds., 2006), discusses strategies for improving the accuracy of gold standard tests and measurements. See also **clinical measurement**.

## Gompertz model

See **proportional hazards models** (parametric survival models).

## Goodness-of-fit

Often referred to by its abbreviation, GoF, a test or a measure of how well a **theoretical distribution** or a specified **model** fits a set of data. An example is the **chi-squared ($\chi^2$) test for goodness-of-fit**, which is used to compare a **frequency distribution** against the corresponding theoretical distribution. As with the standard $\chi^2$ test, it is based on a comparison of **observed** *vs.* **expected frequencies. Degrees of freedom** for the test are calculated as the number of categories or classes in the frequency distribution *minus* the number of parameters that have to be estimated from the data (to give the parameters of the theoretical distribution, if necessary) *minus* 1. The assessment of normality of distribution of a continuous variable is based on a comparison between the values of the observed distribution against the **expected values** were the variable to follow a perfectly **Normal distribution**, with parameters given by the sample mean and standard deviation (see **Normal plot, Shapiro–Wilks test**). With regard to **regression analysis**, a number of test statistics provide an *overall* assessment of how well a model fits the data. These are generally computed from measures of the difference between observed and fitted values (i.e. from the **residuals**), and based on a comparison against the corresponding **saturated model**. The latter fits the data perfectly, albeit at the expense of simplicity and stability (see **parsimony**). Pearson's $\chi^2$ test and the residual deviance test are two such tests, which may be used for a rough preliminary assessment of fit where the outcome variable is a risk or a rate (see AGRESTI, 2007). In both cases, the number of degrees of freedom for the test of fit equals the difference in number of **parameters** between the two models being compared. The validity of these assessments depends on the number of unique covariate patterns (see **deviance statistic**; **Pearson goodness-of-fit statistic**). Small **P-values** indicate poor fit. Large $P$-values cannot give a definitive statement of goodness-of-fit, except in reference to the extra terms in the saturated model. In linear regression, these tests are based on the **residual sum of squares** (see **residual F-test**). The **Hosmer and Lemeshow $X^2$ statistic** may be used to assess the overall predictive ability of logistic regression models, what is known as **calibration**. **ROC curves** may be plotted for the range of predicted probabilities given by the model, which evaluates yet another aspect of GoF, **discrimination**. GoF is not synonymous with overall **statistical significance**. The latter is given by tests of regression, i.e. by the level of significance associated with the estimated coefficient(s) for any given single predictor or group of predictors. Measures such as $r^2$ (**r-squared**) and $R^2$ (**multiple correlation coefficient**, squared), based on the correlation between observed and pre-dicted values for the outcome variable, are sometimes used with linear regression models but are less useful with other types of regression. These measures compare a regression model against a model with no predictors (a **null model**), not against a saturated model. **Regression diagnostics** take the process of **model checking** further by providing a means to evaluate whether the fit of a model is *consistently adequate* for the entire ranges of values of the variables analysed. See KIRKWOOD & STERNE (2003), HAMILTON (1992), HOSMER, LEMESHOW & STURDIVANT (2013), and Greenland, in ROTHMAN, GREENLAND & LASH (eds., 2012), for further details. See also **validation**.

## GRADE approach

From the website (www.gradeworkinggroup.org; accessed 12/2016): "The Grading of Recommendations Assessment, Development and Evaluation (short GRADE) working group began in the year 2000 as an informal collaboration of people with an interest in addressing the shortcomings of grading systems in health care. The working group has developed a common, sensible and transparent approach to grading quality (or certainty) of evidence and strength of recommendations. Many international organizations have pro-vided input into the development of the GRADE approach, which is now considered the standard in guideline development." See also **clinical guidelines**, **hierarchy of evidence**, **critical appraisal**; GUYATT *et al.*, for the GRADE Working Group (2008).

## Graphical displays

Graphs play an important role in **exploratory** and **confirmatory data analyses**, enabling the visualization of the **distribution** of individual variables (their centre, degree of spread or variability and frequency distribution), and also depicting the relationship (**linear** or **non-linear**) between two (or more) variables, to give a ready assessment as to the shape and pattern of any relationship. Graphs that depict distributions include (a) for binary and other categorical variables: **bar charts**, **pie charts**, **stacked bar charts**; (b) for ordinal and quantitative variables: **box-and-whiskers plots, dot plots, error bar charts, stem-and-leaf plots, histograms, frequency polygons, cumulative frequency polygons**. Relationships between quantitative and/or ordinal variables are commonly depicted using **scatterplots**. **Line graphs** and **growth charts**, such as used for serial measurements, time series and growth standards and references, may be used to show the variation over time (or **longitudinal** change) in a given measurement. Where the distribution of a quantitative or ordinal variable is given for different categories or levels of a categorical or ordered categorical variable, boxplots, dot plots, error bar charts and frequency polygons are often used, with the display showing a separate graph for each category in question. In **meta-analyses**, a number of graphical techniques are used to give a visual assessment of the variation (or heterogeneity) among primary studies with respect to estimates of treatment and exposure effect (**forest plot, L'Abbé plot, Galbraith plot**), and to give an indication as to the presence of publication and other types of bias (**funnel plot**). Additional graphs often seen in the literature are **Normal plots, ROC curves** and summary ROC curves (for diagnostic testing and screening), **survival curves** and **difference** *vs.* **average plots** in the context of method comparison studies and the evaluation of regression to the mean. See MUSCATELLO *et al.* (2006) for a randomized controlled trial of graph design interventions, which was carried out to help determine optimized graphical presentations for effective communication of population health statistics. TUKEY (1977) and CLEVELAND (1993; 1994) illustrate graphing and exploratory data analysis aspects. See also HAMILTON (1992; 2012) and MITCHELL (2012a) for an illustration of the use of graphs in statistical analysis, with special focus on **regression analysis**.

## Greenwood's formula

An alternative equation for the **standard error** of the **Kaplan–Meier** or product-limit estimate of survival probability (i.e. the **survival function**). ALTMAN (1991) gives the formula and additional details.

## Group sequential design

See **sequential designs**.

## Growth charts

Graphical or tabular displays of the **longitudinal** changes in some measurement of interest, where the pattern of change over time is growth. Growth curves may be plotted using *actual* (or expected) measurements at the different time points (or ages), or the *changes* observed (or expected) between consecutive measurements. The latter gives a measure of the velocity or rate of change in the measurement in question, which may be constant, or display acceleration and/or deceleration. An example of growth charts are the updated child growth standards by the World Health Organization's Multicentre Growth Reference Study (WHO, 2006). **Smoothing** techniques are employed to fit each growth curve. Growth *references* may also be charted, and describe the growth patterns of a given population. They provide additional information with which to assess child growth in that same population, as growth *standards* are not always attainable. Stunting and low rate of growth are considered to be present when a child or infant is below the 3rd and 25th **percentiles**, respectively, for height- (length-) for-age and height velocity. Stunting (moderate/severe) is also defined as height-for-age that is minus 2 **standard deviations (SD)** below the **median** of the reference population. Underweight (moderate/severe) and wasting (moderate/severe) are defined as weight-for-age that is minus 2 SD below the median of the reference population, and weight-for-height that is minus 2 SD below the median of the reference population. Low birthweight is usually defined as less than 2500 g. Figure G.3a charts the median or 50th percentile weight measurements (in kg) of low birthweight infants (from 0 to 108 months), together with local reference values and WHO weight-for-age standards, in the study by van der MEI *et al.* (2000) on the growth and survival of low birthweight infants in a rural area of Ghana (Agogo, Ashanti Region). 105 infants weighing 1000–2000 g at birth were initially enrolled in the study; follow-up was not complete for all children. Figure G.3b charts median incremental weight gain (velocity, in kg/month) among the same group of children, for different age spans between the ages of 0 to 36 months, together with local reference values, and WHO weight velocity standards for the same age spans. See www.who.int/childgrowth/mgrs/en for growth charts for a number of different indicators (height- or length-for-age, weight-for-age, BMI-for-age, head circumference-for-age, and various velocity indicators), by both **z-scores** (i.e. standardized differences between individual values and a mean or median value, expressed as number of SDs) and **percentiles**. See also HILLS (1974), and COLE (2012).

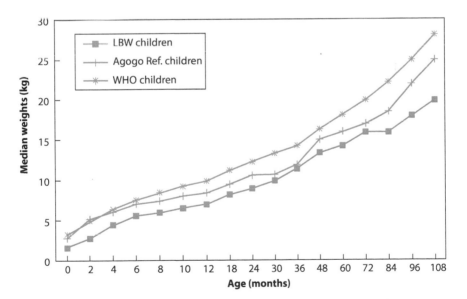

**Figure G.3a** Growth charts: charting of median weight measurements (in kg) and median incremental weight gain (in kg/month) for low birthweight (LBW) (1000–2000 g) infants in a rural area of Ghana. Local reference values and WHO standards for the same ages and age spans are also displayed (initial sample size = 105). (Reproduced from van der Mei J *et al.* (2000). Growth and survival of low birthweight infants from 0 to 9 years in a rural area of Ghana. Comparison of moderately low (1501–2000 g) and very low birthweight (1000–1500 g) infants and a local reference population. *Trop Med Int Health* **5**: 571–7 (with permission).) *(Continued)*

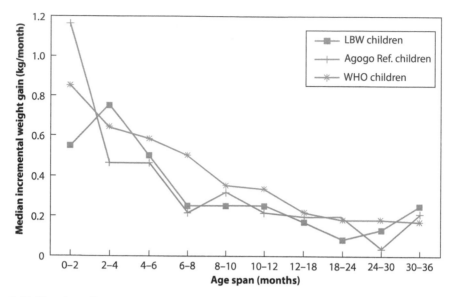

Figure G.3b *(Continued)*

## Growth curve

See **monotonic curve**. Cf. peaked (**non-monotonic**) curve. See also **summary measures**.

## Guttman scale

A cumulative measurement scale made up of a series of ranked questions or statements, whereby agreement with a given statement implies agreement with lower ranked statements. This gives rise to an automatic scoring system that is also informative with regard to precisely which items or statements an individual is in agreement with. Individuals are thus ranked as to their degree of tolerance or acceptance of a particular circumstance, or agreement with a particular viewpoint. See also **Likert scale**, **visual analogue scale**, **composite score**, **ordinal variable**.

## h

The hat statistic. See **leverage**.

## H

The **test statistic** for the **Kruskal–Wallis test**. It may also represent the **harmonic mean**.

## $H_0$

See **null hypothesis**.

## $H_1$

See **alternative hypothesis**.

## Half-life

The time it takes for a substance (such as a drug treatment) to lose half of its biological (pharmacological, physiological, radiological, etc.) activity, or half of its concentration. In physics and chemistry, and in particular where it concerns radioactive substances, these processes can often be described by an **exponential** 'decay' curve, reflecting a process taking place at a constant rate. Under these circumstances, the half-life does not depend on the initial quantity, nor does it change as the quantity decays (that is, it remains the same in respect of any amount of the diminishing quantity). This is due to the so-called 'memory-less' property of exponential processes. By contrast, biological processes are usually dependent on a variety of factors (such as the structure and physiology of the various tissues) and may need to be described by more complex relationships. In such cases, half-life may depend on initial quantity and likely changes with time as the quantity decays.

## Harmonic mean

A **measure** of location or **central tendency** that is usually appropriate when averaging **rates** and speeds. To calculate the harmonic mean ($H$) of $n$ numbers, $x_1, x_2, x_3,..., x_n$, first take the reciprocals of these $n$ numbers (i.e. $1/x_1, ..., 1/x_n$). Next, calculate the arithmetic **mean** of these reciprocals. Finally, the harmonic mean is the reciprocal of the last result obtained:

$$H = \frac{1}{\left[\dfrac{1}{x_1} + \dfrac{1}{x_2} + \dfrac{1}{x_3} + ... + \dfrac{1}{x_n}\right] \div n} = \frac{n}{\dfrac{1}{x_1} + \dfrac{1}{x_2} + \dfrac{1}{x_3} + ... + \dfrac{1}{x_n}}$$

The value of the harmonic mean will be lower or equal, but never greater, then the value of the corresponding **geometric** and arithmetic means. See also **reciprocal transformation**.

## Hat statistic

Synonym for $h$, or **leverage** statistic.

## Hazard function

Or $h(t)$. The set of estimates of instantaneous rate or hazard (changing or constant) over a given time-period. The term is often used interchangeably with **hazard rate**. See also **cumulative hazard function**, $H(t)$, baseline hazard function, $h_0(t)$, and cumulative baseline hazard function, $H_0(t)$ (under hazard rate), **bathtub curve**.

## Hazard rate

In the context of **survival analysis**, the hazard rate (given by the hazard function, $[h(t)]$) is the conditional failure rate at any given time $t$, a non-negative function expressed in units of the reciprocal of time ($1/t$ or $t^{-1}$). It is interpreted as the probability that an individual will experience the event of interest at time $t$, given that he has not experienced it up to time $t$. The hazard rate (also termed instantaneous rate, or force of morbidity or mortality) gives a measure of the rate at which risk (or **cumulative hazard**, $[H(t)]$) is accumulating. With a *constant* hazard rate, the distribution of survival times is **exponential**, and the reciprocal of the hazard rate is the average or mean survival time, i.e. the average time to **failure** or time to event (see **life expectancy**). When using regression models to analyse survival times, the *baseline* hazard at any given time $t$, $h_0(t)$, is the hazard rate when the value for all predictor variables in the model is set to zero. A functional form for the baseline hazard must be chosen when fitting **parametric survival models**, which defines the **probability distribution function**, $f(t)$, for the **survival times**, given the equivalence $f(t) = h(t) \times \exp[-H(t)]$, where $\exp[-H(t)] = S(t)$. In the case of the **Cox regression model**, a semi-parametric model, the baseline hazard function is left unspecified. Rather, it is represented by a **nuisance parameter**, the values of which are directly derived from the data at informative time points. The Cox model does give, however, the *cumulative* baseline hazard function, $H_0(t)$, i.e. the accumulated risk over time, absent of any effect from predictor or explanatory variables. See CLEVES, GOULD & MARCHENKO (2016) for further details. See also **rate**.

## Hazard ratio

A measure of **relative risk** used in **survival analysis**. The hazard ratio ($HR$ or $HR_{CM}$ or Cox–Mantel) is calculated as follows:

$$HR = \frac{O_1/E_1}{O_0/E_0}$$

where $O_0$ is the **observed** number of people with the event of interest in group 0 (for example, the unexposed or control group); $E_0$ is the **expected** number of people with the event in group 0, under the hypothesis (**null hypothesis**) that the two groups being compared experience the same event **hazard**; $O_1$ and $E_1$ as above, for group 1 (for example, the exposed or treatment group). Observed and expected numbers in each group are calculated as a summation across all time strata or **risk sets**. The hazard ratio thus calculated is assumed to remain constant over time. An *HR* of 1 suggests the hazard or 'risk' of the event is the same in the two groups. An *HR* greater than 1 suggests group 1 is more likely to experience the event. The opposite is true for an *HR* less than 1. See Box C.3 (**Cox regression**, p. 82) for an example and interpretation. The formula above is based on the same calculations as for the **logrank** or Cox–Mantel **test**. See also **Mantel–Haenszel method** ($HR_{MH}$), **Peto's method** ($HR_{Peto}$); ALTMAN (1991).

## Health economics (Evaluation of)

See **cost-benefit analysis, cost-effectiveness analysis, cost-minimization analysis, cost-utility analysis, quality-adjusted life-years** (**QALYs**). For a comprehensive overview and illustrative examples see DRUMMOND (1994) and AJETUNMOBI (2002). See also DRUMMOND *et al.* (2015), THOMPSON & BARBER (2000). HIGGINS & GREEN (eds., 2008) give guidance for undertaking systematic reviews of economic evaluations.

## Healthy worker effect

A type of **selection bias** that tends to occur in **cohort studies** investigating the effects of occupational hazards, whereby the **exposed**, i.e. the workers, may be selectively healthier than the general population (comprised of employed and unemployed individuals) from which the **controls** might be selected. This is due to the fact that the workers' employment status itself acts as a filter that tends to favour the healthy and fit over the diseased or incapacitated, leading to the underestimation of occupational **exposure effects**. In such a study, **standardization** still leads to biased estimates of occupational exposure effect in the comparison between the special exposure cohort (the workers) and the unexposed (the general population controls). Care should be taken to select controls from an unexposed (with regard to the exposure of interest) occupational group. See also **volunteer bias**.

## Hedges' adjusted *g*

A standardized measure of the difference between two **means**, often employed in the context of **meta-analysis**. Hedges' *g* is similar to **Cohen's *d***, but includes an adjustment for the overestimation of effect that tends to occur in small sized studies ('small sample bias'). See **standardized difference, standardized measures of effect, effect size, weighted average**. See also **Glass's Delta** (Δ).

## Heterogeneity

Or lack of **homogeneity**. A term usually employed in the context of **meta-analysis**, when estimates from **primary studies** show differences in **magnitude**, and possibly also different sign or **direction**. In the presence of marked heterogeneity, a single, **pooled** summary of these individual study results should not be produced. With moderate heterogeneity, the **DerSimonian and Laird random effects model** may be used to estimate an *average* **treatment** or **exposure effect**. Heterogeneity may be formally assessed with the **chi-squared** ($\chi^2$) **test for heterogeneity** (or ***Q* test**), both in the context of meta-analysis and in the context of **stratification** using the **Mantel–Haenszel method**. Tests of heterogeneity may lack the **power** needed for statistical significance. The inclusion of **interaction** terms is a useful technique for assessing whether homogeneity or heterogeneity of effects may be inferred (BLAND 2015). In addition to the test of heterogeneity, an **index of heterogeneity** ($I^2$) may be calculated, and visual inspection of **forest plots**, **Galbraith plots** and **L'Abbé plots** can aid in the assessment. See Thompson, in EGGER, DAVEY SMITH & ALTMAN (eds., 2001), THOMPSON (1994) and HIGGINS *et al.* (2003), for a discussion of sources of heterogeneity and methodology for its evaluation. BENNETT & EMBERSON (2009) recommend the use of stratification for exploring sources of clinical and statistical heterogeneity. See also BLAND (2015), KIRKWOOD & STERNE (2003), BORENSTEIN *et al.* (2009) and BAX *et al.* (2009). Further details are given under **meta-regression**, which may be carried out to further investigate possible sources of statistical heterogeneity.

## Heteroscedasticity

Lack of uniformity or constancy with respect to a measure of dispersion such as the **variance** or the **standard deviation**. See **assumptions**. Cf. **homoscedasticity**, **overdispersion**.

## Hierarchical model

A statistical **model** that is fitted to data so that their hierarchical structure may be taken into account. Examples of hierarchical levels are the individual level, the research facility level and the country level, in a **multicentre trial**. Typically, units within each level are **clusters** of smaller units, and represent the **random effects** (i.e. the subject-specific and cluster-specific effects at the different hierarchical levels) in a model that is typically specified as having a mixture of random and **fixed effects**. Conceptually, reference is made to *multilevel* and *longitudinal* analysis, where the former implies a multilevel organizational structure gives rise to the data, and the latter, the data stem from repeated measurements or assessments over time. Methods of analysis are similar in both instances, however, due to the clustered nature of the data and inclusion of mixed effects. See GOLDSTEIN (2010) and RABE-HESKETH & SKRONDAL (2012) for a full discussion of concept, theory and application. See also ARMITAGE, BERRY & MATHEWS (2002). Synonymous with **multilevel model**, **random effects model**, **mixed effects model**. See also **clustered designs**, **clustered data**, **longitudinal study**, **longitudinal data**.

## Hierarchy of evidence

In the context of **evidence-based medicine**, the relative weight of **systematic reviews** and different types of **primary studies** when translating research results into clinical practice, where decisions concerning treatments and interventions are made. This acknowledges the fact that certain **study designs** are better suited for providing **unbiased** estimates of treatment effect. The quality and **validity** of any given study must also be evaluated (see **CONSORT statement, critical appraisal**). The suggested hierarchy is as follows (highest-ranking first) (GUYATT *et al.*, for the Evidence-based Medicine Working Group, 1995; GUYATT *et al.*, 2014; GREENHALGH, 1997, 2014):

1. Systematic reviews and meta-analyses
2. Randomized controlled trials with definitive results (confidence intervals that do not overlap the threshold clinically significant effect)
3. Randomized controlled trials with non-definitive results (a point estimate that suggests a clinically significant effect but with confidence intervals overlapping the threshold for this effect)
4. Cohort studies
5. Case–control studies
6. Cross-sectional surveys
7. Case series/reports.

See also **clinical guidelines**, **GRADE approach**; MACHIN & CAMPBELL (2005).

## High-leverage point

See **leverage**.

## High–low graph

A **graphical display**, also known as hi–lo or **range** plot, that shows the minimum and maximum values of a quantitative variable (usually, a **continuous variable**) for values of another

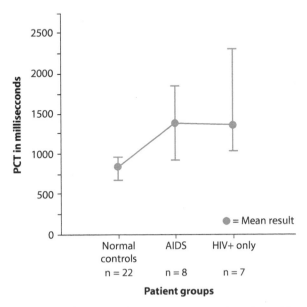

Figure H.1 High–low graph: range (and mean) of pupil cycle time (PCT) in milliseconds among normal controls, AIDS patients, and HIV-positive individuals without AIDS. (Reproduced from Maclean H, Dhillon B (1993). Pupil cycle time and human immunodeficiency virus (HIV) infection. *Eye* **7**: 785–6 (with permission).)

variable (possibly, but not necessarily, a time/age variable). An example is the graph in Figure H.1, in the study by MACLEAN & DHILLON (1993), which was set up to investigate whether ocular autonomic dysfunction is evident in HIV-positive individuals. Pupil cycle time (PCT) measurements (in milliseconds), a non-invasive, reliable method, showed the range of PCT measurements to be considerably wider among HIV-positive individuals (of which 59% met the criteria for an AIDS diagnosis) than among normal controls, which suggests ocular autonomic dysfunction may be present even in the earlier stages of HIV infection. The minimum and maximum values are usually connected by spikes (depicting the range or spread), and the average value in each category (or at different time points) of the variable on the *x*-axis is also commonly shown. In graphs displaying time trends, the spikes are sometimes connected so that both trend and variability are readily expressed. **Box-and-whiskers plots** (also known as boxplots) and **dot plots** are alternative ways of depicting this type of information.

## Higher-order interaction

A **statistical interaction** involving three or more factors or variables.

## Histogram

A **graphical display** of the **frequency distribution** of a **quantitative variable**, most commonly, a **continuous** variable on an **interval/ratio** scale. It differs from a **bar chart** in that the bars are contiguous, as the values on the **x-axis** represent a truly numerical variable, which has been categorized into **class intervals**. Figure H.2 shows the *relative* frequency distribution of serum 25-hydroxyvitamin D (25(OH)D) concentrations among 5907 participants (age ≥40 years) in the US National Health and Nutrition Examination Survey (NHANES, 2001–2004), in the study by MORIOKA *et al.* (2015) seeking to determine whether vitamin D status modifies the association between statin use and musculoskeletal pain. It is a **unimodal distribution** with a mild positive **skew** and therefore with lower

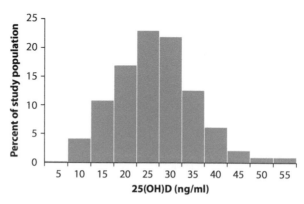

**Figure H.2** Histogram: distribution of serum 25-hydroxyvitamin D (25(OH)D) concentrations (in ng/ml) among 5907 participants in the US NHANES (2001–2004) aged ≥40 years. Mean serum 25(OH)D is 23.6 ng/ml (95% CI from 22.9 to 24.3). The authors report 1281 (21.7%) participants with levels below 15 ng/ml. (Reproduced from Morioka TY *et al.* (2015). Vitamin D status modifies the association between statin use and musculoskeletal pain: A population based study. *Atherosclerosis* **238**: 77–82 (with permission).)

frequencies for higher values of the distribution. A **Normal plot** of these data would likely indicate some departure from the assumption of normality. Note that the **frequency** or count in each class interval (or the relative frequency as in this example) is proportional to the *area* of each bar or rectangle and not to the height of the same, except where all class intervals have equal width. When class intervals have unequal widths, bar *heights* are proportional to the **frequency density**, i.e. the frequency per unit of the quantity in question. Frequency may be expressed as *relative frequency* by dividing the frequency in each class interval by the total number of observations, or as *relative frequency density*, by dividing the relative frequency by the width of the class interval (BLAND, 2015). See also **frequency polygon** (Figure F.3, p. 140).

## Historical controls

As opposed to *concurrent* controls. See **control group**.

## Homogeneity

Depending on context, this term expresses both similarity of **treatment** or **exposure effects**, and similarity among the members of a given group with regard to relevant **risk** or **prognostic factors**. In the context of **meta-analysis**, homogeneity is said to be present when estimates of treatment or exposure effect are found to be similar among the different **primary studies** included. Likewise, in **stratified analyses**, homogeneity refers to constancy of exposure or treatment effects across different strata (see **Mantel–Haenszel method**). **Heterogeneity**, or lack of homogeneity, may be tested or evaluated in a number of ways, which results in the choice of **fixed effect** or **random effects models** as the basis for estimating the *overall* effect across all primary studies or across all strata. In the context of **comparative studies**, homogeneity among study participants can be a desirable or necessary feature of the study, in that it reduces response **variability**. This type of homogeneity may be achieved through strategies such as **restriction**.

## Homoscedasticity

Or equality of **variances**. A term used in the context of *t*-tests and **analysis of variance** to refer to the **assumption** of equal variance (for a given measurement or other quantitative variable) among groups being compared, and in the context of **linear regression** to refer to the assumption that the degree of **variability** in the **outcome variable** is approximately constant across all values of a **predictor variable**. The **F-test** and **Bartlett's test** provide a formal assessment of this assumption. **Variance-stabilizing transformations** are carried out for the purpose of equalizing variances among groups or across the values of a predictor. These are often also **normalizing transformations**. See also **residual mean square**. Cf. **heteroscedasticity** (and Figure B.6, Box-and-whiskers plot, p. 40).

## Hosmer and Lemeshow $X^2$ statistic

A **test statistic** (also referred to as $\hat{C}$ statistic) that evaluates the **goodness-of-fit (GoF)** or predictive accuracy of **logistic regression models**, also known as **calibration**. To perform the test, the probability of the outcome of interest is computed for each observation in the data set, on the basis of the model in question. Observations are then grouped into 'probability or risk of event categories' (e.g. 0–10%, 10%+, 20%+, ..., 90%+, also termed 'deciles of risk') and a $r \times 2$ **contingency table** is produced, with the columns representing the **binary outcome** (yes/no type) and the rows representing 'risk of event categories', as described above. The cells of this table contain the **observed frequencies** for the cross-tabulation. The test statistic is computed from the differences between observed and **expected frequencies** in each cell. A **chi-squared ($\chi^2$) test** with $r - 2$ **degrees of freedom** tests how close expected frequencies are to observed frequencies ($r$ is the number of 'risk of event' categories). Large test statistics, and therefore small **P-values**, indicate poor fit, i.e. poor predictive models. The H&L $\chi^2$ test is an alternative to the residual **deviance** and **Pearson $\chi^2$ GoF tests**. See HOSMER, LEMESHOW & STURDIVANT (2013) for further details.

## Hospital-based case–control study

See **case–control study**, **control group**, **Berkson's fallacy**. Cf. population-based case–control study.

## Hotelling's $T^2$ test

A **significance test** that is an extension of the **independent** samples *t*-test, and is used for comparing two groups with respect to a number of *joint* **outcome variables** (i.e. **multivariate data**), as opposed to just a single (univariate) outcome variable, as is commonly the case. See also **Mahalanobis D²**.

## HR

Abbreviation for **hazard ratio**.

## h(t)

See **hazard rate**/hazard function. For $H(t)$, see **cumulative hazard function**.

## Huber estimator

A **robust estimator** that is sometimes approximated by **weighted least squares (WLS)** regression. Observations are downweighted according to the magnitude of **standardized residuals** (when the latter exceed a given value or *tuning constant*), which allows **outlying** observations to be included in data analyses. Huber weights are often utilized in WLS and **iteratively reweighted least squares (IRLS)**. HAMILTON (1992; 2012) gives additional details.

## Huber–White variance estimate

Synonym for **sandwich variance estimate**. See also **robust method**.

## Hypergeometric distribution

A **discrete probability distribution** that describes the **sampling distribution** of a hypergeometric **random variable**. It is used to provide **exact probabilities** for the observed frequencies in a **contingency table**, as for example, when carrying out **Fisher's exact test**. The hypergeometric distribution gives the probability of $r$ successes or events of interest when samples of size $n$ (or $n$ trials) are taken *without* replacement from a population of a given finite size $N$ in which the number of successes is $k$. It is related to the **binomial** probability distribution, which gives the same probabilities when samples are drawn *with* replacement, and may be approximated by it if the samples drawn are sufficiently small in relation to the size of the population, in which case the probability, $p$, of a success is assumed to remain constant between trials. See also **geometric distribution**.

## Hypothesis

A theory about the real state or condition of a system (for example, a particular population), or about the real effect of a factor or agent (for example, a medical intervention or a detrimental exposure). Research studies often test one or more hypotheses on **study samples**, which allows inferences to be drawn about wider **source** and **target populations**. Under **frequentist inference**, the starting point of hypothesis or **significance testing** is the **null hypothesis**, a hypothesis that denies any effects and any differing patterns or trends to be real. Hypothesis testing provides either lack of evidence to reject the null hypothesis, or supporting evidence to reject the null hypothesis and accept an **alternative hypothesis**, which may be quantified through the process of **estimation**.

## Hypothesis testing

See **significance testing**. Although these two terms are often used interchangeably, they originated from two different and conflicting approaches. The interested reader is referred to GOODMAN (1993) for a discussion.

## $I^2$

See **index of heterogeneity**.

## ICC

Abbreviation for **intraclass** (or intracluster) **correlation coefficient**.

## ICD

Abbreviation for the International Classification of Diseases, which is published by the World Health Organization. The current version, completed in 1992, is ICD-10 (10th revision). ICD-11 is to be released in 2018. See also PORTA (ed., 2014); **classification, misclassification**.

## Imputation

A method that deals with **missing data** by inferring their values from existing data. Simple imputation relies on **regression analysis** to derive a model (on the basis of non-missing observations) that predicts the values of the variable with the missing data. Multiple imputation is a more complex method that involves the computation of more than one set of possible values for the missing data, and the analysis of the resulting data sets. See BLAND (2015) for a detailed description and illustration. See also HAMILTON (2012).

## Inception cohort

A defined, representative sample of patients that is assembled at a common point in the course of a target disorder, ideally, close to its onset, to be **followed up** for the purpose of evaluating **prognosis**, i.e. the probability of **survival** to time $x$, or the average time to death (or, more generally, to **failure**, such as a complication or adverse event). See also **cohort**; Guyatt, in HAYNES *et al.* (eds., 2006).

## Incidence

As opposed to **prevalence**. A measure of the number of *new* cases of a disease that occur during a specified period of time. It may be expressed as **incidence rate** or **incidence risk**, where incidence rate is the number of new cases in reference to the *total time at risk* of a group or population that is followed up (see **person-time at risk** or PTAR), and incidence risk is the number of new cases in reference to the *total number at risk* over the specified period of time. In epidemiological studies, rates are often calculated in reference to person-time at risk (e.g. person-days or person-years at risk). Incidence rates (e.g. annual) are sometimes calculated in reference to the average number at risk during a given period of time (PORTA (ed.), 2014; ROTHMAN, 2012). **Hazard rates** are more clearly defined as *instantaneous* rates, i.e. as giving the probability of a given event over a time interval approaching zero, conditional on not having experienced the event up to the beginning of the same interval. Person-time incidence rates are also instantaneous measures, the unit of time in the denominator being arbitrary rather than an indication that the rate applies to a given time-period such as a year (ROTHMAN, 2012). Rates range from 0 to $+\infty$ and are expressed in units of the reciprocal of time or time$^{-1}$ (e.g. year$^{-1}$). Risks are unitless, ranging in value between 0 and 1, as they express probability of disease.

## Incidence density

Synonymous with **incidence rate** and **hazard rate**.

## Incidence proportion

Synonymous with **cumulative incidence**, **incidence risk** or **risk**.

## Incidence rate

A measure of morbidity or disease occurrence. The **incidence** rate (or simply, **rate**) is the number of new cases of a disease in reference to the total **person-time at risk** (PTAR) during a given period of **follow-up** (note: the denominator is *person-time*, not *people*):

$$Incidence\ rate = \frac{number\ of\ new\ occurences\ of\ a\ given\ disease}{total\ person\text{-}time\ at\ risk}$$

The larger the PTAR, the smaller the **standard error** of a rate will be. The incidence rate is usually multiplied by 1000 and expressed per 1000 person-time at risk (or, if the event is rare, per 10,000 or 100,000). Unlike the incidence risk, which is dimensionless and bound between 0 and 1, incidence rates can take any value from 0 to (at least theoretically) infinity. In fact, the magnitude of the rate depends on the unit of person-time chosen for the denominator. Although it is expressed in units of the reciprocal of time (e.g. year$^{-1}$) and cannot be interpreted as a probability, the incidence rate may give an estimate of the **incidence risk**, provided the calculated risk is less than 20% (ROTHMAN, 2012; KIRKWOOD & STERNE, 2003):

$$Risk \approx incidence\ rate \times time$$

This makes it possible to have an approximate risk estimate in studies where **losses to follow-up** and **competing causes** are present. However, the longer the follow-up period, the worse the approximation of risk by rate. Methods for **survival analysis** should be used to obtain risk estimates in these situations, as the rate of occurrence of the event in question is also likely to change over time; an example would be a **birth cohort** that experiences different mortality rates as time progresses. The reciprocal of the incidence rate may be interpreted as the average 'time to event', or as the average **life expectancy** if the event in question is death, provided the rate of the event remains constant over time. For rates that remain constant over time, the **Poisson distribution** provides the basis for a method of analysis, as the numerator of a rate is a **count**, i.e. the number of observed occurrences of the event in question. See **rate** for more on the relationship between rates and risks. See also incidence **rate difference**, incidence **rate ratio**.

## Incidence rate difference

Or simply, **rate difference**. The difference between the **incidence rates** experienced by the **exposed** and unexposed groups (or control *vs.* treated) in a **follow-up study**. See also **absolute risk difference**, **measures of effect**.

## Incidence rate ratio

Or simply, **rate ratio**. The ratio between the **incidence rates** experienced by the **exposed** and unexposed groups (or treated *vs.* control) in a **follow-up study**. For rare events, the rate ratio is a good approximation to the **risk** and **odds ratios**. See also **relative risk**, **measures of effect**.

## Incidence risk

A measure of morbidity or disease occurrence also known as 'incidence proportion' or 'cumulative incidence'. The **incidence** risk (or simply, **risk**) is the number of new cases of a disease during a specified period of time, in reference to the number of people at risk of contracting the disease at the beginning of the same period:

$$Incidence\ risk = \frac{number\ of\ new\ occurences\ of\ a\ given\ disease}{total\ number\ at\ risk}$$

As a proportion or probability, the incidence risk may range between 0 and 1, and it may also be expressed as a percentage. The incidence risk may be approximated by the **incidence rate** multiplied by length of **follow-up** if the calculated risk is less than 20% (ROTHMAN, 2012). See also **attack rate**, **case-fatality rate**, incidence **risk difference** (or **absolute risk difference**), incidence **risk ratio**.

## Incidence risk difference

Or simply, **risk difference**. The difference between the **incidence risks** experienced by the **exposed** and unexposed groups (or control *vs.* treated) in a **follow-up study**. Synonymous with **absolute risk difference**. See also **measures of effect**.

## Incidence risk ratio

Or simply, **risk ratio**. The ratio between the **incidence risks** experienced by the **exposed** and unexposed groups (or treated *vs.* control) in a **follow-up study**. See also **relative risk**, **measures of effect**.

## Inclusion criteria

See **eligibility criteria**.

## Incomplete block design

A **study design** for an **experimental study** in which incomplete **blocks** are used to provide control for one or more sources of response variability (other than the factor or factors under study). An incomplete block is one that is smaller than the number of treatments under study (e.g. a **randomized block design** in which the patients in each block are fewer than the number of treatments), or one for which the trial periods are fewer than the number of treatments (e.g. a **multiperiod crossover trial** in which none of the blocks or study participants receives all treatments under study). The **balanced incomplete block design** is often utilized. See SENN (2002). Cf. **complete block design**.

## Independence

Or more specifically, independence of observations. Two observations made on the same individual or **study unit** (or on individually **matched** study units) are said to be paired, i.e. *not* independent from each other. Independence is an **assumption** of many statistical methods, for example, the independent samples *t*-test and the **chi-squared test**. In making simple comparisons, non-independence may be dealt with through tests such as the **paired** *t*-test and **McNemar's test**. Data **dependence** in **clustered designs** also requires the use of special methods of analysis. Standard **regression** methods are usually not indicated.

## Independent effect

Two **predictor variables** or exposures that affect a given **outcome** are said to be independent if the effect of each of these predictors remains constant across all levels of the other. Depending on the chosen **measure of effect**, this lack of statistical **interaction** or **effect-measure modification** may also correspond to a lack of **biological interaction**. See also **log-linear model**.

## Independent events

In **probability** theory, two events are said to be independent if the occurrence of one of the events does not affect the probability of occurrence of the other event, such that knowledge of one event gives no information about the other. The probability that they will *both* occur is the product of their individual probabilities of occurrence. For example, if two fair six-sided dice are thrown, the probability of throwing a 'double six' is (probability of throwing a 'six') × (probability of throwing another 'six') = $1/6 \times 1/6 = 1/36$. See also **conditional probability**. Cf. **mutually exclusive**.

## Independent samples *t*-test

See *t*-test.

## Independent variable

See **predictor variable**.

## Index of dispersion

Synonym for variance-to-mean ratio or VMR. The index or coefficient of dispersion is the ratio of the **variance** of a **probability distribution** to its **mean**. If less than 1, the distribution is **underdispersed** (e.g. binomial), and if greater than 1, **overdispersed** (e.g. negative binomial). The Poisson distribution has VMR = 1, i.e. variance equal to the mean. Cf. **dispersion parameter, scale parameter**.

## Index of heterogeneity

A measure of the extent of **heterogeneity** among the primary studies in a **meta-analysis**, with regard to their respective estimates of treatment or exposure effect. The index ($I^2$) is calculated as:

$$I^2 = \frac{Q - df}{Q} \times 100\%$$

where $Q$ is the test statistic for the **Q test** for heterogeneity, and $df$ is the number of **degrees of freedom** for the test. In the absence of heterogeneity, the expected value of $Q$ equals the test's degrees of freedom. $I^2$ is interpreted as the percentage of $Q$ that is not explained by the variation within the studies (BLAND, 2015), i.e. that is due to between-study variation. The range of possible values for $I^2$ is from zero to under 100%, with values close to zero indicating lack of heterogeneity. When expressed as a proportion, it gives the same measure as the **intraclass correlation coefficient** or **ICC**. See HIGGINS *et al.* (2003) for further details. See also **forest plot, Galbraith plot, L'Abbé plot, meta-regression, DerSimonian and Laird random effects model**.

## Indicator variable

A **binary variable**, with values usually coded 0 or 1. See also **dummy variable**.

## Indirect standardization

See **standardization**.

## Individual participant data

Often referred to by its abbreviation, IPD. In the context of **meta-analysis**, data that are available at the individual level, as opposed to data that are summaries for each of the **primary studies** included. Possible advantages over the use of **aggregate data** include better control of **confounding**, and greater ability to evaluate the presence of **heterogeneity** of effect, although methodological and practical challenges are also mentioned by Haynes, in HAYNES *et al.* (eds., 2006). The potential for **publication bias** (as individual data may not be obtainable from all relevant studies) is an additional drawback. EGGER, DAVEY SMITH & ALTMAN (eds., 2001) provide further discussion.

## Induction period

The time-period from exposure to a given **component cause** until the onset of disease. The induction period for a **causal mechanism** can rarely be known, as one cannot be certain of the full sequence of component causes that have interacted to produce a given case of disease. Nonetheless, this period will comprise an initial stage resulting from the action of the first component cause, and it will end immediately following the last acting component cause, at which point the induction period ends and the disease period begins. *Initiators* (using the language of oncological research – ROTHMAN, 2012) may be associated with long induction periods, whereas *promoters*, i.e. causes acting later in the causation timeline, may have comparatively short induction times. The period of disease may itself be divided into the initial or **latency period** (at which point all necessary actions have taken place and disease has been caused, although signs and symptoms of disease have not yet developed), and a period in which disease may be detected either by means of suitable **diagnostic tests** or from its clinical manifestations. It is not always possible to distinguish the induction from the latency period, so a disease with extended latency may appear to have a long induction period. Latency may be reduced with improved disease detection, whereas the induction period may provide an opportunity for detection of intermediary biomarkers, which may be used to classify individuals into 'risk of disease' categories. ROTHMAN also discusses the role of *catalysts* as component causes of disease. See also **natural history of disease**.

## Infant mortality rate

The number of deaths among infants under 1 year of age that occur during a given time-period and in a given geographical region (such as a country), divided by the total number of live births in the same region during the same given time-period. The infant mortality rate is often multiplied by 1000 to be given as a rate per 1000 live births (or more precisely, a ratio), and the time-period chosen is usually 1 year. See also **perinatal mortality rate**, **stillbirth rate**, **neonatal mortality rate**, **child mortality rate**, **mortality rate**.

## Inference

The process of drawing conclusions about **population parameters** on the basis of **sample statistics**. In survey-type studies, the notion of 'population parameter' may be taken quite literally. In other types of study, namely in analytical comparative studies, the idea of 'population parameter' is perhaps best described as an underlying 'true effect' that is expected to be present beyond the study sample from which it is estimated. **Frequentist** and **Bayesian** inference are the two main approaches to statistical inference.

## Influence

See **influential observation**.

## Influential observation

An observation that has undue influence on the value of parameter **estimates**. An arithmetic **mean**, for example, may be unduly influenced by the presence of an outlying observation. **Outliers** may also exert undue influence on **correlation** and **regression coefficients**, causing their magnitude (and sometimes, also, direction) to be distorted (see Figure O.2, p. 249). Influential observations may therefore be overly fitted (they tend to have high **leverage** and large **standardized residuals**), and may not stand out as outliers in plots of **residuals** (see **regression diagnostics**). For each observation in a data set, **Cook's distance** gives a measure of the influence of that observation on a given regression model.

## Information bias

A type of **bias** that may occur in all types of **study design**, due to systematic errors in measuring **exposures** and/or responses (**outcomes**), and which results in under- or over-estimation of effects. Information biases may stem from observer or interviewer errors (for example, *assessment bias* due to lack of **blinding** in a **clinical trial**; *surveillance bias* due to differential follow-up of exposed and unexposed in a **cohort study**), respondent errors (*recall bias* due to differing memory of past exposures between cases and controls in a **case–control study**; *response bias*, again, due to lack of blinding, or due to fear or embarrassment), and instrument errors (such as **diagnostic tests** that *lack accuracy*; inadequate or *invalid* questionnaires; *uncalibrated* measuring tools). For further discussion, see ROTHMAN (2012); **misclassification** (differential and non-differential), **measurement error, measurement bias**. In crossover trials, **treatment–period interactions** may cause patient response to be measured with error in the period(s) into which a previous treatment effect was carried over. See also **ecological bias**. Cf. **selection bias**.

## Informative censoring

See **censoring, selection bias**. See also **differential censoring**.

## Informative loss to follow-up

See **loss to follow-up, selection bias**. See also **differential loss to follow-up**.

## Informed consent

The agreement, usually written, expressed by individuals to be participants in a **clinical trial** and undergo the trial's procedures, following full disclosure to the individual of the trial's objectives, treatments and interventions involved (including the possibility of being assigned to the **placebo** or **control group**), and all known side-effects and **adverse reactions**, regardless of how rarely they are expected to occur. Individuals should also be assured of their right to **withdraw** from a trial at any time if they so decide. Sackett, in HAYNES *et al.* (eds., 2006), recommends a balanced approach to the process of obtaining informed consent, whereby prospective trial participants are adequately informed but not discouraged from participation. POCOCK (1983) discusses legal aspects, the lack of uniform international standards, and the finer points of doctor/patient communication. In the context of **observational studies**, confidentiality, with regard to information obtained from records, questionnaires and interviews, is a key ethical issue (WALD, 2004).

## Instantaneous rate

Synonym for **hazard rate**.

## Instrumental variable

In linear regression, a variable that is **correlated** with a **predictor** (or explanatory) **variable**, but not with the **outcome** (or response) **variable** (except through the predictor). Instrumental variables can help reduce the effect of **measurement error** in explanatory variables, which can bias the estimation of **regression coefficients**, i.e. the estimation of treatment and exposure effects. They are also relevant when important predictors are thought to have been omitted from a regression model, leading to data **dependence**. See also **regression dilution bias**. Cf. **covariate**, **confounding variable**.

## Integer

A whole positive or negative number that does not have a fractional component. Examples are −45, −9, 18, 27, 36 and 0. See also **discrete variable**, **count**.

## Intention-to-treat analysis

Also referred to by its abbreviation, ITT. In the context of **randomized controlled trials**, this term refers to an approach to statistical analysis in which patients remain in the treatment or intervention groups to which they were originally assigned, regardless of whether or not they did indeed receive the allocated treatment, the comparison treatment, additional concomitant treatments or no treatment at all. Including these patients in the treatment group they actually received (or ignoring them altogether) may result in severe **bias**, and may even lead to a spurious reversal of **treatment effect**. To minimize the bias that may result from these **protocol breaches**, patients should be analysed in the groups to which they were randomized. Each **treatment group** is thus comprised of patients who **complied** with the treatment assigned, patients who complied while also taking **concomitant** treatments, patients who **dropped-out** or were **withdrawn** from the trial and patients who 'crossed-over' to receive the alternative treatment, allowing a pragmatic evaluation of treatment effectiveness to be made. As noted by ROTHMAN (2012), intention-to-treat analysis is not without its problems. The **misclassification** of 'exposure' may result in underestimation (or dilution) of treatment effects, which could be a serious matter in studies of safety or harm, if not, perhaps, in studies of efficacy. See also **pragmatic trial**, **effectiveness**. Cf. **perprotocol analysis**.

## Interaction

An interaction between two or more factors or variables is said to exist if the effect of one variable (on a given response or **outcome variable**) is not constant or homogeneous across levels of the other. For example, smoking and obesity are **risk factors** for several diseases. It would seem plausible for the effect of one of these factors, for example smoking, to be greater among people who are obese than among people who are not obese. Thus, adding to the **independent effects** of each of these two risk factors, there could be a 'penalty' for being both a smoker and overweight, the end effect being greater than the sum of the two separate effects. In this instance, the two risk factors have a **synergistic** effect. In other instances, risk factors or exposures may be **antagonistic**, their simultaneous presence diminishing or negating each other's effect. This is more specifically referred to as **biological interaction**, and depending on the chosen **measurement scale** or **measure of effect**, we may also find that a **regression model** that summarizes these relationships may or not necessitate the inclusion of a product term, i.e. **statistical interaction**. For this reason, statistical interaction has been said not to have universal meaning (ROTHMAN, 2012). In regression analysis, a **linear** or a **generalized linear model** with two **main effects** that interact with each other may be written as:

$$\hat{y} = \alpha + \beta_1 x_1 + \beta_2 x_2 + \beta_3 x_1 x_2$$

where $\beta_3$ represents the **regression coefficient** for the interaction or **product term**. Generally speaking, in an **additive model** the sign of the $\beta_3$ coefficient will be positive if the interaction is synergistic, or negative if it is antagonistic (assuming $\beta_1$ and $\beta_2$ are also positive). Where both interaction and **confounding** are present, estimates of effect should be given separately for each **stratum**. Figure I.1 shows the graphical depiction of an interaction, in which two **predictor variables** (body mass index [BMI] in kg/m², and a binary variable, intrauterine exposure to siege – i.e. malnutrition in utero, yes or no) interact to determine the value of a continuous outcome variable (systolic blood pressure in mmHg, in adult women). The graph shows that the increase in systolic blood pressure with increasing BMI is steeper among the exposed (the 'intrauterine' group) as compared to the unexposed (the 'infant' group). Had there been no inter-action, the two regression lines would have been parallel, and the vertical distance between them the estimated difference in systolic blood pressure between the two exposure groups. See **effect-measure modification, additive effect, multiplicative effect, likelihood ratio test**. See also HILLS (1974), COX (1984), HAMILTON (2012), MITCHELL (2012b).

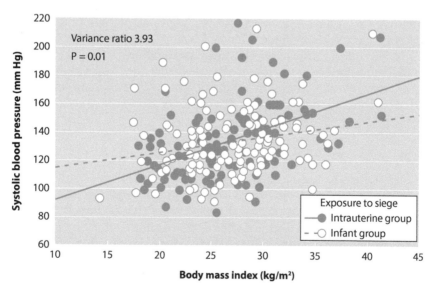

Figure I.1 Graphical display of an interaction: effect of BMI and intrauterine *vs.* as infant exposure to the Leningrad siege of 1941–1944 (and consequent malnutrition) on systolic blood pressure in adult women. (Reproduced from Stanner SA *et al.* (1997). Does malnutrition in utero determine diabetes and coronary heart disease in adulthood? Results from the Leningrad siege study, a cross-sectional study. *Br Med J* **315**: 1342 (with permission).)

## Intercept

In the context of **regression modelling**, the intercept or alpha($\alpha$)-coefficient is a constant value (specific to any given model), which represents the predicted value of the **outcome variable** when the value for all **predictor variables** is equal to zero. It is also denoted by $a$ or $b_0$. In **Poisson** and **logistic** regression, the 'intercept' corresponds to the baseline log rate and log odds, respectively. In **Cox** regression, the intercept is indistinguishable from the quantity that is referred to as the baseline hazard, $h_0(t)$, so Cox regression models do not have a separate intercept. See **centring**, **regression through the origin**, **Egger's test**, **Galbraith plot**. See also **regression coefficient**.

## Interim analyses

In the context of **clinical trials**, interim analyses are statistical analyses carried out at different times before the projected end of a trial, usually in order to assess whether the accumulating data are beginning to demonstrate a beneficial effect of one treatment over the other(s), with sufficient certainty. This prevents additional patients from being randomized to a demonstrably inferior treatment. An important issue with interim analyses is the risk of false-positive findings due to **multiple significance testing**. For this reason, **sequential designs** – group or continuous – are employed, which provide a blueprint for the conduct of periodic data analyses while the trial is still in progress. In the case of group sequential designs, and depending on the number of interim analyses planned, **nominal significance levels** (constant or varying) are specified so that the *overall* chance of a **type I error** is kept at an acceptable level. These nominal significance levels constitute the **stopping rules** for a given sequential trial, and will lead to a decision to halt the trial if at any point the results of a planned interim analysis meet the criteria set out by the rules. Interim analyses raise many issues and should be given careful consideration when designing a trial. See POCOCK (1983) for a fuller discussion and illustrative examples. See also **adaptive designs**.

## Intermediary cause

In the context of disease **causation**, an intermediary cause is a result in the causal pathway between **exposure** and disease. Although it is associated with both exposure and disease, an intermediary cause should not be considered a **confounding factor**. Thus, it is not usually adjusted for when carrying out statistical analyses. See also **surrogate endpoint**.

## International Classification of Diseases

Or International Statistical Classification of Diseases and Related Health Problems. See **ICD**.

## Interobserver agreement

See **agreement**, **kappa statistic**.

## Interquartile range

A measure of the **variability** or dispersion in a set of measurements. The interquartile range (IQR) is the interval between the 25th and the 75th **centiles** (also known as lower and upper **quartiles**), and comprises 50% of the observations in a variable (Figure B.6, **Box-and-whiskers plot**, p. 40). The IQR is a **resistant measure** in that it is not influenced by extreme observations or **outliers**, and is often used for describing data when the **standard deviation** may be unsuitable (for example, with skewed variables and ordinal data). The IQR is usually presented with the **median**, as **descriptive measures**. See also **nonparametric methods**.

## Interrupted time series

See **time series**.

## Interval censoring

See **censoring**.

## Interval estimate

See **estimate**, **confidence interval**.

## Interval variable

A **quantitative variable** that does not possess a true zero and allows negative values. Unlike **ratio variables**, for interval variables the ratio between any two values gives a different result depending on which scale measurements are made. A well-known example of an interval variable is temperature, measured in degrees Fahrenheit or Celsius (centigrade): a 10% increase in temperature from 50°F to 55°F, for example, does not correspond to a 10% increase on the centigrade scale: it corresponds to a 28% increase from 10°C to 12.8°C. Statistical methods for ratio/continuous variables are usually suitable to analyse this type of data. See also **measurement scale**.

## Intervention study

A **clinical trial**, health services research study (for example, a practice-based behaviour-change intervention study) or epidemiological study (a **field trial** or a **community intervention trial**) in which a specific intervention is being evaluated for its **effectiveness**. Clinical trials are usually therapeutic, and focus on treatments and interventions that will improve the outcomes of diseased individuals, whereas intervention studies at the community level are often preventive, and target at-risk groups in a given population. KIRKWOOD & STERNE (2003) discuss alternative evaluation designs that may be used when a randomized, controlled intervention is not feasible, and which allow pre/post, intervention/control, and adopters/non-adopters comparisons to be made, as a means to evaluate the impact of interventions. See HENNEKENS, BURING & MAYRENT (eds., 1987) for an overview. Cf. **observational study**. See also **experimental study**.

## Intraclass correlation coefficient

A measure of **reliability** or agreement for **quantitative measurements**. The intra-class correlation coefficient (ICC) is used when replicate measurements have no time or serial sequence (e.g. two white blood cell counts made on the same blood sample, where we cannot state which is the first and which is the second measurement). The ICC is calculated using a similar but modified method to that used to calculate **Pearson's cor-relation coefficient** (DUNN & EVERITT, 1995). Like the latter, the ICC has an ideal value of 1 (it ranges from 0 to 1), but is more appropriate for assessing agreement. When the measurement in question takes only two values or categories, the ICC is equivalent to the **kappa statistic**. It also yields similar results to the weighted kappa statistic. Alternatively, the ICC may be calculated using a cluster **random effects** model, as the ratio of the estimated between-subject variability ($\sigma_b^2$) to the total observed variability, the latter also including an error or within-subject component, $\sigma_w^2$ (KIRKWOOD & STERNE, 2003):

$$ICC = \frac{\sigma_b^2}{\sigma_b^2 + \sigma_w^2}$$

Thus, the ICC may be interpreted as the proportion of total variability not due to measurement error, but due to true variability. BLAND (2015) gives an alternative method for calculating the ICC, based on **one-way ANOVA** (analysis of variance) with 'subject' as a factor, where the residual or within-subject **mean square** is used to esti-mate within-subject variance, and the between-subject mean square is used to derive the between-subject variance. As with the **correlation coefficient**, the ICC should only be calculated from **random samples**, where the values for neither measurement have been pre-determined. In addition to measuring reliability, the ICC may also be used to measure the amount of clustering present when planning for, and analysing data from **clustered designs**, where the cluster **design effect** must be taken into account. Again, this is measured as the ratio of between-cluster variability to total variability (where total variability has an error or within-cluster component, in addition to the between-cluster component), usually termed *intracluster* correlation coefficient. In this context, an ICC of 0 is indicative of lack of clustering, whereas an ICC of 1 is indicative of highly clustered observations (i.e. lack of within-cluster variation). Researchers are encour-aged to publish cluster-specific measures and ICC estimates, in order to facilitate future research (BLAND, 2015). See ELDRIDGE & KERRY (2012) for a detailed discussion. See also **index of heterogeneity** ($I^2$).

## Intracluster correlation coefficient

See **intraclass correlation coefficient**.

## Intraobserver agreement

See **agreement, kappa statistic**.

## Inverse normal

The inverse normal for any given value of a **continuous variable** is the value from a theoretical **Normal distribution** (with the same **mean** and **standard deviation**) that corresponds to the same **quantile** in the **cumulative frequency distribution** of the variable. Plotting a variable against its inverse normal allows a visual assessment of normality of distribution (see **Normal plot**). Cf. **z-score** or standard normal deviate.

## Inverse normal plot

See **Normal plot**.

## Inverse variance method

A **pooling** method that combines **estimates** of absolute or relative effect, for both binary and continuous outcomes, to produce a single summary, which is a **weighted average** across the different **primary studies** in a **meta-analysis** (or the different **strata** of a **confounding variable** in an observational study). Weights are in *inverse* proportion to the variance of the estimates, i.e. in *direct* proportion to their **precision**. Relative effect measures for binary outcomes (including hazard ratios for 'time to event' data) are combined on the **log scale**. See Deeks, Altman & Bradburn, in EGGER, DAVEY SMITH & ALTMAN (eds., 2001) for formulae and illustrative examples. The inverse variance method (and, likewise, the **Mantel–Haenszel method** and **Peto's method**) is employed under the assumption of a **fixed effect**, as, to quote HILLS (1974, p. 161) "…weighting by accuracy [precision] is only relevant when combining different estimates of a common 'true value'." Cf. **DerSimonian and Laird random effects model**.

## IPD

Abbreviation for **individual participant data**.

## IRLS

Abbreviation for **iteratively reweighted least squares**.

## Iteratively reweighted least squares

Also referred to by its abbreviation, IRLS. A type of **weighted least squares (WLS)** regression that is carried out through a succession of iterations and re-estimation of weights, until convergence is reached, in similar fashion to **maximum likelihood estimation**. When starting values are obtained by **ordinary least squares (OLS)** (at iteration 0), high-leverage **influential** observations may not be properly downweighted as they will not have large residuals (HAMILTON, 1992). IRLS may be employed with binary and other types of outcome other than continuous. See also **robust method, meta-regression**; HAMILTON (2012).

## J-shaped curve

A depiction of a **non-linear relationship** between a quantitative, ordinal or ordered categorical **risk factor** and risk or probability of disease (or death), whereby the lowest levels of exposure are associated with an increased risk as compared to low to moderate levels of exposure to the risk factor in question. As extent of exposure increases from this point, a sharp or more gradual increase in risk occurs, giving the characteristic J-shape (in other words, a J-shaped curve has one *turn point*). The opposite pattern characterizes a *reverse J-shaped curve*: highest risk for low levels of a given factor (likely, a **preventive factor**), lowest risk at moderate to high levels of the factor, with the highest levels of the factor again experiencing an increase in risk (Figure J.1b – SEMPOS *et al.*, 2013). A J-shaped curve has been described for the relationship between ethanol intake, blood pressure measurements and serum cholesterol levels and risk of cardiovascular disease (CVD). Under this pattern of relationship, alcohol abstainers seem to have greater risk of CVD than light to moderate drinkers, and very low blood pressure and cholesterol levels likewise do not appear to

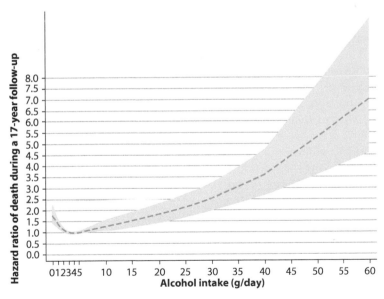

Figure J.1a J-shaped curve: the hazard ratio (*HR*) of all-cause mortality by self-reported alcohol consumption (in g/day), adjusted for age, education, marital status, smoking, BMI, fitness, diabetes, and previous ischaemic heart disease. Hazard ratios are calculated in reference to an alcohol intake of approximately 4 g/day (thus, *HR* of 1). (Reproduced from Midlöv P *et al.* (2016). Women's health in the Lund area (WHILA) – Alcohol consumption and all-cause mortality among women – a 17-year follow-up study. *BMC Public Health* **16**: 22.)

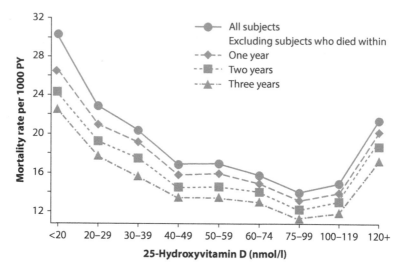

**Figure J.1b** Reverse J-shaped curve: the association between mortality rate (all-cause, per 1000 person-years (PY), and adjusted for age, sex, race/ethnicity and season) and serum 25-hydroxyvitamin D concentration (in nmol/l), modelled using cubic splines, in the 15-year follow-up of the US NHANES (National Health and Nutrition Examination Survey) III through 2006 (n = 15099 age ⩾20 years; 3784 deaths observed). (Reproduced from Sempos CT *et al.* (2013). Is there a reverse J-shaped association between 25-hydroxyvitamin D and all-cause mortality? Results from the US nationally representative NHANES. *J Clin Endocrinol Metab* **98**: 3001–9 (with permission).)

confer protection. This is in contrast, for example, with exposure to cigarette smoke and risk of CVD and lung cancer, where non-smokers experience the lowest risk of disease and mortality rates. Research studies have alternatively found J-shaped relationships to have, rather, a **U-shaped** pattern. In either case, interpretation of these effects requires careful consideration of possible harms *vs.* potential benefits. Figure J.1a (MIDLÖV *et al.*, 2016) illustrates the J-shaped relationship between self-reported alcohol intake (in g/day) and all-cause mortality (expressed as hazard ratios by alcohol consumption), in a follow-up study involving 6353 women aged 50–59 years, in the Lund area in Sweden (participation rate was 64.2%, 6916 women, of whom 563 were excluded due to incomplete data). Average duration of follow-up was 17 years, and 579 deaths were registered by the end of the study period. **Hazard ratios** are adjusted for sociodemographic and lifestyle factors, diabetes and previous ischaemic heart disease. See also di CASTELNUOVO *et al.* (2006); **dose-response relationship**. Cf. **exponential curve**.

## J-shaped distribution

The **distribution** of a continuous variable with an extreme *negative* (J-shaped) or *positive* **skew** (reverse J-shaped). Figure J.2a (SUREDA *et al.*, 2014) shows the extreme positive skew (toward high values) of the distribution of salivary cotinine concentrations (in ng/ml) among a representative sample of the non-smoking adult population in Barcelona exposed to secondhand smoke, following the introduction of the Spanish smoke-free legislation in 2006, which was later extended in 2011. This is in contrast with the less extreme positive

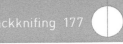

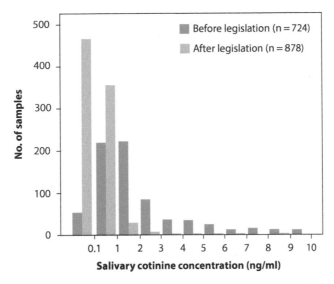

**Figure J.2a** A reverse J-shaped distribution: extreme positive skew of the distribution of salivary cotinine concentrations (in ng/ml) among the non-smoker adult population of Barcelona (*n* = 878), after the introduction of smoke-free legislation in Spain. Also shown is the less extreme lognormal distribution of salivary cotinine (*n* = 724) before the legislation. (Reproduced from Sureda X *et al.* (2014). Impact of the Spanish smoke-free legislation on adult, non-smoker exposure to secondhand smoke: cross-sectional surveys before (2004) and after (2012) legislation. *PLoS One* **9**: e89430.)

skew of the distribution before the introduction of the legislation. The former is an example of a reverse J-shaped distribution, a J-shaped distribution being its mirror image, with a skew toward low values (Figure J.2b – COX *et al.*, 2013). The percentage of non-smokers with cotinine concentrations below the quantification limit of 0.1 ng/ml increased from 7.3% before the legislation (2004–2005) to 53.2% after the legislation (2011–2012). In contrast with a **lognormal distribution** (for example, the 'before legislation' distribution), a **logarithmic transformation** will not convert a reverse J-shaped distribution into an approximately **Normal distribution**, although it may make it more symmetrical. See also **exponential distribution**.

## Jackknifing

A method for validating or assessing the overall **goodness-of-fit** (**GoF**) and adequacy (**regression diagnostics**) of a **model** (MOSTELLER & TUKEY, 1977). With this method, a single **study sample** (of size *n*) is used to both derive and validate the model, as opposed to using an external or **validation sample**. To prevent an overoptimistic assessment, a **residual** for each observation is calculated from a model that excludes that same observation, i.e. from a model based on a sample of size *n* – 1. The residuals thus obtained are then analysed in a number of ways to provide the GoF assessment and regression diagnostics. Jackknifed residuals are sometimes referred to as studentized residuals. The mean of the different **estimates** obtained from each of the *n* samples of size *n* – 1 is termed the *jackknife estimate*. The method may also be used to obtain an estimate of the **variance** (or

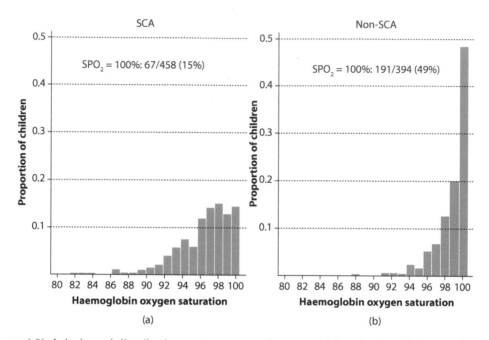

**Figure J.2b** A J-shaped distribution: extreme negative skew of distribution of daytime haemoglobin oxygen saturation (SpO$_2$, in %) in Tanzanian children with (a), and without (b), sickle cell anaemia (SCA). (Reproduced from Cox SE *et al.* (2013). Hematological and genetic predictors of daytime hemoglobin saturation in Tanzanian children with and without sickle cell anemia. *ISRN Hematol* **2013**: 472909.)

precision) and **bias** of an **estimator**. The variance estimate is calculated as the sum of the squared differences between each of the estimates obtained from each of the $n$ samples (as described above, where each sample has size $n - 1$) and the jackknife estimate, all multiplied by $(n - 1)/n$. The estimate of bias is the difference between the jackknife estimate and the estimate obtained from the original size $n$ sample, multiplied by $(n - 1)$. **Confidence intervals** may be constructed on the basis of these different quantities. HAMILTON (1992) compares jackknifing, as a method to estimate the variance and bias of an estimator, to **bootstrapping**, a resampling method that may be employed for the same purpose. Jackknifing should be used preferably when the data do not include **outliers**. See also **standardized residual**.

## Jittering

Random variability that is introduced when plotting **bivariate relationships**, to prevent observations sharing the same $(x, y)$ coordinate from being plotted on the exact same spot. The jittering, or slight scattering of observations around their shared coordinate (along the **x-axis**), gives a better sense of the number of observations sharing that same coordinate, and overall, a better sense of the total **sample size** and of a variable's **distribution** according to the values of another variable. This technique is particularly useful when the variable represented on the x-axis is a **categorical** or **ordered categorical variable**, as illustrated in Figure J.3 (LECLERCQ *et al.*, 2005).

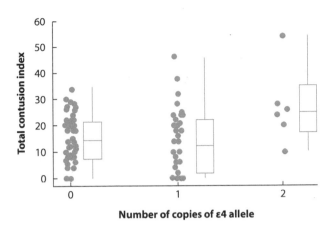

**Figure J.3** Random jitter along the *x*-axis: dotplot of total contusion index in patients with trau-matic brain injury with 0, 1 or 2 copies of the apolipoprotein E (*APOE*) ε4 allele (the latter is strongly associated with presence of cerebral amyloid angiopathy or CAA). Within each group, jittering separates data points with the same value for the *y*-variable. Boxplots are also shown. (Reproduced from Leclercq PD *et al.* (2005). Cerebral amyloid angiopathy in traumatic brain injury: association with apolipoprotein E genotype. *J Neurol Neurosurg Psychiatry* **76**: 229–33 (with permission).)

# K

## Kaplan–Meier method

A method for estimating the cumulative probability of survival at different time points over a given period of time (what is known as the **survival function** or [$S(t)$]), in studies where **censoring** is present and duration of **follow-up** varies among study participants. Calculations for the Kaplan–Meier method are based on **risk sets**, and are carried out as follows: firstly, a probability of survival is calculated each time, and at the *exact times*, an event of interest occurs (cf. **life table method**, where probabilities are calculated for *time intervals*, i.e. the time variable is grouped). The cumulative probability of survival *up to and including* that point in time is then calculated by multiplying the probability of survival *at* time $t$ by the probability of survival *up to* time $t$ (given by the cumulative probability of survival at the time of occurrence of the previous event). The cumulative probabilities thus obtained over the duration of follow-up may be used to construct the **Kaplan–Meier survival curve**, just as life table estimates of cumulative survival probability are also used to construct survival curves. The set of estimates of cumulative survival probability may also be used to derive the **cumulative hazard function**, $H(t)$, i.e. the cumulative hazards at those same time points along the follow-up period. See ALTMAN (1991), KIRKWOOD & STERNE (2003), DAWSON & TRAPP (2004) and CLEVES, GOULD & MARCHENKO (2016) for examples and further details. See also **logrank test**, **Greenwood's formula**, Nelson–Aalen estimator (under cumulative hazard function).

## Kaplan–Meier survival curve

A **survival curve** that is constructed using the estimates of cumulative survival probability (i.e. the **survival function**) obtained with the **Kaplan–Meier method**. The curve has a characteristic 'step' appearance due to the way in which survival probabilities, and therefore, cumulative survival probabilities, are calculated, with the probability of survival remaining constant between events, only dropping to coincide with the occurrence of a new event (Figure K.1, **$y$-axis** gives the values of the survival function, [$S(t)$]). This is the graphical display of the data analysed under **Cox regression** (Box C.3, p. 82). **Censored** observations should ideally be marked on the curve at the times at which they occur. The number of individuals still at risk can be shown at regular time intervals along the $x$-axis. A **confidence interval** for the survival curve(s) may also be presented (see **Greenwood's formula**). The survival curves of two or more separate groups can be formally compared with the **logrank test** (see Box L.2, p. 201) or the **Mantel–Haenszel $\chi^2$ test**. With no censored observations, the **Wilcoxon rank sum test** may be used to test the null hypothesis that **median** survival is similar in the two groups (DAWSON & TRAPP, 2004). See also **life expectancy**; BLAND (2015).

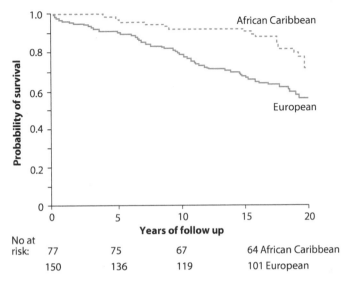

No at
risk:

| | | | |
|---|---|---|---|
| 77 | 75 | 67 | 64 African Caribbean |
| 150 | 136 | 119 | 101 European |

Figure K.1 Kaplan–Meier survival curve: differences in probability of survival (all-cause mortality) between African Caribbeans and Europeans in a 20-year follow-up study of a non-insulin dependent diabetes mellitus patient cohort (London, UK, 1975–1995). (Reproduced from Chaturvedi N et al. (1996). Differences in mortality and morbidity in African Caribbean and European people with non-insulin dependent diabetes mellitus: results of a 20 year follow up of a London cohort of a multinational study. Br Med J **313**: 848–52 (with permission).)

## kappa statistic

Also known as Cohen's kappa. A measure of **agreement** for **categorical variables**. kappa (κ) may be used to assess the extent of agreement between two (or more) raters, or between two alternative classification or diagnostic methods. As with the coefficient of **reliability (R)**, κ measures chance-corrected proportional agreement, i.e. the **proportion** of agreement over and above what might be expected by chance alone:

$$\kappa = \frac{observed\ agreement - chance\ agreement}{1 - chance\ agreement}$$

$$= 1 - \frac{observed\ disagreement}{chance\text{-}expected\ disagreement}$$

Chance agreement is calculated using the same method as for calculating **expected frequencies** for **contingency tables**. The expected frequencies for cells denoting agreement are then added up and divided by the total number of observations to give the proportion of agreement that is attributed to chance. κ takes the value of one (1) when there is perfect agreement; zero represents agreement no better than by chance alone, and negative values, agreement worse than expected by chance. With **ordered categorical variables**, the weighted kappa statistic may be calculated, which takes partial agreement into account. An incorrect approach to measuring agreement is to test for the presence of an **association**; it is in fact possible to have a strong association and zero agreement. These are two separate concepts and methods such as the **chi-squared test** or **rank correlation** are not appropriate to test for or measure agreement. kappa is dependent on the **bias** between raters (or methods), i.e. the degree of systematic disagreement between the raters in a study, and also on the proportion of subjects in each category. It is therefore difficult to give precise values of κ that reflect poor, moderate or good agreement. The number of classifying categories affects the value of kappa, which will be lower with increasing number of categories. See also **coefficient of concordance**. See **intraclass correlation coefficient** (**ICC**) for another measure of reliability for quantitative measurements. See ALTMAN (1991), BLAND (2015), DUNN & EVERITT (1995) and KIRKWOOD & STERNE (2003) for illustrative examples and additional details.

## Kendall's tau

A **non-parametric correlation coefficient** that is calculated by computing the number of concordant and discordant pairs, based on the **ranking** of each observation under each of the two variables in question. The coefficient, τ or tau, is calculated as the proportion of concordant pairs *minus* the proportion of discordant pairs. Unlike **Spearman's** rho, tau is a useful measure of the **strength of association** between the two variables (BLAND, 2015), similarly to **Pearson's** *r*. Kendall's correlation coefficient is particularly appropriate for use with small **sample sizes**. The statistical significance of Kendall's tau may also be tested as an alternative to the **chi-squared test for trend** when analysing a binary outcome across the ordered categories of an exposure. This is in addition to its use in measuring the correlation between **ordinal** and/or **interval/ratio** variables, and between ordinal (or interval/ratio) and **ordered categorical** data. See BLAND (2015) for further discussion and methodology, including how to deal with tied rankings. See also **rank correlation, Begg and Mazumdar test, meta-regression, DerSimonian and Laird random effects model**.

## Kernel smoothers

See **smoothing**.

## Kolmogorov–Smirnov test

A **non-parametric significance test** that is used to evaluate **goodness-of-fit** (**GoF**). The test is usually carried out to compare an empirical **frequency distribution** against a given **theoretical distribution** (for example, a Normal, lognormal, or exponential distribution), and to test for distributional differences between **samples** from different populations. In each instance, the comparison is made between the empirical **cumulative frequency distribution** and the theoretical cumulative distribution function, or between the empirical cumulative frequency distributions. The **test statistic** is given by the maximum absolute difference between these functions. See FLEISS (1999) for further details. See also **Shapiro–Wilk** and **Shapiro–Francia test**.

## Kruskal–Wallis test

A **non-parametric significance test** that is used to compare two or more independent groups with respect to the **distribution** of a quantitative or ordinal variable. The test is based on the **ranks** given to the values of the variable in question, and produces a **test statistic**, $H$. Under the **null hypothesis** that the groups all come from populations with the same **median** value, $H$ follows a **chi-squared distribution** with $k-1$ **degrees of freedom**, where $k$ is the number of groups being compared. This test is an extension of the **Mann–Whitney $U$-test**, which is indicated when there are just two groups, and may be carried out when the **assumptions** for **analysis of variance** (more specifically, **one-way ANOVA**) cannot be met.

## Kurtosis

A measure of the **density** in the tails of a **unimodal continuous distribution** (empirical or theoretical), as compared with what would be expected were the variable **normally distributed** with same mean and variance. **Distributions** that are more pointed than the corresponding Normal distribution are called **leptokurtic**, and have tail densities lower than expected, i.e. a positive kurtosis. Distributions that are flatter than the corresponding Normal distribution are called **platykurtic** and have a negative kurtosis with tail densities higher than expected. The Normal distribution is said to be **mesokurtic** and has a kurtosis of zero (or 3, depending on the method of calculation). See also **skewness**, **Normal plot**.

## L'Abbé plot

A graphical method that is used to evaluate **heterogeneity** of effect among the different **primary studies** included in a **meta-analysis**, and which may be employed with **binary outcomes** (L'ABBÉ, DETSKY & O'ROURKE, 1987). For each individual study, the **risk** or **odds** in the **exposed** or **treatment group** is plotted on the *y*-**axis** against the risk or odds in the **control group** on the *x*-**axis**, as shown in Figure L.1 (BAX *et al.*, 2009). The area of each plotted circle is proportional to the **weight** of the corresponding study. A L'Abbé plot often shows the **regression line** of treatment *vs.* control results (with greater between-study heterogeneity corresponding to greater scatter around this line), in addition to a central diagonal line that represents absence of **treatment** or **exposure effect** (i.e. no difference in risk of outcome between exposed and control groups); both are shown in Figure L.1. See also **forest plot**, **Galbraith plot**, **index of heterogeneity**, **meta-regression**.

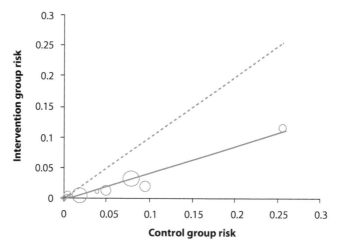

**Figure L.1** A L'Abbé plot: lack of scatter around the solid regression line suggests homogeneity of effect (central diagonal dotted line represents absence of effect). (Reproduced from Bax L *et al.* (2009). More than numbers: the power of graphs in meta-analysis. *Am J Epidemiol* **169**: 249–55 (with permission).)

## Lack-of-fit *F*-test

See **residual *F*-test**.

## Ladder of powers

See **transformations**.

## Lagged regression

Regression analysis that includes as **predictor variables** past values of the outcome or predictor variables. See **autocorrelation, cross-correlation, autoregressive model** (time series), **transition model** (longitudinal data), **ARMAX model** (time series) and standard regression methods.

## Large sample method

Or asymptotic method. A method of statistical analysis that assumes the **sampling distribution** of **test statistics** to follow a given **theoretical distribution** (such as the **standard Normal distribution** or a **chi-squared distribution**) when the **null hypothesis** is true. Likewise, it assumes the sampling distribution of **estimates** to follow a Normal distribution. Such tests and methods become more accurate as **sample size** increases, even if usual **assumptions** about the data being analysed are not met. See also **central limit theorem, approximation**.

## Last observation carried forward

Also referred to by its abbreviation, LOCF. A method for replacing **missing data** in a **longitudinal study**. For any given study participant for whom data are missing, these are assumed to have the same values as at the time of the last recorded observation for that individual. In other words, the last observation is carried forward to fill in the missing data. This method has been criticized for making unrealistic assumptions about non-variability of response over time. Simple and multiple **imputation** methods are considered preferable to the use of LOCF.

## Latency period

The length of time in the **natural history of a disease** during which the disease may be detected by means of pertinent **diagnostic tests**, while the patient, however, remains asymptomatic. See **induction period** for additional details.

## Latent variable

A variable that cannot be measured or observed directly, but only indirectly through measurable or observable variables with which it is thought to be closely associated. In **factor analysis**, for example, latent variables are the factors postulated to explain correlations between measurable variables. The latter provide an indirect measure of the unmeasurable factor. In regression analysis, **random effects** models are also referred to as latent variable models. These effects represent unobserved between-subject or between-cluster heterogeneity. SKRONDAL & RABE-HESKETH (2004) discuss and illustrate the concept and pervasiveness of latency, propose a number of approaches to its modelling, and present a unifying general model framework. Proposed models include latent class or **cluster models**, **multilevel** and **longitudinal models**, **factor models** and structural equation models or SEM (see HAMILTON (2012) for an overview of SEM). See also **composite score**.

## Latin square

An array for treatment **allocation** that allows for two **blocking** factors in an **experimental study**, commonly, 'subject' and 'observer', or 'subject' and 'study period'. The levels of one factor are represented by the rows, with the columns representing the levels of the second factor. The **treatment** (i.e. the factor of interest in the study) to be administered at each combination of the two blocking factors is usually represented by Roman letters (e.g. A, B, C and D), or sometimes, numerals (1, 2, 3, 4, for example). **Multiperiod crossover trials** make use of a particular type of Latin square in which each treatment follows each of the other treatments the same number of times, and each treatment pair sequence occurs only once (if there is an odd number of treatments, a second Latin square that is the mirror image of the first one is used, with treatment pair sequences occurring twice between the two squares). See FLEISS (1999) for details of the complete **randomization** procedure. A Latin square design is a **complete block design**. Lack of **interaction** between the factors in the study, i.e. blocking and treatment factors, is assumed.

## Lead-time bias

In the context of **screening** or early diagnosis, a type of **bias** that is due to detection of disease at presymptomatic stages, without, however, the possibility of offering a better treatment than that which is offered to symptomatic patients. When estimating length of **survival**, patients diagnosed at an early stage will appear to have longer survival compared to patients who are diagnosed at a later stage (perhaps when they become symptomatic). This, however, may be indicative only of the 'zero-time shift' in the time of diagnosis, and is one of the reasons evidence of the **effectiveness** of screening programmes must come from **randomized controlled trials** (HAYNES *et al.* [eds., 2006]). WALD (2004) suggests the use of age-specific **mortality rates** rather than length of survival, as a strategy for avoiding both lead-time and **length-time bias**. See also **induction period, latency period**.

## Least squares estimation

A method of **regression analysis** that is carried out to find the line of best fit, i.e. the line (or **model**) that best describes the relationship between a **quantitative outcome** and one or more **predictor variables**. The method seeks to minimize the sum of squared **residuals**; in **simple linear regression**, these are the vertical distances from each observation to the regression line. Residuals are analysed in a variety of ways to evaluate the fit and adequacy of regression models. Least square residuals are expected to be **independent** and **normally distributed**, with constant variance (**homoscedasticity**) across the values of the predictor(s). **Maximum likelihood estimation** provides an alternative method of fitting regression models, in particular where residuals cannot be normally distributed. See also **ordinary least squares (OLS)**, **weighted least squares (WLS)**, **iteratively reweighted least squares (IRLS)**.

## Left censoring

See **censoring**.

## Length-time bias

In the context of **screening** or early diagnosis, a type of **bias** that results from greater probability of early diagnosis among patients with long preclinical stages of disease (e.g. patients with slow-growing tumors). Due to the positive association between duration of preclinical and clinical stages of disease, early diagnosis may sometimes appear to lead to longer survival. WALD (2004) suggests using age-specific **mortality rates**, rather than length of survival, as a strategy for avoiding both length-time and **lead-time bias** in studies evaluating the **effectiveness** of screening programmes. In addition, and as discussed also by HAYNES *et al.* (eds., 2006), it remains important that evidence of effectiveness should come from a **randomized controlled trial**. See also **induction period**, **latency period**.

## Leptokurtic

A theoretical or empirical **distribution** that is more pointed than the corresponding theoretical **Normal distribution**. These distributions have a positive **kurtosis**, i.e. tail densities that are lower than expected for a Normal distribution or a normally distributed variable. The logistic and Cauchy distributions are examples of continuous theoretical distributions that are leptokurtic. See also **mesokurtic, platykurtic**.

## Level of significance

See **significance level**.

## Levene's test

A **significance test** that is carried out to compare the **variances** of two or more groups, with respect to a given **quantitative variable**. The test does not require the variable in question to have a **Normal distribution**. A common application of Levene's test is in checking the assumption of **homoscedasticity**, which may be necessary when performing an **analysis of variance** to compare different groups with respect to a mean measurement or quantity, and when carrying out an independent samples *t*-test. See also *F*-test, **Bartlett's test**.

## Leverage

In the context of **regression analysis**, a measure of the extent to which the value of an observation is extreme, in respect of a given **predictor variable** or set of predictors, i.e. the extent to which a data point is an **outlying** observation on the X variable space.

Observations displaying high leverage (outliers in *x*) have the potential to **influence** the slope of a regression line, or, more generally, the estimated magnitude of regression coefficients, depending on the value of the *y* or **outcome variable**. The leverage or hat statistic, *h*, is closely related to **Mahalanobis distance**. See Figure O.2 (p. 249) for a graphical illustration of the effects of outliers in *y*, high-leverage points, and influential points. See also **regression diagnostics, standardized residual**. See HAMILTON (1992) for additional details.

## LHH

Abbreviation for **likelihood of being helped** *vs.* **harmed**.

## Liang–Zeger regression analysis

See **generalized estimating equations (GEEs)**.

## Life expectancy

The average length of **survival** from beginning of **follow-up**. It is calculated from a **life table** as follows:

$$\text{Life expectancy} = \tfrac{1}{2} + \Sigma(\text{number of time units in an interval} \times \text{cumulative chance of survival in the same interval})$$

where the **sigma notation**, $\Sigma$, represents summation across all time intervals, and the quantity ½ is a **continuity correction**. A life expectancy estimate may be obtained also from the **Kaplan–Meier survival curve**: it is the median survival time, provided the curve drops to 50% probability of survival. With a constant hazard, life expectancy is given by the reciprocal of the **hazard rate**.

## Life table method

A table that is used to record the **survival** (and failure) experience of a group of people or **cohort**, over a specific **follow-up period**. The following information is presented (KIRKWOOD & STERNE, 2003):

1. time, which is commonly expressed as *time from beginning of follow-up*, or as *age*. Time is divided into intervals, and for each time interval (or age group) a number of summaries may be obtained as detailed below;
2. *number alive at the beginning* of the interval (or number in each age group). The number alive is the number at risk before correcting for losses to follow-up;
3. *number of events* (e.g. deaths) during the interval;
4. *number lost to follow-up* during each time interval;
5. *number at risk* is then calculated as:

$$\text{number at the beginning} - (\text{number lost}/2);$$

6. and *risk of dying* (or of any other event) during each time interval is calculated as:

(number of deaths)/(number at risk);

7. from which *chance of surviving* a given time interval is calculated as:

1 – risk of dying during the interval;

8. and finally, *cumulative chance of surviving* from beginning of follow-up (i.e. chance of surviving this time interval *given* that one has survived the previous time interval), which is:

cumulative chance of surviving to end of previous interval × chance of surviving present interval

The cumulative chance of surviving each of the various time intervals may then be used to construct a life table **survival curve**. It may also be used to estimate **life expectancy**. The life table method is adequate if the time intervals are relatively short (DAWSON & TRAPP, 2004). Where this is not the case, bias may be introduced given the assumption that losses to follow-up have occurred mid-way through the time intervals. The **Kaplan–Meier method** is an alternative approach to constructing a survival curve.

## Likelihood

The **probability** of observing a given set of **data** given the value of a **parameter** (or set of parameters), i.e. given a particular **model** seeking to explain the relationships between the **variables** in the data set. See also **maximum likelihood estimation, likelihood function, log likelihood, likelihood ratio test**. Cf. posterior distribution under **Bayesian inference**.

## Likelihood function

In the context of **maximum likelihood estimation**, the likelihood function is an equation that gives the probability of a set of data given a particular set of **model parameters**. The exact form of this equation depends on the underlying **probability distribution** for the **outcome variable**. A plot of the value for the likelihood (on the **y-axis**) against a range of possible values for the parameter of interest (on the **x-axis**) typically shows a bell-shaped, unimodal curve, with its peak at the maximum likelihood estimate (MLE) for the parameter (i.e. the value of the parameter that maximizes the value obtained from the likelihood equation). The calculation of the likelihood value is based on the **conditional probability** of each observation in the data set, i.e. the probability of each of the outcomes observed given the model and given the actual values of the **predictor variables** for each observation. Each different set of model parameters produces a different likelihood value: the larger the likelihood, the greater the probability of the data observed coming from the specified model. See CLAYTON & HILLS (1993), and HOSMER, LEMESHOW & STURDIVANT (2013) for an in-depth discussion. A comprehensive overview is given by KIRKWOOD & STERNE (2003). See also **likelihood, log likelihood, (log) likelihood ratio function, likelihood ratio test**.

## Likelihood of being helped *vs.* harmed

A measure of the relative magnitude of the **NNT** or **number needed to treat** *vs.* the **NNH** or **number needed to harm**, for a given treatment or intervention. It is calculated as the ratio of their reciprocals:

$$LHH = \left( \frac{1}{NNT} \right) \div \left( \frac{1}{NNH} \right)$$

STRAUS *et al.* (2010) give modifications to the basic formula that better reflect an individual patient's risk profile and values. See also **patient expected event rate** (**PEER**).

## Likelihood ratio function

The **likelihood function** may be redefined as a likelihood ratio (LR) function, by expressing the likelihood value for any given value of a **parameter** of interest as a ratio to the likelihood at the MLE (**maximum likelihood estimate**) for the same parameter. When likelihood is expressed as **log likelihood**, the log likelihood ratio is the difference between the two log likelihoods. At its maximum, the LR has a value of 1, and the log LR has a value of 0 (zero). The log likelihood ratio may be plotted for different values of the parameter of interest, with different cut-offs for log likelihood ratio corresponding to different **supported ranges** (or, by approximation, **confidence intervals**) for the value of the parameter. The shape of the likelihood ratio function is the same as the shape of the likelihood function. The plot of the log likelihood ratio function is often approximated by a **quadratic function** calculated from the sample estimate and standard error, which will be accurate if the data are normally distributed, and a good approximation where sample sizes are sufficiently large. Where there is more than one parameter, reference is made to 'profile' log likelihood ratios. KIRKWOOD & STERNE (2003) discuss statistical **significance tests** based on alternative computations of the log likelihood ratio, namely the **likelihood ratio test**, **Wald test**, and the score test. The first two are widely used to test the significance of predictors in regression models, with the likelihood ratio test having generally greater applicability.

## Likelihood ratio test

A **significance test** used in the context of **Cox** (regression for survival times), **logistic** (regression for proportions/binary outcomes) and **Poisson regression** (regression for counts and rates), to test the **statistical significance** of one or more **predictor variables**. The **test statistic** for the likelihood ratio test (LRT) is $G$, a statistic that is related to the **deviance statistic**, $D$. To test the significance of a given variable, two **nested models** are fitted, with and without the variable in question. The **log likelihood** for the model that includes this variable is larger (less negative) than that for the model that excludes the variable. The LRT evaluates whether inclusion of this particular variable is worthwhile, i.e. whether the **fit** of the model (as measured by the change in the value of the log likelihood) worsens significantly when the model is simplified and the variable is excluded. Under the **null hypothesis**, the LRT test statistic follows a **chi-squared distribution** with **degrees of freedom** equal to the number of predictors (i.e. parameters) whose significance is being tested. When a model with one or more predictors is compared to a model with no predictors (a **null model**), the likelihood ratio test is equivalent to the overall **F-test**, which is carried out to test the joint significance of all predictor variables in a multiple linear regression model. When nested models are compared, the LRT is equivalent to the partial *F*-test. As an extension of the above, the likelihood ratio test may also be used when evaluating the presence of **interactions**, departures from **linear trends**, **cluster** effects and **collinearity**. See CLAYTON & HILLS (1993), AGRESTI (2007), KIRKWOOD & STERNE (2003) and HOSMER, LEMESHOW & STURDIVANT (2013) for further details. See also **maximum likelihood estimation**, **generalized linear model**, **Akaike's information criterion (AIC)**, **Bayes' factor (BF)**.

## Likelihood ratios

In the context of **diagnostic testing**. Table 4 shows the layout of the results of a hypothetical diagnostic test:

Table 4  Layout of results from a dichotomous diagnostic test

|  |  | Disease | | |
| --- | --- | --- | --- | --- |
|  |  | Present | Absent | Total |
| **Test result** | **Positive** | *a* | *b* | *a + b* |
|  | **Negative** | *c* | *d* | *c + d* |
|  | **Total** | *a + c* | *b + d* | *a + b + c + d* |

Several quantities may be estimated from such a table: **sensitivity** and **specificity**, which express the test's accuracy or performance, and the test's **predictive values**, which express its usefulness in practice. The likelihood ratio (LR) compares the likelihood of a positive result among patients *with* the disease in question, to the likelihood of the same positive result among patients *without* the disease:

$$LR+ = \frac{\text{likelihood of +ve test result among diseased}}{\text{likelihood of +ve test result among non-diseased}} = \frac{a/(a+c)}{b/(b+d)} = \frac{\text{sensitivity}}{\text{false-positive rate}}$$

For a negative test result, the LR compares the likelihood of this test result in patients with the condition relative to the likelihood of the same test result in patients without the condition:

$$LR- = \frac{\text{likelihood of -ve test result among diseased}}{\text{likelihood of -ve test result among non-diseased}} = \frac{c/(a+c)}{d/(b+d)} = \frac{\text{false-negative rate}}{\text{specificity}}$$

An *overall* measure of a test's accuracy is given by the **diagnostic odds ratio**, i.e. LR+/LR−. Likelihood ratios have some advantages over the other measures mentioned above: they are not affected by changes in **prevalence** of disease and may be used when test results are grouped into more than two categories. Another useful property is the fact that LRs may be converted into **post-test odds** and **post-test probabilities** of disease if the **pretest probability** of disease is known (see Box P.5, p. 274). WALD (2004) makes a distinction between a LR that is calculated for a *group* (as in the formulae above), and a LR that is calculated for an *individual*, which in turn allows the calculation of individualized post-test odds and post-test probabilities of disease. See Box P.5 (p. 274) for a nomogram on which post-test probabilities can be read-off for different pretest probability and LR combinations. See also **SnNout**, **SpPin**.

## Likert scale

An **ordinal measurement scale** that provides a semi-quantitative means of assessing subjective responses, such as degree of pain experienced, quality of life, patient satisfaction with services provided, etc. The ordinal scale is typically comprised of five or six levels, from 'strongly disagree', coded 1, to 'strongly agree', coded 5 or 6, or a similar variation. The subjective response is often a **latent variable**, which one may be attempting to measure by means of the various component items or subscales of a composite rating scale. Scores for each of the component items may be added (as is the case with the APGAR score) or averaged, which results in a **composite score**. See also **Guttman scale**, **visual analogue scale**.

## Limits of agreement

In the context of **method comparison studies,** the extent of **agreement** between two raters or two different methods with respect to a **quantitative measurement** may be expressed as the limits of agreement (given in the same units as the measurement in question), as follows:

95% limits of agreement = mean difference between methods ± 1.96 (standard deviation of the differences)

where 1.96 is the 2.5% **percentage point** of the **standard Normal distribution**. Note this is *not* a **confidence interval**, but rather an expression of the **variability** of observed disagreement. The calculation of the **standard deviation (SD)** of the differences is given under **repeatability**. A graphical display such as the **Bland–Altman plot** is a useful tool for evaluating both extent of agreement and presence of systematic features characterizing any existing disagreement, such as, for example, greater disagreement for higher or lower average values of the measurement in question. See BLAND (2015) and KIRKWOOD & STERNE (2003) for further details and illustrative examples. A related concept is that of **reliability**, measured (for quantitative variables) by the **intraclass correlation coefficient (ICC)** or by the index of reliability, *R*.

## Line graph

A **graphical display** of change over time in a given outcome, measurement or characteristic, which may be measured at the individual, group or population level. This type of graph is particularly useful to illustrate change patterns in **serial measurements** and **time series**. With all graphical displays, and in this case in particular, it is important to avoid distortions in the representation of the data, which can occur, for example, when the variation in outcome takes place over a relatively narrow range of values on the *y*-axis. If only this range

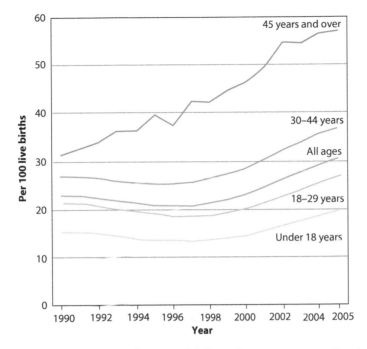

Figure L.2 Line graph for a time trend: rates of delivery by caesarean section in the US, 1990–2005, by maternal age. (Reproduced from National Center for Health Statistics. Health, United States, 2008 With Chartbook. Hyattsville, MD: 2009.)

of values is given for the y-axis, changes over time may appear considerably more dramatic than they actual are. A possible solution is to insert a truncation to represent the range of y values over which no events or measurements were recorded. Figure L.2 shows the trends in caesarean delivery rates in the US by maternal age, over the period 1990–2005 (US National Center for Health Statistics, 2009). It can be seen that in any particular year, caesarean delivery rates increase with age. In addition, for all age groups except 45 years and older, a slight downward trend up until the mid-1990s was followed by steady increases thereafter, with rates in 2005 roughly 28–37% higher than the rates in 1990. For the older age group, the rate has generally increased steadily and somewhat steeply (but with some upward and downward fluctuations), and in 2005 it was approximately 85% higher than in 1990.

## Linear mixed effects model

Synonym for **multilevel** or **random effects model** for a **continuous** outcome variable.

## Linear regression model

In a narrow sense, a regression **model** that predicts a **quantitative,** often **continuous,** outcome, from one (**simple regression** – see Figures O.2 and P.6, pp. 249 and 279) or more (**multiple regression** – see Figure A.1, p. 11) **predictor variables**. Model fitting is usually by the method of **least squares**. See **generalized linear model** for an expanded definition of linear model, which relates to **maximum likelihood estimation; curvilinear regression, non-linear regression**.

## Linear relationship

A term that describes a relationship between two variables where increments in one of the variables are associated with increments (or decrements) in the other variable, which results in a fairly straight positively (or negatively) sloped linear association. The variables involved are often, but not necessarily, **quantitative variables**: a linear trend may also exist where the mean of a quantitative measurement or the **proportion** with a given binary outcome increases or decreases linearly across values of an **ordinal variable**, or levels of an **ordered categorical variable**. A **dose–response relationship** is sometimes characterized by a linear trend. A linear relationship should not be assumed, but rather assessed through **exploratory data analyses** and possibly formal **significance tests**. In **regression models**, two assessments are of interest when evaluating linearity of effect (KIRKWOOD & STERNE, 2003): the presence of a linear effect (for which the null hypothesis is that no such effect exists), and the presence of an effect that deviates from a linear relationship. Here, the null hypothesis is that the relationship is linear. **Dummy variables** and **quadratic terms** may be included in regression models in order to explore alternative shapes for the relationship. See also **chi-squared test for trend, Cuzick's test, correlation**. Cf. **non-linear relationship**.

## Linear transformation

See **transformations**. Cf. non-linear transformation.

## Link function

In the context of **generalized linear models**, a link function is an equation that gives a **transformation** of the **predicted outcome**, so that models that do not produce **Normal** errors or **residuals** may still be specified as **linear models**. Common examples of link functions are the logit function (**logistic regression**, binomial errors), the log function (**Poisson regression**, Poisson errors) and the identity function, which is implicit when predicting untransformed **interval/ratio variables** through **simple** or **multiple linear regression**.

## LL

Abbreviation for **log likelihood**.

## ln

Or alternatively, $\log_e$. A logarithm to base $e$ (where $e$ is the irrational natural number equal to 2.7182818…). For a value between 0 and 1 on the **arithmetic scale**, the corresponding logarithm to base $e$ is a negative number. However, logs cannot be calculated for negative numbers. The ln of 1 is equal to zero, i.e. $\ln(1) = \log_e(1) = 0$. The log of zero is not defined as there is no number $x$ that satisfies the equation $e^x = 0$. On the other hand, $y^0$ is always taken to be equal to 1. A logarithm may be converted back to the corresponding value on the arithmetic scale through **exponentiation**, i.e. by applying the **antilog** function. Two important arithmetic equivalences involving logarithms have wide application in statistical analysis (for example, in interpreting the regression coefficients from **generalized linear models**). They are as follows:

$$\log(a \times b) = \log(a) + \log(b)$$

and,

$$\log(a \div b) = \log(a) - \log(b)$$

where log, in this instance, refers to either $\log_e$ or $\log_{10}$. See also **$\log_{10}$, logarithmic scale, logarithmic transformation**.

## Locally weighted regression

A **smoothing** method that uses local subsets of data (i.e. neighbouring data values in the predictor variable space) to explore **non-linear relationships** through the use of **polynomials** (CLEVELAND, 1979; CLEVELAND & DEVLIN, 1988). Weights may be used in similar fashion to **iteratively reweighted least squares** to downweight influential outlying observations. The method does not require a regression **model** to be specified. The resulting line is commonly referred to as the 'smooth', and the noise component is referred to as the 'rough'. The acronyms 'lowess' and 'loess' are often used to refer to this method. See also **spline regression**. See ARMITAGE, BERRY & MATHEWS (2002) and HAMILTON (2012) for illustrative examples.

## LOCF

Abbreviation for **last observation carried forward**.

## Loess

Or local regression. See **locally weighted regression**.

## Log likelihood function

See **likelihood function**. The log likelihood (LL) function is simply the **ln** or **$\log_e$** of the likelihood function, and is used preferentially due to computational advantages.

## Log likelihood ratio

See **likelihood ratio function**.

## Log-linear model

A **generalized linear model** for a **count outcome variable**, which predicts a **logarithmic transformation** of the count (or frequency) variable as a linear function of the **predictor variables** included in the model. The effect on the original scale is therefore **multiplicative**. A common application of log-linear modelling is the analysis of **multidimensional tables**, where the observed outcome for each cell of the multiway table is a frequency. The **null hypotheses** to be tested with a sequence of **nested models** range from *mutual* *independence* to *mutual association*. For example, in a three-way table, the null hypothesis of mutual association assumes a fixed pattern of association for each two-way cross-tabulation of the variables at each level of the third variable, i.e. absence of a three-way **interaction**. At a more basic level, the marginal totals or **main effects** of each factor are also of interest. Log-linear modelling for contingency tables is equivalent to **Poisson regression** with all **categorical predictors**. See AGRESTI (2007) for further details and illustrative examples. In a wider sense, the term 'log-linear model' may be applied to any linear model that predicts the logarithm of risks, rates, odds and hazards (see **exponential model**; Greenland, in ROTHMAN, GREENLAND & LASH [eds., 2012]).

## Log-log plot

See **exponential curve, curvilinear regression**.

## Log-logistic model

See **accelerated failure time models** (parametric survival models).

## Log-normal model

See **accelerated failure time models** (parametric survival models).

## Log odds

The logarithm to base $e$ of the **odds**, i.e. the **logit**. See **logistic regression**.

## $log_{10}$

A logarithm to base 10. The $log_{10}$ of 100 is 2, and the **antilog** of 2 is 100 given that $10 \times 10 = 100$ (i.e. $10^2 = 100$). The $log_{10}(1000) = 3$ since $1000 = 10^3$, and the antilog of 3 is given by $10^3 = 1000$. As with logarithms to base $e$ (**ln**), logarithms to base 10 may only be calculated for positive numbers. The $log_{10}$ of 1 is zero and the $log_{10}$ of zero is not defined. See also **logarithmic scale, logarithmic transformation, exponentiation**.

## Logarithmic scale

A quantitative, **continuous** scale in which equidistant increments reflect a *constant ratio* rather than a *fixed difference*. If we imagine the logarithmic representation of a ruler with range 0 cm to 1000 cm, the distance between 1 cm and 10 cm is the same as between 10 and 100 cm, or between 100 and 1000 cm, as the ratio between all these values is the same, i.e. $10/1 = 100/10 = 1000/100 = 10$. Likewise, the distance between 2 and 4 is equal to the distance between 4 and 8, and equal to the distance between 300 and 600, i.e. $4/2 = 8/4 = 600/300 = 2$. **Back-transformation** to the original units of a measurement (on the **arithmetic scale**) is done by **exponentiating** the values on the log scale. The logarithmic scale has a number of useful applications in statistical analysis, including the calculation of **geometric means** for positively **skewed** variables, the ability to equalize the

**variances** of two groups being compared by means of a ***t*-test** and the ability to specify **regression models** for binary outcomes, rates and counts as **linear**. To quote BLAND (2015, p. 71), "…Multiplicative relationships may become additive, curves may become straight lines and skew distributions may become symmetrical." BLAND (2015) points out the need for caution in interpreting the logarithmic scale. In the example given, a steep decline in incidence or mortality rate over time, where these are expressed on the log scale, cannot be interpreted as a steep decline when considering these measures on the original scale, as the rate of decline is shown to change from an initial steady decline to a steeper decline later on. See also **ln**, **log$_{10}$**, **logarithmic transformation**.

## Logarithmic transformation

A data **transformation** that converts the observed values of a **quantitative variable** into the corresponding values on a **logarithmic scale** (natural or to base *e*, **ln**, or to base 10, **log$_{10}$**). This can be particularly useful when dealing with positively **skewed** variables. The logarithmic transformation has the effect of stretching out the lower end of the original scale and compressing the upper end (KIRKWOOD & STERNE, 2003; BLAND, 2015), thus changing the distribution of the variable in question from one which is asymmetrical and skewed toward higher values, to one which may be more symmetrical about its centre and which may display the desirable properties of a **Normal distribution**. Such a variable is said to have a **lognormal distribution**. When the value of one or more observations pertaining to the same variable is equal to zero, an amount is usually added to the value of *all* observations, which is usually also subtracted when results are back transformed. The value ½ is a reasonable choice in many situations, though the magnitude and range of the original values should be considered when making this determination. The log transformation is both **normalizing** and **variance-stabilizing**. Stable variances or **homoscedasticity** is an **assumption** required by parametric methods such as the *t*-test and analysis of variance. The transformation is also useful in meeting the assumption of a **linear relationship**, as required by simple linear regression, as an example. See also **antilog/exponentiation**, **non-linear relationship**, **generalized linear model**. The **square root** and **reciprocal transformations** are alternative transformations for positively skewed variables.

## log$_e$

Alternative notation for **ln** or logarithm to base *e*.

## Logistic regression

A method of **regression analysis** with application in the analysis of binary outcomes, which are commonly summarized as proportions or **risks**, and as **odds**. Thus, the *observed* **outcome variable** in logistic regression is a **binary variable** (e.g. yes/no; alive/dead). The *predicted* outcome however, is not a binary variable or a risk, but the logit transformation of the latter (i.e. the natural logarithm of the **odds**):

$$Logit = \log_e[odds] = \log_e\left[\frac{p}{1-p}\right]$$

where $p$ is the **probability** or risk of the event in question. A logistic model is a **generalized linear model** where the predicted logit is a linear function of the variables in the model. This **transformation** of the predicted outcome prevents a model from predicting impossible values for $p$, i.e. outside the range 0 to 1. From the predicted logit, the predicted probability ($p$) of the outcome may be calculated for any given observation. Logistic regression is often carried out to analyse data from unmatched or frequency matched **case–control studies**, since **odds ratios** (**OR**) may be readily obtained by exponentiating the estimated regression coefficients for the different **predictor variables**. The method is especially useful when dealing with **confounding**, with the advantage over **stratification** of being able to include continuous **covariates** as predictors. If data are individually **matched**, **conditional logistic regression** should be used, as an extension of **McNemar's test** for paired (non-independent) proportions. Repeated binary responses in **longitudinal studies** and other **clustered designs** may be analysed using **generalized estimating equations** (**GEEs**) and **random effects** models. **Polytomous logistic regression** and **ordered logistic regression** are used for **nominal** and **ordered categorical** outcomes. See also **overdispersion/ beta-binomial regression**. An example of a logistic regression analysis is given in Box L.1. See AGRESTI (2007), HOSMER, LEMESHOW & STURDIVANT (2013), KIRKWOOD & STERNE (2003) and HAMILTON (1992) for further discussion.

## BOX L.1

Based on data from Kahigwa E *et al.* (2002). Risk factors for presentation to hospital with severe anaemia in Tanzanian children: a case–control study. *Trop Med Int Health* **7**: 823–30 (with permission).

Prospective case–control study carried out between July and October 2000 in south-eastern Tanzania, to investigate risk factors for presentation to hospital with severe anaemia in children under 5 years of age, in order to facilitate the design of anaemia control programmes. Severe anaemia was defined as packed cell volume (PCV) <25%, based on mortality risk. There were 216 cases of severe anaemia aged 2–59 months, and 234 age-matched controls (**frequency matching**). More than half of the cases (55.6%) were infants under the age of 1. A number of sociodemographic and child factors were found to be significantly associated with severe anaemia, notably, *Plasmodium falciparum* parasitaemia (OR = 4.3; 95% CI: 2.9–6.5). Multivariable logistic regression showed the following to be independent risk factors for admission with severe anaemia: health expenditure in the last 6 months >5000 TSh, malnutrition (measured by a reduced mid upper arm circumference, MUAC), living more than 10 km away from the hospital, history of previous blood transfusion, and *P. falciparum* parasitaemia:

| Predictor variables | OR | 95% CI |
|---|---|---|
| **1** Increased health expenditure in past 6 months | 2.2 | 1.3–3.9 |
| **2** Malnutrition (reduced MUAC) | 2.4 | 1.3–4.3 |
| **3** Distance from hospital >10 km | 3.0 | 1.8–4.9 |
| **4** Previous blood transfusion | 3.8 | 1.7–9.1 |
| **5** Asexual *P. falciparum* parasitaemia | 9.5 | 4.3–21.3 |

*continued.....*

*continued.....*

> *Interpretation:* All predictors are dichotomous, yes/no type variables. For *P. falciparum* parasitaemia, the odds ratio was 9.5 (larger than under the univariable regression), and thus the odds of severe anaemia on admission were almost ten times higher for children with asexual parasitaemia than for those without. The 95% confidence interval indicates that the odds could be higher by a factor of only 4.3 or by a factor of 21.3. Note that the 95% CI for the OR is not symmetrical around the point estimate. The value '9.5' is the **antilog** of the regression coefficient for '*P. falciparum*' in the logistic regression model.

## Logit transformation

The natural **logarithm (ln)** of the **odds**. See **logistic regression**. See also **arcsine square root** transformation, **complementary log-log** transformation, **probit** transformation.

## Lognormal distribution

A positively **skewed** distribution that displays a **Normal distribution**, following a **logarithmic transformation** of its values. Variables with a lognormal distribution are often analysed on the transformed scale, with the results presented in the original scale after a **back-transformation**. For example, the arithmetic **mean** of the log values may be calculated, **exponentiated** and reported as a **geometric mean**. An example is given in Figures L.3a and L.3b, from the community based cross-sectional study by DAS *et al.* (2010) on the relationship between plasma homocysteine levels and a number of lifestyle factors, in India (Assam, North Eastern Region). Plasma total homocysteine levels were measured over the period 2002–2005 in 970 healthy volunteers of both genders (51.3% male and 48.7% female), with ages ranging between 35 and 86 years. Fifty five percent of the study sample was found to have hyperhomocysteinemia, with mean plasma total homocysteine of 18.4 µmol/l. Figure L.4 shows the distribution of **survival times** for 449 patients with

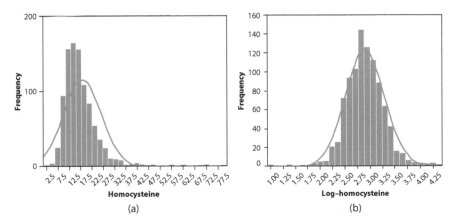

Figures L.3a and L.3b Lognormal distribution before and after a logarithmic transformation: distribution of plasma total homocysteine (in µmol/l untransformed) in 970 healthy volunteers from Assam, north eastern India. The theoretical Normal curve is shown superimposed on each histogram. (Reproduced from Das M *et al.* (2010). A community based study of the relationship between homocysteine and some of the life style factors. *Indian J Clin Biochem* **25**: 295–301 (with permission).)

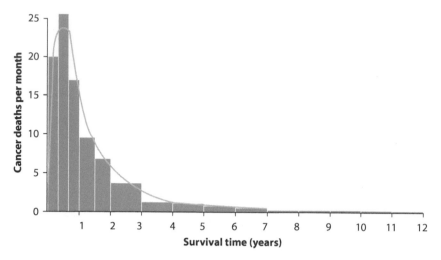

Figure L.4 Lognormal distribution: distribution of survival times (in years) for 449 patients with cancer of the larynx. Data are from selected hospitals reporting to regional cancer registries in England and Wales. The theoretical lognormal curve is shown superimposed on the histogram. (Reproduced from Mould RF *et al.* (1976). Distribution of survival times of 12,000 head and neck cancer patients who died with their disease. *Br J Cancer* **34**: 180–90 (with permission).)

cancer of the larynx. The study by MOULD *et al.* (1976) is one of many studies determining the probability distribution (lognormal or otherwise) of survival times among cancer patients. See also **probability distribution**. Cf. **exponential distribution**, (reverse) **J-shaped distribution**.

## Logrank test

Or alternatively, **Cox–Mantel $\chi^2$ test**. A **non-parametric significance test** that is carried out to compare the survival experience of two or more independent groups, as expressed by their **survival curves**. The test is carried out by computing the expected number of events in each group as the summation of the number of **expected** events at different time intervals (the 'strata'), the upper limit of each of these intervals being defined by the exact times at which an event has occurred (see **risk set**). The overall **chi-squared test statistic ($X^2$)** is based on the difference between observed and expected number of events in each group. The number of **degrees of freedom** for the test is the number of groups *minus* 1. The observed and expected number of events thus calculated may be used to compute a measure of **relative risk** between any two exposure or treatment groups, the **hazard ratio (*HR*)**. ALTMAN (1991, p. 373) notes that the expected number of events (*E*) in each group is "[...] better thought of as a measure of the extent of exposure of the subjects rather than the expected number of events. The reason is that under some unusual circumstances *E* can be larger than the sample size." The test can be **stratified** to adjust for **confounders**, but in these situations, regression methods for survival data (e.g. **Cox regression**) may be preferable. A logrank test for **trend** may also be performed. See Box L.2 for an illustrative example. Both the logrank and the **Mantel–Haenszel $\chi^2$** test for survival curves are unweighted. Other tests give distinct weights to the contributions of the different failure times to the test statistic and relax the assumptions of **proportional hazards** and similar **censoring** patterns.

## BOX L.2

**Logrank test for equality of survivor functions** (from Figure K.1, **Kaplan–Meier survival curve**, p. 181. Based on data from Chaturvedi *et al.* (1996). Differences in mortality and morbidity in African Caribbean and European people with non-insulin dependent diabetes mellitus: results of a 20 year follow up of a London cohort of a multinational study. *Br Med J* **313**: 848–52):

| Ethnic group | Events (deaths) | |
| --- | --- | --- |
| | Observed (O) | Number followed |
| AFRCRB | 16 | 77 |
| EUR | 59 | 150 |

Number of expected events (E) in each group: not given, but test and HR estimate based on comparison O vs. E.

$X^2$ statistic$_{(df=1)}$ = 9.55; $P$ = 0.002     HR = 0.41 (95% CI: 0.23–0.73)

*Interpretation:* The difference between the observed and expected number of deaths in each group is sufficiently large, which results in a statistically significant *P*-value. This is equivalent to the unadjusted analysis under **Cox regression** (Box C.3, p. 82). The 95% confidence interval (CI) for the hazard ratio (*HR*) supports the assertion that overall risk of death among African Caribbeans with non-insulin dependent diabetes is lower than among Europeans.

## Longitudinal data

Data that arise from measurements or assessments made at different time points in a **longitudinal study**. The analysis of longitudinal data depends on the nature of the **outcome variable** (e.g. continuous, binary or count variable), on the structure and completeness of the repeated observations over time, on their **correlation structure**, on the pattern of **missing data** ('missing at random' or 'missing *completely* at random'), on the possible inclusion of **time-varying covariates** and on the purpose of the analysis. Studies of **growth** and **change** are typically conducted on the basis of **repeated measurements** over time, which may be analysed using data reduction methods (**summary measures**), **repeated measures ANOVA**, multilevel models for continuous outcomes (**linear mixed effects models**) and **autocorrelation models**. SINGER & WILLETT (2003) point out that three or more waves of data are necessary for a proper evaluation of change that circumvents both the problem of **measurement error** and **regression to the mean**, and allows the evaluation of the pattern of change within each study participant to be made. Binary outcomes and counts may too be analysed using **marginal**, **random effects** (multilevel), and **transition models**, which estimate, respectively, the effect of predictor variables on average responses, the effect of predictors on individual responses and the effect of past responses on present response. Whereas data **dependence** in random effects models is assumed to be due to unexplained between-subject heterogeneity, in transition models it is assumed to be due to time or serial dependence. In the study of event occurrence, methods for the analysis of **survival times** are often indicated, where survival time or time to 'failure' measures time to the (often single) event of interest. In this instance, "[…] time is an object of study in its own right and we want to know whether, and when, events occur and how their occurrence varies as a function of predictors. Conceptually, then, *time is an outcome"*, rather than a predictor (SINGER & WILLETT, 2003, p. vi – preamble). See ARMITAGE, BERRY & MATHEWS (2002), and SKRONDAL & RABE-HESKETH (2004) for an overview. See also DIGGLE *et al.* (2002) and RABE-HESKETH & SKRONDAL (2012) for an in-depth presentation.

## Longitudinal study

An **observational** or **experimental study** that is usually carried out as a **prospective**, **follow-up study**, during which individuals may be observed or interviewed at several points in time, leading to the recording of **repeated measurements** or assessments on the **outcome** of interest, and sometimes also on explanatory or **predictor variables**, as is the case with **time-varying covariates**. Studies of **growth** and studies of **change** typically generate repeated measurements over time, which may be analysed using data reduction methods (see **summary measures**), or, alternatively, using more complex methods that take into account the **clustered** nature of the data. An advantage of longitudinal studies, as compared to **cross-sectional studies**, is the ability to distinguish between within-subject and between-subject effects, i.e. between changes over time within individuals and differences between individuals at the baseline time cross-section, what is termed 'age' and 'cohort' effects in certain contexts (DIGGLE *et al.*, 2002). Longitudinal studies may be carried out also to measure the frequency or **risk** of occurrence of an event of interest over a given period of follow-up. Often, in this type of study, the occurrence of events is measured in reference to **person-time at risk**, leading to the computation of **rates**, or, alternatively, time to event is measured, requiring special methods for the analysis of **survival times**. **Censoring** and **missing data**, due to losses to follow-up, withdrawals and failure to competing causes, are of particular concern with longitudinal studies. **Cohort studies, clinical trials** and other **intervention studies** are examples of study designs that may give rise to **longitudinal data**. A longitudinal study may also be conducted **retrospectively**, in which case there is no follow-up in the usual sense of the term, although an equal attempt is made at establishing a temporal relationship between **exposure** and disease from information contained in occupational and other historical records. See also SINGER & WILLETT (2003) and RABE-HESKETH & SKRONDAL (2012).

## Loss to follow-up

A situation whereby an individual has ceased his or her participation in a research study, and researchers have lost the ability to contact that individual in order to ascertain the eventual outcome and any other pertinent information. In **follow-up studies** (including **randomized controlled trials**), individuals lost to follow-up may be included in **sensitivity analyses**, which are performed on the basis of a number of assumptions for the **missing** or right-**censored** outcomes. Loss to follow-up may be *informative* or *non-informative*, depending on whether its occurrence is associated with greater probability of a particular outcome (POCOCK, 1983). It may also be *differential* or *non-differential*, depending on whether it affects all treatment or exposure groups in a differing or similar manner. **Selection bias** may stem from informative losses to follow-up, in particular if also differential. Cf. surveillance bias (**information bias**).

## Lower quartile

The 25th **centile**. See **interquartile range**.

## Lowess

Or locally weighted scatterplot smoothing. See **locally weighted regression**.

## LR

Abbreviation for **likelihood ratio**.

## LRT

Abbreviation for **likelihood ratio test**.

## MA

Or MA($q$). Abbreviation for **moving average model**; alternatively, model for moving average error process with MA($q$) disturbance.

## Magnitude of effect

The size of a **measure of effect**. For absolute and relative differences (risk and rate differences, excess relative risk, relative risk reduction, attributable fraction), magnitude is measured as distance from zero (or 0%). For ratios (risk ratio, rate ratio, odds ratio, hazard ratio), magnitude is measured as distance from 1. See also **effect size** (for standardized measures of effect), **direction of effect**, **strength of association**.

## Mahalanobis D²

A measure of the multidimensional distance between two data points (or one data point and the mean of a set of variables). Mahalanobis distance finds its application in the analysis of **multivariate data** (i.e. multiple outcomes), as for example, **discriminant analysis** and other multivariate **classification** methods. It is also closely related to the **leverage** statistic, $h$. See also **Hotelling's $T^2$ test**, **regression diagnostics**.

## Main effect

The **independent effect** of each of the treatments, exposures and other risk or prognostic factors included in a **regression model**. A main effect estimate is an **adjusted estimate** in regard of all other predictor variables included in the analysis. In other words, a main effect estimate is a weighted average across the levels or values of the other cofactors or covariates. In addition to main effects, it is also possible to obtain estimates of **interaction effects**. These terms, main effect and interaction effect, are often used in the context of **factorial designs** (in which the aim is to estimate both types of effect), and in the context of **multivariable regression** and **two-way ANOVA** (analysis of variance). In the latter context, **balanced designs** allow the estimation of main effects that are truly independent of the effect of the other factor. See also **biological interaction**.

## Mallow's $C_p$

The statistic that is the basis for **all-subsets model selection**. For each model, $C_p$ is calculated on the basis of its **residual sum of squares**, number of **parameters** ($p$) and total number of observations ($n$), and in reference to the residual variance or **mean square** of the model that includes all predictors. The model with the lowest value for $C_p$ (with $C_p \approx p$) is the one selected as providing the best balance between fit and simplicity, i.e. **parsimony**. See HAMILTON (1992) for further details. Cf. adjusted $r^2$ and $R^2$ (see **r-squared** and **multiple correlation coefficient**, squared), **Akaike's information criterion (AIC)**.

## Mann–Whitney *U*-test

A **significance test** that is carried out to compare two groups with respect to the distribution of a **quantitative** or **ordinal variable**. The **null hypothesis** is that there is no tendency for members of one population to exceed members of the other. The test is a **non-parametric** alternative to the independent samples *t*-test and is indicated when the **assumptions** of Normality and homoscedasticity cannot be met. For paired data, the **Wilcoxon matched pairs signed rank test** and the **sign test** should be used. The Mann–Whitney *U*-test is based on a **ranking** or ordering of the data and not on the actual data values. The Wilcoxon rank sum *T*-test for independent samples is equivalent to the Mann–Whitney *U*-test. See BLAND (2015) for further details and an illustrative example.

## MANOVA

A **multivariate** extension to **analysis of variance (ANOVA)**. MANOVA is often used in psychological research, to test for group differences with regard to sets of measurements or profiles, as opposed to the use of ANOVA to test for group differences with regard to single measurements. MANOVA provides the **significance test** for linear **discriminant analysis**.

## Mantel–Haenszel $\chi^2$ test

A **significance test** that is carried out to compare different exposure or treatment groups with respect to the **risk**, **rate** or **odds** of a given outcome, while adjusting for the presence of a **confounder**. After **stratification** by the categories of the confounding variable, results in each stratum are **pooled** to produce a single **test statistic** across all strata. The number of **degrees of freedom** for the test is always one. A $\chi^2$ test for **heterogeneity** may also be performed to test the hypothesis of no interaction between exposure and confounder. This is equivalent to the $Q$ test for heterogeneity that is used in the context of **meta-analysis**. See also **Mantel–Haenszel method**. See KIRKWOOD & STERNE (2003) for formulae and illustrative examples.

## Mantel–Haenszel $\chi^2$ test for survival curves

A **significance test** for comparing **survival curves** that is equivalent to the **logrank test**. This variation of the test is based on a comparison between observed and expected number of events among the *treated* or *exposed*, across all time strata or **risk sets**. The **test statistic** follows the chi-squared ($\chi^2$) distribution with 1 degree of freedom, as two groups are being compared. See also **Mantel–Haenszel method** for the hazard ratio. See ALTMAN (1991) for formulae and an illustrative example.

## Mantel–Haenszel method

A **pooling** method that combines **estimates** of absolute or relative effect from several **two-by-two tables**, to produce a single summary that is a **weighted average** across the individual tables. These represent the different **strata** of a **confounding variable** and the single summary is an **adjusted estimate** of **exposure** or **treatment effect**. The analysis of results from **observational studies** (**cohort** and **case–control**) and **meta-analysis** are common applications of the method. Weights are in proportion to the size of each stratum (or to the size of each primary study in a meta-analysis). The method gives similar results to the **inverse variance method**, but is limited to the analysis of binary outcomes. It is considered preferable to the latter when data are sparse (BRADBURN *et al.*, 2007). Relative effect measures (risk, rate and odds ratios) are combined in the original, untransformed scale, allowing for sparseness of data and the possibility of zero counts or frequencies (HILLS, 1974). See Deeks, Altman & Bradburn, in EGGER, DAVEY SMITH & ALTMAN (eds., 2001), and ROTHMAN (2012) for formulae and illustrative examples. See also **Peto's method**, **Mantel–Haenszel $\chi^2$ test**.

## Mantel–Haenszel method for the hazard ratio

A special application of the **Mantel–Haenszel method** of **stratification**, in which the strata are defined by the exact times at which an event has occurred (see **risk set**). The aim is to calculate a **pooled** estimate of the **hazard ratio** across all time strata (denoted by $HR_{MH}$), as follows:

$$HR_{MH} = exp\left[\frac{O_1 - E_1}{V}\right]$$

where $O_1$ and $E_1$ are the summation of the **observed** and **expected** number of events among the *treated* or *exposed*, across all time strata, $V$ is the summation of the **variances** of the expected numbers, also across all strata, and *exp* is the **exponentiation** or antilog function. As with other commonly used methods of **survival analysis**, the hazard ratio is assumed to be constant over time, although the **hazard rates** in the comparison groups are allowed to vary. With rare events, this method may be preferable to the method based on the **logrank test** ($HR_{CM}$ or Cox–Mantel). See ALTMAN (1991) for formulae and an illustrative example. A **significance test** may be carried out using the **Mantel–Haenszel $\chi^2$ test** for survival curves, to test the null hypothesis of a hazard ratio of 1. See also **Peto's method** ($HR_{Peto}$).

## Marginal model

Synonymous with population-averaged model. A **regression** model for the analysis of **longitudinal data**, in which marginal or group-level responses alone are estimated. These are the expected or average responses for individuals sharing the same value for a given **predictor variable**. Individual-level responses and trajectories, commonly referred to as subject- and cluster-specific effects, are not modelled (cf. **conditional model**). Marginal models are often fitted through **generalized estimating equations (GEEs)**. Valid **inference** requires the introduction of an approximate **correlation structure** for within-subject or within-cluster observations and estimation of **robust standard errors**. These models are particularly useful in the analysis of **counts** and **binary outcomes**, and may be viewed as the "… natural analogues for correlated data of GLMs (**generalized linear models**) for independent data." (DIGGLE *et al.*, 2002, p. 127). Alternatively, a **random effects** (conditional) or a **transition model** may be fitted, depending on the research question at hand

and additional assumptions for the data. For **continuous outcomes**, marginal and conditional models are generally equivalent. See also AGRESTI (2007).

## Marginal totals

Also, marginal distribution. The row and column subtotals in a **contingency table**, reflecting the **independent** distributions of the variables that are cross-tabulated. See also **conditional probability**.

## Markov chain model

See **autoregressive model** (time series), **transition model** (longitudinal data).

## Masking

See **blinding**.

## Matched case–control study

A **case–control study** in which selection of **controls** is achieved through *individual* **matching** (as opposed to *frequency* matching). The purpose of individual matching is mainly to increase **efficiency** in the presence of **confounding**, although this increase in efficiency is only achieved with strong confounders. Where this is not the case, the possible gains generally do not compensate for the additional logistical requirements. KIRKWOOD & STERNE (2003) discuss another situation in which individual matching may be necessary, and that is when the **source population** cannot be enumerated. This situation arises when selecting controls for hospital-based case–control studies, where the hospital or health facility in question is likely to have a wide **catchment area**, as is the case when a hospital receives referrals from beyond its immediate geographical surroundings. Selection of neighbour controls for cases seen at such facilities presents a way of dealing with this difficulty. As with study designs involving some type of pairing, the analysis of matched case–control studies must take this feature into account. At a very basic level, and with no other risk factors involved and one control per case, the comparison cases *vs.* controls may be carried out with **McNemar's test**. With several controls per case, the **Mantel–Haenszel method** may be used, but **stratification** will be by case–control sets, which does not allow further stratification according to the strata of potential confounders. **Conditional logistic regression** allows multiple controls per case and one or more confounding variables to be included, both categorical and quantitative. Both stratification and conditional logistic regression are used to remove the **selection bias** introduced by matching (ROTHMAN, 2012). With *frequency* matching, standard methods of analysis may be used. The matching variable, however, must be included in the analysis, i.e. it must be **adjusted** for (KIRKWOOD & STERNE, 2003).

## Matched pairs design

A **study design** in which the comparison groups arise by individually **matching** study participants in regard of a variable or factor of interest that is thought related to the response variable. Examples are the **matched case–control design**, and studies in which an individual receives a different treatment in each eye or in each of two different skin areas. Matched pairs designs give rise to **paired data**. See also **before–after comparison**, **crossover design**.

## Matched pairs *t*-test

See **paired *t*-test**.

## Matching

The selection of **controls** in **cohort** and **case–control studies**, with the view to ensure a similar distribution of important **risk factors** (frequently, age and gender) in the two study groups (exposed and unexposed, or cases and controls). In cohort studies, the purpose of matching is to prevent the occurrence of bias through **confounding**. In case–control studies, matching actually may distort the association between disease and **exposure** (ROTHMAN, 2012). This is due to the fact that **selection bias** is introduced, and the distribution of exposure in the control group no longer estimates that in the **source population**. The effect of matching will be to bias the estimate of exposure effect toward the null effect value. The role of matching in case–control studies is to make control of confounding more **efficient**. However, **stratification** must be used *in addition* to the matching, in order for the bias caused by the confounding variable to be removed. In fact, the matching variable should be controlled for, even if it is not a confounding variable, provided it is associated with the exposure variable; this unnecessary matching leads to **overmatching** and loss of efficiency. KIRKWOOD & STERNE (2003) suggest that matching not be used unless the matching variable is strongly related to both exposure and disease. A possible drawback of matching in case–control studies is that the effect of the matching variable itself cannot usually be estimated. Matching can be (a) individual or pairwise, or (b) by **stratum**, group or frequency. If matching is at the *individual* level, results are analysed by stratifying by individual match (i.e. each matched pair is a stratum), which precludes further stratification according to the strata of additional confounders. **Conditional logistic regression** may be a preferable method of analysis in these situations. For *frequency* matching, the **Mantel–Haenszel method** allows stratification by more than one confounder. However, **logistic regression** may also be employed to circumvent the problem of non-informative strata; the matching variable(s) must be included. Individual matching is sometimes necessary as a strategy for selecting controls in hospital-based case–control studies, if the source population cannot be enumerated. Neighbourhood and member of household or family member controls are usually selected. CLAYTON & HILLS (1993) point out that use of matching in these situations minimizes the occurrence of selection bias. See Rothman, Greenland & Lash, in ROTHMAN, GREENLAND & LASH (eds., 2012), for further discussion. See also **density sampling**.

## Maternal mortality rate

A measure of the risk of dying from causes associated with (direct obstetric deaths), or aggravated by (indirect obstetric deaths) pregnancy and childbirth. Calculated as the number of deaths from complications of pregnancy, delivery or postpartum that occur in a given population and over a given time-period, divided by the number of live births in the same population over the same period of time (usually 1 year), and usually expressed per 1000 or 100,000. It is therefore a ratio, rather than a true rate. The WHO definition of a maternal death is the death of a woman (from the above causes) while pregnant or within 42 days of the end of the pregnancy, regardless of duration or site. See also **mortality rate**, **birth rate**, **fertility rate**. Additional details are given by PORTA (ed., 2014).

## Maximal model

A **regression model** that includes a large number of the relevant **predictor variables** to a particular data analysis, plus some of the **interactions** between them, without however resulting in the estimation of as many parameters or coefficients as there are observations, as is the case with a **saturated model**. See also scale parameter (under **overdispersion**), **null model**.

## Maximum likelihood estimate

Often referred to by its abbreviation, MLE. In the context of **maximum likelihood estimation**, the particular value of a **parameter** that maximizes the corresponding **likelihood function**.

## Maximum likelihood estimation

An alternative method to **least squares estimation**, which is used to fit **logistic, Cox** and **Poisson** regression models (see **generalized linear model**). The method seeks to find model **coefficients** that maximize the **likelihood function**, i.e. the probability of the data observed given that certain values are chosen as the model's parameters (CLAYTON & HILLS, 1993). This is done through an iterative process of fitting and re-estimation of coefficients or parameters, until convergence is achieved. The parameter values that maximize this probability are said to produce the maximum likelihood model for the data, and are referred to as the **maximum likelihood estimates** or **MLE**. The statistical significance of the **predictor variables** included is usually assessed with the **likelihood ratio test**, or with the **Wald test** if testing a single predictor. See also **iteratively reweighted least squares**.

## McNemar's test

A **significance test** that is a variation of the **sign test**, and is carried out to compare **paired binary data**. Table 5 shows the layout of the results of a hypothetical study comparing a novel diagnostic test against the accepted gold standard. Measures such as sensitivity and specificity give the diagnostic accuracy of the novel test. The table highlights the number of discordant pairs (assumed to be fixed), on which McNemar's test is based. The corresponding **confidence interval** is based on the total sample size (ALTMAN, 1991). The **test statistic** is calculated as:

$$X^2 = [(|b - c| - 1)^2]/(b + c)$$

and follows the **chi-squared distribution** with one **degree of freedom** when the **null hypothesis** is true. Note that some define the test statistic slightly differently, with the numerator simplified to $(b - c)^2$ on the right-hand side of the equation, i.e. without sub-tracting the **continuity correction** of 1, which when applied has the effect of reducing the difference between **observed** and **expected frequencies** (in the discordant pairs cells); this produces a more conservative **P-value**. A requirement for the validity of the test is that the total number of discordant pairs is at least 10. BLAND (2015), and KIRKWOOD & STERNE (2003) give additional methodology for interval estimation and significance test-ing. Alternative methods for analysing paired binary data include **diagnostic test** statistics, as mentioned above, estimation of the difference between paired **proportions**, estimation of the **odds ratio** as a measure of association for paired binary data, **conditional logistic regression** (especially in the context of matched case–control studies) and assessment of **agreement** through a measure such as the kappa statistic. See also **Stuart–Maxwell test**.

Table 5  Layout of the results of paired binary data for McNemar's test

|  |  | Gold standard test | |
|---|---|---|---|
|  |  | Positive result | Negative result |
| **Novel test** | Positive result | *a* | *c* |
|  | Negative result | *b* | *d* |

## Mean

A measure of the centre of a **quantitative distribution**. The mean is a reliable measure of centre or '**average**' if the variable being summarized has a **symmetrical** distribution. When the distribution is asymmetrical, the simple arithmetic mean does not provide a fair summary for the bulk of the data, since it is influenced by extreme observations or **outliers** (Figure G.2, Geometric mean, p. 147). However, if the mean is to reflect all data points, not just typical data points, the arithmetic mean is the most informative summary measure for skewed data, as pointed out by ALEXANDER (2012) and THOMPSON & BARBER (2000). The formula for calculating the arithmetic mean is:

$$\bar{x} = \frac{sum\ of\ individual\ observations}{sample\ size} = \frac{\Sigma x_i}{n}$$

where $\bar{x}$ is the mean (read '*x* bar'), and the upper case Greek letter sigma, $\Sigma$, indicates summation across the $x_i$s or individual observations. Other types of mean include the **geometric mean** and the **harmonic mean**, while the **median** and the **mode** are additional **measures of central tendency**. The **standard deviation (SD)** is also commonly presented to describe the spread of individual observations around the mean.

## Mean squared error

The **variance** of an unbiased **estimator**, often denoted by the abbreviation MSE. An esti-mator is said to be **unbiased** if the mean of its **sampling distribution** equals the true value of the **parameter** that is being estimated. The variance is then the average squared distance each sample **estimate** is from the theoretical mean, and the square root of the MSE is the standard deviation of the sampling distribution, i.e. the **standard error** of the sample estimate. In the case of a **biased** estimator, the mean squared error is given by (variance + square of the bias). See also **sandwich variance estimate**. See HAMILTON (1992) for further details. The term 'mean squared error' is also used to refer to the **residual mean square** or residual variance of a measurement, in the context of **analysis of variance**.

## Mean squares

In the context of **analysis of variance**, the residual mean square (within-groups) and the mean square due to the factor (or due to regression, between-groups) are each computed by dividing the respective **sums of squares** by the corresponding number of **degrees of freedom**. The residual mean square ($MS_{residual}$) gives an estimate of the common variance of the measurements, under the assumption of **homoscedasticity** or equality of variances among the different groups. The ratio 'mean square due to regression' to 'residual mean square' gives the **test statistic** for the variance-ratio or ***F*-test** (see Box O.3, One-way ANOVA, p. 246). In **two-way ANOVA** balanced designs with replication, the total sum of squares is partitioned into the following components: the sum of squares for each of the **main factors** in the analysis (for example, treatment group and gender); the sum of squares due to the **interaction** between the main factors; and the **residual** or within-groups sum of squares. **Significance testing** of these effects (main factors plus interaction) is carried out by computing a test statistic that is the ratio of the relevant mean square to the residual mean square (after dividing each sum of squares by the appropriate number of degrees of freedom). Where there is no replication, a within-groups sum of squares cannot be calculated, and the interaction sum of squares is taken as the residual component. The balanced design without replication is an extension of the **paired *t*-test**, where the pairing involves three or more sets of measurements. KIRKWOOD & STERNE (2003) give details also for **repeated measures ANOVA**. See also **root mean square error** (RMS error).

## Measurement

A data value that arises by using a standardized measuring tool to read off the amount or intensity of a quantifiable variable such as, for example, length, distance, temperature, colour saturation, weight, haemoglobin, serum cholesterol, blood pressure. Measurements are typically **continuous** quantitative variables on an **interval/ratio scale**, although assessments made on an ordinal scale (ranks and scores) may be considered semi-quantitative measurements. These data are usually summarized and analysed using parametric methods such as the arithmetic **mean** and the **standard deviation**, ***t*-tests**, **analysis of variance**, **correlation** and **linear regression**, in particular where the variable(s) in question display an approximately **Normal distribution**. To this end, data **transformations** may be applied. Cf. **count**, which arises by counting the number of occurrences of an event or attribute.

## Measurement bias

A systematic error that is incurred when taking and/or recording **quantitative measurements**. This type of measurement error often arises in the context of **method comparison**

**studies** as a discrepancy between measurements made by different raters, methods or tools. In the context of **calibration** studies, biased measurements may still be useful if the bias or discrepancy between the methods involved can be quantified. In addition to the **mean** bias estimate, **limits of agreement** (usually 95% limits of agreement) may be calculated. See also **clinical measurement, information bias**. Cf. **measurement error**.

## Measurement error

A **random error** that is made when taking and/or recording **quantitative measurements**. Measurement error or inconsistency is often due to natural biological variability. The consequence of measurement error with respect to a quantitative *exposure* is **regression dilution bias**, which causes the **association** between exposure and outcome to be underestimated. This is equivalent to the effect of non-differential **misclassification** of exposure status. When the error is in respect of a quantitative *outcome*, the issue is the lack of **precision** of estimates of association or exposure effect. These may be under- or overestimated depending on a number of factors (see **regression to the mean** in comparative studies). FROST & THOMPSON (2000) and KIRKWOOD & STERNE (2003) discuss methodology for correcting for regression dilution bias, and measurement error in multiple regression models. BLAND (2015) suggests two ways of evaluating measurement error, by quantifying the amount of *within-subject* variability as expressed by the **repeatability** of the measurement, and by estimating a measure of **reliability**, the **intraclass correlation coefficient** or **ICC**. See also **clinical measurement, information bias**. Cf. **measurement bias**.

## Measurement scale

The nature and range of the values taken by a given **variable** that contains information on counts, measurements, characteristics or events. The most concise measurement scale is the **binary** or dichotomous scale, which has a qualitative nature and takes only two possible values. This is the scale on which 'yes/no' outcome and exposure variables are measured. An extension of the binary scale is the **nominal** or polychotomous scale, also qualitative, but with a larger number of possible values. The values taken by binary and nominal variables are simply codes representing different **categories** and have no numerical meaning. An example of this type of scale is 'ethnic group'. Where the categories have an intrinsic ordering (e.g. variables recording the severity of subjective symptoms) the result is an **ordered categorical variable**. **Ranks** and scores are said to be on a semi-quantitative **ordinal** scale. Examples are 'degree of pain' measured on a **Likert scale** or **visual analogue scale**, or the ranks given by a **Guttman scale**. **Interval** and **ratio** scales are truly quantitative or numerical. The range of possible values on an interval scale could be, at least in theory, from $-\infty$ to $+\infty$. Thus, a zero value on an interval scale does not represent the absence of a quantity or measurement. Temperature measured in °C or °F is a typical example of a measurement on an interval scale. Ratio scales, on the other hand, have true zeros: 0 kg, 0 cm, 0 beats per minute, 0 mmHg, all represent an absence of the feature that is being measured. Interval/ratio variables are usually **continuous**, i.e. their measurements may take any value within a given range (however, the **precision** of most measuring tools is somewhat limited). Quantitative variables may also contain information on **discrete counts**, such as number of children per classroom, number of practice visits, number of cigarettes smoked, etc. The choice of statistical method to analyse a body of **data** depends on the scale on which the variables concerned are measured, among other factors. BLAND (2015) and KIRKWOOD & STERNE (2003) provide comprehensive guides to choosing the appropriate methodology for the various types of data. See also **composite score**, **arithmetic scale**, **logarithmic scale**.

## Measures of association

Statistical measures that summarize the **association** between any two variables, typically, exposure and disease or treatment and outcome. Commonly used measures of association are the **risk ratio**, the **odds ratio**, the **rate ratio** and the **hazard ratio**, also termed **relative risk** measures (KIRKWOOD & STERNE, 2003). These measures express the **strength** (and direction) **of association** between the factors involved, in contrast to **measures of impact**, which express *net* and *proportional* effect. The **correlation coefficient** is a measure of association for quantitative and ordinal variables. For the relationship cross-tabulated in a **contingency table**, the **contingency coefficient** and **Cramér's V** provide a measure of the strength of association, while the **chi-squared test statistic** ($X^2$) and corresponding $P$-value test the null hypothesis of **independence**. See **measures of effect** for additional details.

## Measures of central tendency

Statistical summaries that give the location of the centre of a **distribution**, as expressed by the arithmetic, geometric and harmonic **means**, by the **median**, or by its **mode** (modal value) or modal category. These descriptive measures are often presented alongside **measures of dispersion**, which give the degree of spread or variability around the location measure.

## Measures of dispersion

Statistical summaries that give the degree of spread or variability around a **measure of central tendency**. **Parametric** measures include the **variance** and **standard deviation**, the **coefficient of variation**, and ranges based on percentage points of theoretical distributions. **Non-parametric** measures include the **interquartile range**, and any ranges based on centiles of the actual distribution.

## Measures of effect

Statistical measures that summarize the **absolute** and **relative effects** of treatments and exposures in **comparative studies**. *Absolute* effects are given by *differences* in measures of disease occurrence (risk and rate differences), while *relative* effects are given by their *ratios* (risk, rate, hazard and odds ratios, also known as **measures of association**). An additional measure of relative effect may be obtained in the case of harmful exposures, the **excess relative risk**, which relates the risk (or rate) difference between the exposed and unexposed groups to the risk (or rate) in the unexposed. The excess relative risk may thus be defined as a *relative* or *proportional difference*. Other relative differences such as the attributable and preventable fractions are commonly referred to as **measures of impact** (or more specifically, of *relative* impact). ROTHMAN (2012) discusses the appropriateness of absolute and relative measures of effect, to convey, in summary, the public health impact of an exposure and the strength of its association with the disease in question. Effect measures can vary in both **magnitude** (is it a **strong** effect/is it **clinically significant**?) and **direction** (is exposure/active treatment protective or harmful?), the variation in direction being reflected in the sign of an absolute effect measure, or in a ratio that is greater or less than 1. Greenland, Rothman & Lash, in ROTHMAN, GREENLAND & LASH (eds., 2012), make a further distinction between measures of *effect* and measures of *association*, in that the former terminology is reserved for situations that, through careful study design, approximate the counterfactual ideal of perfect **comparability**, whereas measures arising in the presence of **confounding** (whether ratios or differences) may only be referred to as measures of association, since a **causal relationship** cannot be inferred under these conditions. See also **standardized effect measures**, **effect size**, **exposure effect**, **treatment effect**. See Deeks & Altman, in EGGER, DAVEY SMITH & ALTMAN (eds., 2001), for a discussion on the choice of measures of effect in the context of **meta-analysis**.

## Measures of impact

Statistical measures that express the impact of treatments and exposures among people at risk of developing a given disease or adverse outcome, or among a population experiencing a given prevalence of exposure. Measures of impact are typically derived from simple **measures of effect** (such as differences and ratios), and allow us to quantify in *absolute* or *relative* terms *how many* people or *what proportion* of the exposed (or of the population) might be impacted on by removal of an exposure or adoption of a given treatment policy. KIRKWOOD & STERNE (2003) present a number of measures in reference to observational studies and clinical trials/intervention studies. Among the former is the **attributable risk** or absolute risk increase, and the **attributable fractions** with reference to both the **exposed** population and the overall **population**. With regard to clinical trials and other intervention studies, the **efficacy** (also termed preventable fraction or relative risk reduction) may be calculated, in addition to the **number needed to treat** (**NNT**) and the **number needed to harm** (**NNH**).

## Median

A **non-parametric measure of the centre** of a **distribution**. As opposed to the **mean**, the median is considered a **resistant measure**, given that it is not affected by the presence of **outliers** (see Figures S.4a and S.4b, p. 337). When data are sorted according to increasing values of the variable of interest, the median is the middle value, i.e. the value that divides the data in half: 50% of the observations have values lower than the median and 50% have values higher than the median (Figure B.6, **Box-and-whiskers plot**, p. 40). With an even number of observations, the median is the average of the two central values. The median is also referred to as the 50th **centile**. When the median is used as the measure of centre (for example, to describe a variable with a **skewed** distribution), the spread of the observations may be expressed by the relevant centiles, and commonly by the **interquartile range** (**IQR**). BLAND (2015) gives a **large sample method**, albeit only approximate, for calculating **confidence intervals** for the median and other centiles.

## Megatrial

A **clinical trial** involving a large number of patients, usually many thousands. These trials require very large **sample sizes** since they focus on the **effectiveness** of treatments that may have small relative effects, but nonetheless, the potential for considerable impact given their use in treating common diseases. Megatrials are often conducted as collaborative, **multicentre** efforts, involving a number of different countries. See also **measures of impact**.

## Mesokurtic

Mesokurtic **distributions** are those with a **kurtosis** of zero. Examples include the **Normal distribution** and, when probability of 'success' = probability of 'failure' = 1/2, the **binomial distribution**. See also **leptokurtic** and **platykurtic**.

## Meta-analysis

A statistical method that combines the results from the individual studies included in a **systematic review**, producing a quantitative summary or **pooled estimate** across the different studies. For binary outcomes, methods such as **Mantel–Haenszel's**, **inverse variance** and **Peto's** are used to compute these summaries. When the outcome is a continuous measurement, **weighted mean differences** (which are overall measures of the difference between means) may be computed, or alternatively, **standardized differences** may be calculated for each of the studies and then summarized using the inverse variance method. Meta-analysis is often used to pool results from **randomized controlled trials**, and has the virtue of increasing the **'sample size'** available to estimate the benefits of a given treatment. It may, however, be used also to pool results from other types of study, as, for example, studies that investigate **risk factors** for disease or evaluate the performance of **diagnostic tests**. Issues around meta-analysis include, among others, **publication bias**; **heterogeneity** of effect (which requires causes of statistical heterogeneity be investigated and decisions made on whether to adopt a **fixed effect** or **random effects** approach); and use of **individual participant data** (if obtainable) *vs.* data summaries (**aggregated data**) from the different studies included. Readers are referred to EGGER, DAVEY SMITH & ALTMAN (eds., 2001), HIGGINS & GREEN (eds., 2008) and BORENSTEIN *et al.* (2009) for a full discussion. KIRKWOOD & STERNE (2003) and BLAND (2015) present a comprehensive summary of relevant issues. Figure F.1 (**Forest plot**, p. 135) shows a typical graphical display for the results of a meta-analysis. See also **standardized measures of effect**, **L'Abbé plot**, **Galbraith plot**, **funnel plot**, **cumulative meta-analysis**.

## Meta-regression

A technique that is used to evaluate the results of a **meta-analysis** as to possible causes of observed statistical **heterogeneity**. The aim is to identify study characteristics that pertain to the possibility of **publication bias** (language of publication, inclusion or not in a major search application, relationship between size of study and magnitude of effect, etc.), methodological quality issues (concealment of allocation, avoidance of measurement error, choice of measure of effect, etc.), and clinical heterogeneity (differences in overall severity of illness of trial participants, differences in age and gender distribution, differences in respect of comorbidities, differences in treatment regimens, etc.). The latter is of central importance for the correct interpretation and applicability of the results of meta-analyses (THOMPSON, 1994; Thompson, in EGGER,

DAVEY SMITH & ALTMAN [eds., 2001]). Meta-regression may be viewed as an extension of Egger's regression intercept method for funnel plot asymmetry (**Egger's test**), by simply including additional predictors in the model as specified above. The process is carried out as an **iteratively reweighted** regression, in which both tau squared ($\tau^2$, the estimated variance of the distribution of treatment effects – see **DerSimonian and Laird random effects model**) and the regression coefficients are re-estimated until convergence is achieved. As with regression analysis in general, a reasonable **sample size** (in this case, a reasonably large number of primary studies) is necessary for valid results. BENNETT & EMBERSON (2009) recommend the use of **stratification** for exploring sources of heterogeneity in systematic reviews. See also Sterne, Egger & Davey Smith, in EGGER, DAVEY SMITH & ALTMAN (eds., 2001), THOMPSON & HIGGINS (2002), BORENSTEIN *et al.* (2009) and BLAND (2015); **forest plot, funnel plot, Galbraith plot, L'Abbé plot, index of heterogeneity ($I^2$), Kendall's tau.**

## Method comparison studies

In the context of **clinical measurement**, method comparison studies are carried out to evaluate the extent of **measurement bias** between two different methods or tools. For example, one may wish to determine how well a new computerized method of measuring blood pressure compares with measurements obtained using a standard mercury sphygmomanometer. The specific question is 'what is the average discrepancy between the two methods?' The protocol for comparing methods in this way often includes studies of **repeatability** for each of the methods/tools in question, following which a measure of the average bias or **reproducibility** between the methods is obtained with **limits of agreement** also calculated. Note that the **correlation coefficient** is not indicated here, as it is not a measure of **agreement** but rather a **measure of association** (of linear association, to be exact). In addition to estimating the average bias or difference (and carrying out significance testing using, for example, the **paired *t*-test**), graphical methods such as the **Bland–Altman plot** (BLAND & ALTMAN, 1986) are essential for a better understanding of how the methods compare and how best to analyse the data.

## MID

Abbreviation for **minimally important difference**.

## Mid *P*-value

A modified **P-value** that is calculated preferentially when applying **exact statistical methods** to analyse **discrete** outcomes. Due to the discrete nature of the sampling distribution of the **test statistic** in these circumstances, exact P-values, for example, will be too *conservative*, and tests will require larger test statistics before the desired level of significance may be reach (in other words, the probability of incurring a **type I error**, i.e. of failing to accept the **null hypothesis** when it is true, can be much smaller than test results indicate). Mid P-values are calculated by subtracting half the probability of the observed outcome from the exact P-value, which reduces the magnitude of the same and increases the **significance level** of the results. **Continuity corrections** are applied for the opposite reason, i.e. to produce test results that are more conservative. See AGRESTI (2007).

## Minimally important difference

Or its abbreviation, MID. The smallest **treatment** (or exposure) **effect** that would be considered of sufficient **clinical** (or public health) **significance**. See Sackett, in HAYNES *et al.* (eds., 2006). A comprehensive review and discussion of methods to specify the target difference for a randomized controlled trial is given by COOK *et al.* (2014). See also **power**, **precision**, **sample size** (required).

## Minimization

A quasi-**random** method of **allocating** patients to the different treatments under study in a **clinical trial**. The rationale behind minimization is the need to produce **comparable** treatment groups, in regard of any relevant (and measurable) **prognostic factors**. The method is useful when dealing with small **sample sizes**, where **simple randomization** may produce unbalanced groups. See also **baseline characteristics, stratified randomization**. See POCOCK (1983) for further details and an illustrative example. Sackett, in HAYNES *et al.* (eds., 2006), compares the relative advantages of minimization and randomization.

## Misclassification

An error that is made when assessing or recording events or characteristics measured on a **categorical scale**, which results in an individual being classified under the wrong **exposure** or **disease** category. In comparative studies, misclassification may be differential (biased), if it occurs to a greater extent in one of the comparison groups, or non-differential (random), if it affects all groups with equal probability. **Recall bias** is an example of an **information bias** due to differential misclassification of *exposure*, which is prone to occur in **case–control studies**. Differential misclassification of *disease* may occur in **follow-up studies**, when the more intensive surveillance of one of the exposure or treatment groups results in greater probability of disease detection in that same group (**surveillance bias**). Non-differential misclassification with regard to a dichotomous exposure has the effect of underestimating **exposure effect** if there is one (overestimation may occur with more than two exposure categories). This is due to the fact that misclassification approximates the exposure groups, akin to a certain percentage of individuals in each exposure group having swapped its exposure membership. Non-differential misclassification of disease status in case–control studies tends to have a similar effect, known as **regression dilution bias**. Rothman, Greenland & Lash, in ROTHMAN, GREENLAND & LASH (eds., 2012), discuss the effects of non-differential misclassification of disease status in follow-up studies, which may result in underestimation of effects, depending on whether the misclassification is as a result of under- or overascertainment, and an absolute or relative measure of effect is being estimated. Overestimation of effect is also possible in the specific case where classification errors with regard to disease *and* exposure are not independent. The consequences of differential misclassification of exposure and disease are less predictable: exposure effects may be underestimated or, more often, overestimated. The authors also discuss strategies for avoiding misclassification in epidemiological research, and point out the pervasiveness of non-differential misclassification, which should be suspected in studies showing little or no effect as magnitude of effect might just be underestimated. See also **classification**. The consequences of random measurement error with regard to a quantitative exposure are discussed under **measurement error** and regression dilution bias; with regard to a quantitative outcome, under measurement error and **regression to the mean**. See also ROTHMAN (2012), GRIMES & SCHULZ (2002).

## Misclassification rate

Or error rate. See **classification table**.

## Missing data

Data that are (or should have been) measurements and observations made in the course of a research study and which are not available for analysis. Often, this is in reference to **censored outcomes**, due to **withdrawal** from participation or **losses to follow-up**. The problem of missing data is of particular concern in **longitudinal studies**, in which **repeated measurements** or assessments are recorded over time. A number of strategies may be employed in these situations, including filling in for missing values (with averages calculated from the study sample, with stochastic or error-added mean values or with the last recorded measurement or observation for a study participant – termed **last observation carried forward**), **imputation** and the use of **summary measures**. Spurious precision, dilution of effect and bias are some of the possible consequences of using these various strategies, which multiple imputation is better able to avoid. Generally speaking, consequences of missing data include, among others, loss of power and precision, introduction of selection and information biases, and the inability to calculate risk-based measures (rates may still be calculated). See BLAND (2015) for a comprehensive overview. Additional information and resources may be found at www.missingdata.org.uk.

## Misspecification

In the context of **regression analysis**, a **model** is said to be misspecified if it has been incorrectly formulated to describe the relationships between **outcome** and **predictor variables** in a given body of data. The misspecification may concern the need to **transform** variables from their original scale to, perhaps, a logarithmic or some other scale (usually, as a variance-reducing or as a **variance-stabilizing** measure), or an incorrect **assumption** regarding the shape of the relationship between outcome and predictors. The problem of misspecification is sometimes compounded by the omission of relevant predictor variables in causing **overdispersion**. It is assumed a model is correctly specified before proceeding to evaluate **goodness-of-fit** (**GoF**) and perform **regression diagnostics**.

## Mixed effects model

A **regression model** that includes both **fixed** and **random effects**. Synonymous with **hierarchical model**, **multilevel model**, **random effects model**.

## MLE

Abbreviation for **maximum likelihood estimate**.

## Mode

The value most commonly observed for a given **variable**, as, for example, the modal age among patients newly diagnosed with breast cancer. Variables whose **distribution** has a single peak, such as those with an approximately **Normal distribution**, are termed **unimodal**. A multimodal distribution often reflects a mix of populations in the study sample (see Figure B.3, **Bimodal distribution**, p. 32). When the variable in question is **categorical** or a **categorized continuous variable**, reference is made to the *modal category* or *class interval* as being the category or class with the highest **frequency**. See also **measures of central tendency**.

## Model

In the context of **regression analysis**, a model is an equation that summarizes the relationship between a response, dependent or **outcome variable**, and one or more **predictor** (independent or explanatory) **variables**. With a single independent variable, the general form of the equation is:

*Predicted outcome* = $\hat{y}$

$$= a + bx$$

$$= \text{constant value} + (\text{rate of change in } y \text{ per unit of } x) \times (\text{value of } x)$$

where $\hat{y}$ (read 'y hat') is the predicted or **fitted value** for the outcome variable; $x$ is the observed value of the independent variable; $a$ is the **intercept**; and $b$ is the **regression coefficient**. The difference between observed and predicted $y$ values is the **residual**. A **multiple regression** model is an extension of the single independent variable model (**simple regression**), and may include two or more independent variables. In the example that follows (Box M.1), a quantitative outcome variable (**linear regression**) is modelled by a quantitative predictor, and by a **categorical variable** representing treatment group (this is the same illustrative example as under **ANCOVA**, p. 11). See **generalized linear model** for regression methods for binary, count and rate outcomes.

### BOX M.1

From **Figure A.1**, p. 11.

Figure A.1 shows the graphical display of an analysis of covariance for the comparison of acupuncture *vs.* a placebo needle in a randomized trial of the effects of both treatments on patients with rotator cuff tendonitis. The outcome variable is post-treatment pain score, and the quantitative predictor is pretreatment or baseline pain score (here, higher scores reflect a better outcome) (original study by KLEINHENZ *et al.* [1999]; reported results by VICKERS & ALTMAN [2001]).

The equation that summarizes the relationship between post-treatment pain score, as the outcome, and treatment group and pretreatment pain score, as the predictors, can be written as:

*Predicted follow-up score* = 24 + 0.71 × *baseline score* + 12.7 × *treatment group*

*continued...*

*continued...*

*Interpretation:*

1  Positive-sign relationship with 'treatment group': the regression coefficient for the treatment group coded as '1' is positive; on average, follow-up pain score is 12.7 score points higher in the acupuncture group compared to the placebo needle group (this is the vertical distance between the parallel lines on Figure A.1). ('Treatment group' is entered into the analysis as a **dummy variable**, coded **0** for the placebo needle group, and **1** for the acupuncture group. Note that in this study, higher scores reflect a better outcome, i.e. less pain.)

2  Positive-sign relationship with 'baseline score': follow-up pain score goes up (i.e. improves) by 0.71 score points for each unit increase in baseline pain score.

3  Intercept or base value for follow-up pain score: 24.

## Model checking

The process of evaluating the **goodness-of-fit** and **regression diagnostics** of a regression model, following **model selection**, **model specification** and **model fitting**. The analysis of **residuals** plays a central role in this process. See HAMILTON (1992; 2012), ARMITAGE, BERRY & MATHEWS (2002), HOSMER, LEMESHOW & STURDIVANT (2013), CLEVES, GOULD & MARCHENKO (2016) and Greenland, in ROTHMAN, GREENLAND & LASH (eds., 2012). See also **validation** (external validation, cross-validation, jackknifing); **bootstrapping** (which may be used to carry out resampling analysis, for a further assessment of **sampling error**, i.e. the extent to which random variability could have influenced the results obtained).

## Model fitting

The process of estimating the **parameters** or coefficients in a **regression model**, following **model selection** and **model specification**. See also **least squares estimation, maximum likelihood estimation, model checking**.

## Model selection

The process of determining which **predictor variables** to include in a **regression model**. See also **parsimony, stepwise regression, all-subsets model selection, collinearity, overdispersion, causal model, predictive model, model specification, model fitting, model checking**.

## Model specification

The process of determining the functional form or shape of the relationship between **predictors** and **outcome variable** in a **regression model**. **Transformations** are sometimes necessary in order to attain a linear relationship. See also **misspecification, linear regression, curvilinear regression, non-linear regression, model selection, model fitting, model checking**.

## Monotonic curve

A curve depicting a **non-linear relationship** that does not change **direction**, although its rate of change may show acceleration and deceleration. **Exponential** (Figure E.2, p. 125), negative exponential, and **sigmoid** (Figure S.3, p. 332) **curves** (also termed 'growth curves' or sometimes 'decay curves') are well-known examples. Cf. **non-monotonic curve**.

## Monte Carlo methods

Methods based on repeated simulations, commonly referred to as trials, which are performed in order to find solutions to intractable statistical problems. Monte Carlo methods are sometimes used to evaluate the performance of **bootstrapping**, and the two methods are contrasted under the latter. See HAMILTON (1992), BLAND (2015) and Stata Online Reference Manual ([simulate] and [permute] commands) for further details.

## Morbidity

Synonymous with illness or disease, this term is often used in reference to 'measures of morbidity', namely, **prevalence** (disease frequency or burden of disease) and **incidence** (disease occurrence as rate or as risk of disease). The term 'comorbidity' refers to the presence of one or more illnesses in addition to the target disease, which is often an important determinant of treatment response and prognosis.

## Mortality

This term is used in reference to the occurrence of death and its distribution and determinants, as expressed by crude and overall **mortality rates**, age-specific mortality rates, cause-specific and case-fatality rates, infant and child mortality rates and maternal mortality rates. **Standardization** is often utilized when comparisons are made between populations, or in reference to the age structure or to the death rates of a standard population.

## Mortality rate

The number of deaths occurring during a given time-period, in a given geographical area (such as a country), divided by the total population size in the same area, at the mid-point of the time-period. The mortality rate is often multiplied by 100,000 to be given as a rate per 100,000 of the relevant population. The time-period chosen is often 1 year (if not, the denominator of the rate is 'total population size × length of time-period'). A stated mortality rate without making reference to cause, or without specifying the age group to which it pertains or a standard for comparison, is referred to as **overall** mortality rate (all causes; may be **age-specific**) and **crude** mortality rate (as opposed to age-**adjusted** or **standardized**). See also **cause-specific death rate, case-fatality rate, maternal mortality rate, demographic indicators, population pyramid, standardization**.

## Moving average

A **smoothing** technique often used in the analysis of **time series**, which is performed by replacing each observation with a **weighted average** of the observation and its neighbours. The technique may be used to eliminate **cyclic variation** so that trends may be emphasized (EVERITT, 2006, p. 154). The 'memory' of the given observation is carried through for a given number of time-lags (depending on the span of the smoother), but not beyond.

## Moving average model

Or MA($q$), i.e. $q$th-order moving average model; alternatively, model for moving average error process with MA($q$) disturbance. See **autoregressive model**.

## MSE

Abbreviation for **mean squared error**.

## Multicentre trial

A **clinical trial** that is conducted simultaneously at more than one health facility, or possibly, in a number of different countries. Multicentre trials require close coordination to ensure all participating centres follow the same trial **protocol**. Random allocation of patients to the trial's interventions may be carried out from a central coordinating location or, alternatively, may be conducted in a **stratified** manner, by centre. **Subgroup analyses** are sometimes carried out for an assessment of treatment effect within each centre. See POCOCK (1983) and SENN (2008) for an overview.

## Multidimensional table

A **contingency table** that results from the cross-tabulation of three or more categorical variables. **Log-linear modelling** is commonly used in the analysis of these data.

## Multilevel data

Synonym for **clustered data**.

## Multilevel generalized linear model

Or generalized linear mixed model. A **generalized linear model** that includes **random cluster effects**. See **multilevel model**.

## Multilevel model

Synonymous with **hierarchical model**. A **regression model** for multilevel or **clustered data** (GOLDSTEIN, 2010). At each level, observations within each cluster (e.g. each individual, or each general practice) are usually not independent, and **dependence** is accounted for by including one or more random terms that give the cluster-specific effects. Where the **outcome variable** in a multilevel model is a **continuous variable**, the model is an extension of a **linear regression model**. With **counts** and **categorical** outcomes, the model is an extension of a **generalized linear model**. A limitation of this method is the large number of clusters required (BLAND, 2015). See RABE-HESKETH & SKRONDAL (2012) for a full discussion, and ARMITAGE, BERRY & MATHEWS (2002), SKRONDAL & RABE-HESKETH (2004), AGRESTI (2007) and HAMILTON (2012) for an overview; the gllamm.org website offers resources and references to worked examples. Additional details are given under **random effects** model. See also **longitudinal data**, **repeated measurements analysis**.

## Multimodal distribution

As opposed to a **unimodal distribution**, a multimodal **distribution** is characterised by having two or more peaks, which often reflects the presence in a study sample of individuals from distinct populations with regard to the feature or variable in question. See also **bimodal distribution**, **mode**.

## Multinomial distribution

The **probability distribution** for the frequencies in each category of a **nominal variable**. The **binomial** distribution is a special case of the multinomial distribution for which only two outcomes are possible. See also **Poisson distribution**, **polytomous logistic regression**.

## Multinomial logistic regression

Synonym for **polytomous logistic regression**.

## Multiperiod crossover design

A **study design** that extends the two-period **crossover design** to the comparison of more than two different treatments. A multiperiod crossover trial may be carried out as a **complete** or **incomplete block design**. In the former case, each **block** (i.e. each individual) receives all treatments under study, a different treatment in each of the trial's periods. The 'treatment sequence' × 'trial period' array for treatment **allocation** forms a **Latin square**, in which the number of periods equals the number of blocks. As each treatment appears only once in each sequence, the number of treatments equals also the number of trial periods. Within a Latin square, individuals are **randomized** to unique treatment sequences so that in any given period, each of the treatments is administered to just one individual and each individual receives all treatments under study across the different trial periods. This affords the ability to control both individual **variability** and **period effects**. Every possible treatment pair sequence occurs only once. Latin squares may be replicated as needed, to accommodate the total sample size (i.e. the total number of blocks) in a trial. Randomization should be carried out independently in each square. FLEISS (1999; p. 282) shows a number of Latin squares that are suitable for the multiperiod crossover design, including the following Latin square for a study design comparing four different treatments. Details of the complete randomization procedure are also given. See POCOCK (1983) and SENN (2002) for discussion of the suitability of this study design to certain types of research, among other relevant issues. See also **balanced incomplete block design**.

|  | Trial period |  |  |  |  |  |  |  |  |
|---|---|---|---|---|---|---|---|---|---|
|  | 1 | 2 | 3 | 4 |  | 1 | 2 | 3 | 4 |
|  | 1 | 1 | 2 | 4 | 3 | 1 | A | B | D | C |
| Treatment sequence | 2 | 2 | 3 | 1 | 4 | ≡ | 2 | B | C | A | D |
|  | 3 | 3 | 4 | 2 | 1 | 3 | C | D | B | A |
|  | 4 | 4 | 1 | 3 | 2 | 4 | D | A | C | B |

## Multiple-comparison procedures

Special tests that are carried out following a **statistically significant one-way analysis of variance** (or **analysis of covariance**), to further investigate which pairwise comparisons are statistically significant. Commonly employed are Duncan's multiple range test, Fisher's Least Significant Differences test, Tukey's Honestly Significant Differences test, the Tukey–Kramer test, Scheffé's test and the Newman–Keuls sequential procedure. These procedures are designed to keep **alpha**, the probability of a **type I error**, at some stipulated **level of significance** for the entire set of pairwise comparisons, so that the probability of one or more type I errors does not exceed the value of alpha, the familywise error rate. Some of these procedures are also employed in estimating simultaneous **confidence intervals**. A criticism of multiple-comparison procedures is the corresponding increase in probability of **type II errors**. See POCOCK (1983), BLAND (2015), FLEISS (1999). See also **multiple significance testing**, **Dunnett's correction**, **Bonferroni's correction** (which produces more conservative results, as does Scheffé's test).

## Multiple correlation coefficient

An overall measure of association that is obtained following a **multiple linear regression** analysis. The multiple correlation coefficient, $R$, gives the **strength of association** between outcome and predictor variables, and is calculated as the **correlation** between the **observed values** of an **outcome** (or $y$) **variable** and the values fitted or **predicted** by a model. However, and unlike the correlation coefficient that is obtained for a *univariable* or simple linear regression, $r$, a **directional** sign cannot be meaningfully attached to the multiple correlation coefficient, as two or more predictors are involved in the multivariable relationship. The significance of $R$ is given by the overall variance-ratio or **F-test** (ARMITAGE, BERRY & MATHEWS, 2002). The square of $R$, $R^2$, gives a crude estimate of how well a model fits the data, and is generally interpreted as measuring the proportion of total **variance** in the outcome variable that is explained by the predictors in a model. **Eta squared ($\eta^2$)** and **omega squared ($\omega^2$)** are related measures that may be calculated in the context of **analysis of variance**. See ALTMAN (1991). See also **Pearson's r, r-squared ($r^2$)**, adjusted **r-squared**, **partial correlation coefficient**, **standardized measures of effect**.

## Multiple outcomes

Or multiple endpoints, which arise when two or more **outcome variables** are measured in a research study. Methods for **multivariate data** and **repeated measurements** may be appropriate to analyse multiple outcomes. More commonly, such data are analysed by carrying out **multiple significance testing** (with each outcome analysed separately using

**univariate** methods), which increases the probability of incurring **type I errors**. A possible strategy is to choose higher **nominal significance levels** for each of the separate analyses, so that *overall* **statistical significance** may be kept at an acceptable (but lower) level. See also **Bonferroni correction**. POCOCK (1983) discusses additional approaches.

## Multiple regression analysis

An extension of **simple regression analysis** that allows for two or more **predictor variables** to be included in a regression **model**, such as a **linear, logistic, Poisson** or **Cox** model. We consider multiple (or *multivariable*) linear regression here and discuss the other types of regression under **generalized linear model**. The general form of the equation is:

$$\hat{y} = a + b_1 x_1 + b_2 x_2 + b_3 x_3 + ...$$

where $\hat{y}$ (read 'y hat') is the predicted value of the **outcome variable**; $x_1, x_2, x_3,$ ... are the observed values of the predictor or independent variables; $b_1, b_2, b_3,$ ... are the estimated **regression coefficients** for each independent variable; and $a$ is the **intercept** or constant. Categorical variables are included as **dummy variables**. The regression coefficient for each independent variable defines its relationship with the predicted outcome (see Box M.1, p. 219). Statistical analyses carried out by **analysis of variance** (ANOVA) and **analysis of covariance** (ANCOVA) may be replicated using multiple linear regression. Inclusion of predictors that are strongly associated with the outcome variable (e.g. baseline measurements on the outcome variable) contributes to the greater **precision** of coefficient estimates. See also **categorized continuous variable** for a discussion of the treatment of continuous predictors in multiple regression models.

## Multiple significance testing

Repeated **significance testing** on the same body of data. **Subgroup analyses** are a common example, where first an overall test of statistical significance is performed, with subsequent tests carried out within subgroups of individuals sharing similar characteristics. For example, in the ISIS-2 trial (Box A.1, p. 3) comparing aspirin versus no aspirin for the management of acute myocardial infarction, one may be interested in making this comparison within different age groups, since aspirin could be effective if used for instance, in younger patients, but not in older patients. If three age groups are defined, three significance tests will be performed, the chances of a **type I error** increasing with the number of tests carried out. Likewise, **multiple outcomes** may give rise to a similar problem, and the **Bonferroni** and other test **corrections** are often applied in order to decrease the probability of declaring results to be statistically significant when in reality the relevant **null hypothesis** is true. See also **nominal significance level**. POCOCK (1983) discusses the issue of multiplicity of data. See also BLAND & ALTMAN (2011).

## Multiplicative effects model

As opposed to **additive effects model**. A **model** in which the combined effect of two or more **predictor variables** is the product of their independent or **main effects**. Multiplicative models are usually specified as linear models, with some **transformation** of the **predicted outcome variable** as a linear function of the independent variables in the model. For example, **logistic regression** models are multiplicative models in which the predicted outcome – the logit, which is on the **logarithmic scale** – is calculated by *adding* the individual effects of each independent variable in the model. Alternatively, the effect of each predictor is obtained by **exponentiating** the corresponding **regression coefficient**, and the combined effect of different predictors is calculated by *multiplying* these **back-transformed** coefficients (see **generalized linear model**). When assessing **biological interaction** using multiplicative models, it should be noted the former is measured as a departure from *additivity* of **absolute effects**. Thus, the choice of a multiplicative model is not equivalent with the underlying relationship being multiplicative, i.e. with the presence of biological interaction. See HILLS (1974) and ROTHMAN (2012) for further discussion.

## Multistage sampling

A **sampling** method in which the selection of **study units** is done in more than one stage, going from the relevant top hierarchical level in a **population** to the lowest. For example, patients may be selected through a two-stage sampling procedure as follows: a **random sample** of general practices (the first-stage units) in a given area is taken and a given number of patients, the second-stage units, are subsequently sampled (also at random) from the selected practices. If first-stage units have different sizes, the method should be performed with 'proportional probability to size' with replacement, in order to give second-stage units the same probability of being selected. Multistage sampling differs from **cluster sampling**, in which all second-stage units within the first-stage units sampled are selected. However, in both situations, the **clustered** nature of the data must be taken into consideration when calculating **sample size** requirements and choosing methods for statistical analysis.

## Multivariable regression

A regression analysis in which the value of the outcome variable is predicted on the basis of two or more independent or **predictor variables**. Synonym for **multiple regression**. Cf. univariable or **simple regression; multivariate methods**.

## Multivariate analysis of variance

See its acronym, **MANOVA**.

## Multivariate methods

A term sometimes used in reference to statistical methods such as **multiple regression**, which allow the effect of several **predictor variables** to be assessed simultaneously. In a stricter sense, the term refers to methods used to analyse two or more **outcome variables** simultaneously. Examples of the latter are **cluster analysis, discriminant analysis, factor analysis** and **principal components analysis**. Cluster and discriminant analysis are **classification** methods that group *observations*, whereas factor and principal components analysis are data reduction methods that combine *variables* into composite variables. These may be used as independent or dependent variables in subsequent data analyses.

The analysis of **repeated measurements** may be viewed as a special application of multivariate methods. See HAMILTON (1992) and BLAND (2015) for a comprehensive overview of components and factor analysis. HAMILTON (2012) gives details and illustrative examples of cluster analysis. For a comprehensive overview and presentation, see ARMITAGE, BERRY & MATHEWS (2002), EVERITT (2009) and AFIFI, MAY & CLARK (2011). Cf. **multiple** or multivariable **regression**.

## Mutually exclusive

Two or more events or characteristics that cannot occur or be present simultaneously. This is the case with the cells in a **contingency table**: any given observation must be in one cell and one cell only and count toward that cell's tally or observed frequency. See also **probability, independent events, conditional probability**.

# N

## N-of-1 trial

A **clinical trial** conducted on a single individual patient, in the absence of evidence on which to substantiate treatment decisions for that same patient. Ethical considerations and patient compliance are important, as with any medical investigation. N-of-1 trials are, for obvious reasons, more limited than larger clinical trials, but can still be useful if conducted scientifically. This involves some form of **controlling, randomization** and **concealment** of treatment allocation (with regard to the order in which the treatments are to be administered), and **blind** assessment of responses, in addition to repetition of observation. GUYATT *et al.* (2014) and STRAUS *et al.* (2010) recommend the use of period pairs, in which the treatment in question and a placebo or alternative treatment are both administered in random order. These two-period trials are repeated until evidence of benefit or lack thereof emerges. N-of-1 trials are in many ways similar to **crossover trials**, not only because patients act as their own controls, but also because they raise the same practical issues and have similar limitations. See SENN (2002; 2008), STRAUS *et al.* (2010) and GUYATT *et al.* (2014) for further details and discussion. See also **hierarchy of evidence**.

## Natural history of disease

The sequence of periods or stages of a disease, from the initial exposure to the different components of a **causal mechanism**. These include the **induction period**, the **latency period** (or presymptomatic period) and the symptomatic period. Each of these phases may have variable length, which determines whether the disease in question has an acute or insidious onset, rapid or slow progression, acute or chronic symptomatic phase, etc. Treatments and interventions tested in **clinical trials** aim to bring about favourable disease outcomes by influencing the course of diseases at crucial points in their natural history. The induction period may offer opportunities for disease prevention if effective **screening** programmes can be implemented.

## NB model

See **negative binomial regression**.

## Negative binomial distribution

The **probability distribution** of the number of trials required in order to observe $r$ 'successes'. **Count variables** that display greater variability (i.e. **overdispersion**) than is assumed under the **Poisson distribution** may be appropriately described by the negative binomial distribution. Likewise, when Poisson counts arise from **clustered designs**, the within-clusters count variable is assumed to follow the Poisson distribution, and the random between-cluster variability the gamma distribution. A related distribution is the

**binomial**, the probability distribution of the number of successes out of a given (fixed) number of trials. See also **dispersion parameter, negative binomial regression**. The **geometric distribution** is a special case of the negative binomial distribution. See DIGGLE *et al.* (2002), ARMITAGE, BERRY & MATHEWS (2002), and AGRESTI (2007).

## Negative binomial regression

A regression method for **overdispersed count variables**. Negative binomial models include a random term that reflects between-subject (or between-cluster) differences (GARDNER, MELVEY & SHAW, 1995) or heterogeneity, and are an alternative to the over-dispersed Poisson model. Alternatively, **zero-inflated Poisson regression** may be used if overdispersion is mainly due to an excess of zero counts. A *zero-inflated* negative binomial model may be indicated if overdispersion is due to unexplained heterogeneity and an excess of zero counts. **Clustered designs** may add variability to an already overdispersed count variable, and models with additional **random effects** may be indicated here. Both zero-inflated Poisson and zero-inflated negative binomial models are specified as two-part models, with a **logistic regression** part that models the proportion of zero count observations, and a Poisson or negative binomial part that models non-zero counts (but predicts zero counts also). Negative binomial regression may be viewed as fitting **random effects** models, or **generalized linear models** with an additional parameter (the **dispersion parameter**). See AGRESTI (2007), DWIVEDI (2010) and ALEXANDER (2012) for further details and illustrative examples. See also **negative binomial distribution**.

## Negative correlation

See **correlation**.

## Negative exponential

See **exponential distribution; exponential curve, non-linear regression**.

## Negative predictive value

See **predictive values**.

## Negative skew

See **skewness**.

## Negative study

A study that yields non-**statistically significant** results. This, however, does not exclude the possibility of **clinical significance** if a study is too small to offer **precise** estimates of effect. On the other hand, a negative study that is carried out by proper standards is as relevant to the understanding of the question at hand as any **positive study**. CHALMERS (1985) advocates against the use of the term 'negative trial', due to it encouraging selective publication favouring 'positive trials' (**publication bias**). See also *P-value*.

## Nelson–Aalen estimator

See **cumulative hazard function** or $H(t)$. See also **Kaplan–Meier method**.

## Neonatal mortality rate

The number of neonatal deaths occurring during a given time-period, in a given geographical region (such as a country), divided by the total number of live births in the same region during the same time-period. The neonatal mortality rate is often multiplied by 1000 to be given as a rate per 1000 live births, and the time-period chosen is usually 1 year. A neonatal death is the death of an infant under 28 days of age. See also **stillbirth rate**, **perinatal mortality rate**, **infant mortality rate**.

## Nested case–control study

A **case–control study** nested in a **prospective cohort study**. In such a study, **cases** are newly diagnosed, **incident** cases of disease, as opposed to existing cases. The nesting of case–control studies in cohort studies allows an estimation of **exposure effect** at an earlier time, due to their greater **efficiency**. Selection of **controls** is usually through **density sampling**. Occupational cohorts often provide the framework for the nested case–control study, and selection of a concise study sample from such a cohort allows a more in-depth collection of the necessary information to the aims of the study (ROTHMAN, 2012). Cohort studies, however, can provide estimates of exposure effect that are based on risk and rate measures. WALD (2004, p. 21) describes the nested case–control design as "a cohort study from an epidemiological perspective, but with some of the economies of a standard case–control study." ROTHMAN (2012) suggests case–control studies may generally be viewed as being nested in a **source population** that can be defined, even if it cannot always be enumerated. See CLAYTON & HILLS (1993) for further details. The use of **matching** and counter-matching as a strategy for improving the efficiency of estimation is discussed.

## Nested model

A **model** that includes only a subset of the **predictor variables** included in the model on which it is nested. The **outcome variable** and the number of **observations** remain the same in the two models. **Significance tests** such as the partial **F-test** and the **likelihood ratio test** may be carried out to compare nested models. See also **saturated model**.

## Net benefit

A comparative measure of **diagnostic test** performance, which may be calculated as an alternative to comparing the **AUC** (or **area under the curve**) for two different **ROC curves**. It has the advantage of focusing on clinically relevant test result **thresholds**, and taking **misclassification** (i.e. false-positive and false-negative diagnoses) costs and **prevalence** of disease into account. MALLETT *et al.* (2012) give additional details and a formula for its calculation. HALLIGAN, ALTMAN & MALLETT (2015) discuss the relative advantages and disadvantages of both measures (net benefit and ROC AUC) in the context of diagnostic imaging, where assessments based on observer rating scales are often supplemented with computer-aided detection or CAD.

## Newman–Keuls sequential procedure

See **multiple-comparison procedures**.

## NNH

Abbreviation for **number needed to harm**.

## NNT

Abbreviation for **number needed to treat**.

## Nominal significance level

A **statistical significance** threshold that is stipulated for each of a number of **multiple significance tests** to be carried out on the same body of data. The aim is to reduce the probability of false-positive significant results (i.e. **type I errors**) by carrying out the different individual tests at a more stringent, higher level of significance than the desired *overall* level of significance. For example, if the overall probability of a type I error is set at **alpha** ($\alpha$) = 0.05, nominal levels may be stipulated at $P = 0.01$ or at some other more extreme level of significance than 0.05, depending on the number of separate tests to be carried out. See also **multiple outcomes, subgroup analyses, Bonferroni correction, Dunnett's correction, sample size** (required); POCOCK (1983) and ARMITAGE, BERRY & MATTHEWS (2002) in the context of **interim analyses**.

## Nominal variable

A **categorical variable** whose categories have no implicit ordering (e.g. eye colour, nationality, blood group). See also **binary variable, measurement scale**.

## Nomogram

A **graphical** representation of the relationship between a number of variables, all of which are depicted on the same two-dimensional surface. Nomograms allow the computation of functions involving the variables in question. By joining together any given values for two of the variables, the corresponding value(s) of (an)other variable(s) can be read off where the joining line intersects the depiction of that (those) variable(s). Examples of nomograms are given in Box P.2 (**PEER**, p. 255), Box P.5 (**Post-test probability**, p. 274), and Box P.6 (**Power**, p. 276).

## Non-collapsibility

A phenomenon that is observed when the estimate of **exposure effect** for a cohort changes in the direction of the **null value** when stratified results are collapsed into a single two-by-two table. This may happen when the measure of effect is the **odds** or the **rate ratio**, though not the **risk ratio** as the combined measure across strata is calculated as a **weighted average** of the stratum-specific effect measures (Greenland & Rothman, in ROTHMAN, GREENLAND & LASH [eds., 2012]). As noted by Greenland & Rothman, non-collapsibility is a separate phenomenon from **confounding**, not so much a bias but a mathematical artefact. AGRESTI (2007) discusses collapsibility conditions for three-way and multiway tables and logistic models. Cf. **Simpson's paradox**.

## Non-differential censoring

See **censoring**.

## Non-differential loss to follow-up

See **loss to follow-up**.

## Non-differential misclassification

See **misclassification**.

## Non-inferiority trial

Equivalence and non-inferiority trials are discussed under **active control equivalence study** (**ACES**).

## Non-informative censoring

See **censoring**.

## Non-informative loss to follow-up

See **loss to follow-up**.

## Non-linear regression

A method of **regression analysis** in which a **non-linear relationship** is summarized by means of a model, which, unlike in **curvilinear regression**, cannot be specified as linear following the transformation of the outcome and/or predictor variable (due to additive errors or **residuals**). HAMILTON (1992) gives examples of **monotonic** and **non-monotonic curves** resulting from non-linear models, which include **exponential** growth and decay curves, negative exponential curves (describing constrained growth or restrained decay), **sigmoid** or S-shaped curves (see Figure S.3, p. 332), and two-term exponential curves. Non-linear models are fitted through 'trial and error' **iteration**. See also ARMITAGE, BERRY & MATHEWS (2002), HAMILTON (2012).

## Non-linear relationship

A term that describes a relationship between two variables where increments in one of the variables are associated with increments and/or decrements in the other variable, which results in a non-linear association. The variables involved are often, but not necessarily,

**quantitative variables**: a relationship may also be described where the mean of a quantitative measurement or the proportion with a given binary outcome increases or decreases in some non-linear fashion across values of an **ordinal variable**, or levels of an **ordered categorical variable**. Frequently referenced non-linear relationships include the **exponential** (growth or decay), negative exponential and S-shaped or **sigmoid curve** (**monotonic curves**), and the two-term exponential, **J-shaped**, and **U-shaped** or **quadratic curve** (**non-monotonic curves**). Non-linear relationships involving continuous variables may be modelled through **curvilinear** and **non-linear regression**. The former is based on a suitable **transformation** of the outcome and/or predictor variable that linearizes the relationship between them. Examples include **polynomial** and **fractional polynomial** regression with power-transformed predictor variables, and semi-log and log-log models resulting from the **logarithmic transformation** of outcome and/or predictor variable (see **exponential curve**). More generally, the transformation to be effected depends on the distribution of the variables in question, and the pattern of their association. A preliminary assessment is often made following visual inspection of a **scatterplot**. MOSTELLER & TUKEY (1977) and KIRKWOOD & STERNE (2003) give a general guide for simple monotonic curves (see **Tukey and Mosteller's bulging rule**). With **generalized linear models**, which have a built-in transformation of the predicted outcome (such as 'log rate' or the 'logit'), transformation of a continuous predictor may or may not be necessary for a linear relationship with the predicted outcome. These assessments should be carried out using the transformed, not the untransformed $y$-variable. **Categorization** (of a continuous predictor) and **smoothing** techniques may be employed to explore a non-linear relationship. See also **linear relationship, dose response relationship, cyclic variation**. See HAMILTON (1992) for further details.

## Non-linear transformation

See **transformations**.

## Non-monotonic curve

A curve depicting a **non-linear relationship** that changes **direction** one or more times at given inversion or 'turn points'. **Quadratic** (Figure Q.1, p. 292), two-term exponential, and **J-shaped curves** (Figures J.1a and J.1b, pp. 175 and 176) are well-known examples. Cf. **monotonic curve**.

## Non-parametric methods

Statistical methods for the analysis of data that do not conform to the requirements or **assumptions** of **parametric methods**. Commonly used non-parametric methods are the **Mann–Whitney $U$-test**, the **Wilcoxon matched pairs signed rank test**, the **Kruskal–Wallis test** and **rank correlation**. These methods are often based on the **ranks** given to the values of the observations in a quantitative variable, rather than on their actual values, and are also appropriate for the analysis of **ordinal data**. Data **transformations** (for example, to a logarithmic scale) may be an alternative to using non-parametric methods. Limitations of non-parametric tests are a focus on **significance testing**, 'low sensitivity' to real differences or effects and the fact that many do not allow for adjustments to be made for **confounders** (KIRKWOOD & STERNE, 2003). See also BLAND (2015) for an overview and illustrative examples. See **locally weighted regression (smoothing)** and **spline regression** for non-parametric methods of regression analysis. HAMILTON (2012) and ARMITAGE, BERRY & MATHEWS (2002) give further details and illustrative examples. See also **resistant estimate, robust method**.

## Non-respondent bias

See **volunteer bias**.

## Normal distribution

Also commonly known as Gaussian distribution. A continuous **probability distribution** that is completely defined by two parameters: the **mean**, reflecting its centre, and the **standard deviation (SD)**, reflecting the spread of individual observations around the mean. It is sometimes written with initial capitalization of the word Normal, to differentiate this from the word 'normal' in ordinary non-statistical usage. Figure N.2a shows the **histogram** of a variable with an *empirical* Normal distribution, and the shape of the corresponding *theoretical* **Normal curve**. The Normal curve (Figure N.1) has a typical bell shape and is perfectly symmetrical about its centre. Unlike **discrete random variables** for which **exact probabilities** can be obtained for any particular value, for **continuous random variables** the probability of any given value is extremely low (zero, for practical purposes) and probabilities are calculated instead for an interval or range of values. Given the mathematical properties of the Normal curve, we can calculate, for example, the probability of obtaining a measurement below (or above) any given value, provided the variable in question follows an approximately Normal distribution, and we can also calculate, albeit indirectly, the probability between any two values. Tables of the Normal distribution give these probabilities for the 'standard Normal distribution' (i.e. a Normal distribution with mean 0 and standard deviation 1). Table 6 gives the probabilities for select percentage points (**critical values**) of the standard Normal distribution. For Normal distributions with different values for the mean and standard deviation,

**Table 6** Select percentage points of the standard Normal distribution: values in the body of the table are the critical values of *z* for different levels of statistical significance (i.e. probability)

| P-value or α | Percentage points of the standard Normal distribution | |
| --- | --- | --- |
| | One-sided | Two-sided |
| **0.5 (50%)** | 0.00 | 0.67 |
| **0.1 (10%)** | 1.28 | 1.64 |
| **0.05 (5%)** | 1.64 | 1.96 |
| **0.01 (1%)** | 2.33 | 2.58 |
| **0.005 (.5%)** | 2.58 | 2.81 |
| **0.001 (.1%)** | 3.09 | 3.29 |

The critical value for two-sided statistical significance at any given α level corresponds to the critical value for one-sided significance at the α/2 level (e.g. 1.96 is the 5% critical value for two-sided significance and the 2.5% critical value for one-sided significance). Degrees of freedom are not applicable.

the same probabilities may be obtained by converting the original measurements into **z-scores** (i.e. measurements expressed in units of SD). **Parametric methods** are often based on the properties and/or **assumption** of a Normal distribution for one or more of the variables being analysed. The **central limit theorem** confers this distribution a central role in statistical inference. See also **approximation, Normal plot**.

## Normal distribution curve

Figure N.1 shows a theoretical Normal curve with **mean** of 0 and **standard deviation** of 1, i.e. the standard Normal curve. At any given point on the *x*-axis, the height of the curve is given by the **probability density** (on the *y*-axis).

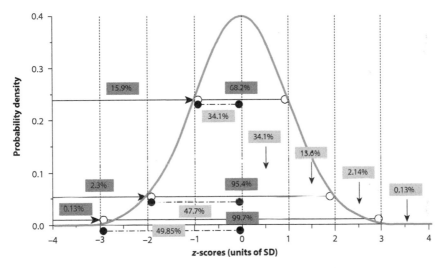

**Figure N.1** Standard Normal curve (mean = 0, standard deviation = 1). Light shaded boxes to the right give the incremental probabilities at 1 SD, 2 SD, 3 SD, and above 3 SD from the mean. Dark shaded boxes in the centre give probabilities for central ranges (O—O) (-1 SD to +1 SD, -2 SD to +2 SD, and -3 SD to +3 SD). Light shaded boxes to the left give one-sided probabilities within 1 SD, 2 SD, and 3 SD from the mean (●—●). One-sided probabilities in the tails of the distribution are shown to the far left (i.e. probabilities below -3 SD, -2 SD, and -1 SD) (drawn using MedCalc Statistical Software).

The total area or probability under the standard Normal curve (i.e. between the curve and the horizontal axis) is 1 (or 100%), and for any given value the area or probability below that value may be calculated. As the curve is symmetrical around 0 (zero), the area below any given negative sign value is equal to the area above the corresponding positive sign value, i.e. the probabilities on the left half/lower tail of the curve are the same as the probabilities on the right half/upper tail (see Table 6, p. 234). If the values of a **normally distributed** variable are rescaled to be converted into standard normal deviates or **z-scores**, its distribution now approximates the standard Normal distribution and the properties of this distribution may be used to calculate the probability of values below, above and between any given value(s) of the variable's distribution. See also **test statistic, critical value**.

## Normal i.i.d. errors

Normally, independently, and identically distributed errors or **residuals**. See **ordinary least squares**. The term 'white noise errors' is used in the context of **time series**, to refer to errors that are uncorrelated between different time points, and specifically, that are independently and identically distributed, with mean zero and constant variance across all time-lags. If also normally distributed, these will be 'Normal i.i.d.'. A white noise process is *stationary*, i.e. it has stable properties/parameters across all time points.

## Normal plot

A **graphical display** that is used to make a visual assessment as to whether the distribution of a given **quantitative variable** may be approximated by a **Normal distribution**. The basic concept behind Normal plots is that of **cumulative frequency distribution (CFD)**, an **S-shaped** function for Normal variables. The Normal plot (a variation of the CFD plot) is a plot of observed *vs.* **expected values** (or empirical *vs.* theoretical **quantiles**), and it will be a straight line if the variable is normally distributed (ALTMAN, 1991). Normal plots are especially useful with small study samples, as histograms provide a satisfactory way of assessing normality with larger samples. BLAND (2015) gives two variations of the Normal plot: the Q-Q or quantile-quantile plot, and the P-P or standardized Normal probability plot. Q-Q plots may be drawn with *expected values* as **z-scores** (or standard Normal deviates), or with *expected values* as the **inverse normal** of the observed values. For the P-P plot, the *observed values* are standardized to mean 0 and SD 1 (i.e. to z-scores) and plotted against the cumulative Normal probabilities. Figures N.3a and N.3b show examples of Q-Q plots for a variable that is normally distributed (Figure N.2a), and for a variable displaying a positive **skew**, i.e. with greater frequency of lower values than higher values (Figure N.2b). The vertical (*y*) axis represents the values of the variable in the original scale, and the horizontal (*x*) axis gives the inverse normal for the same variable (i.e. the corresponding quantiles under the **assumption** that the variable follows a perfectly Normal distribution, given its **mean** and **standard deviation**). If the variable in question has an approximately Normal distribution, the plot results in a fairly straight line along a diagonal line of equivalence. A concave curve results from variables with a positive skew, and a convex curve from

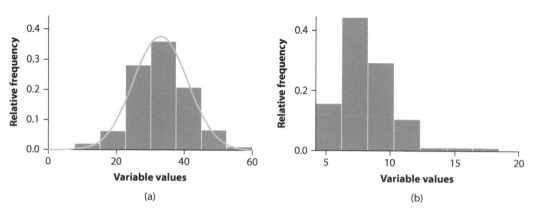

**Figures N.2a and N.2b** Histogram: (a) variable with an approximately Normal distribution; (b) variable with a positively skewed distribution (drawn using Stata Statistical Software).

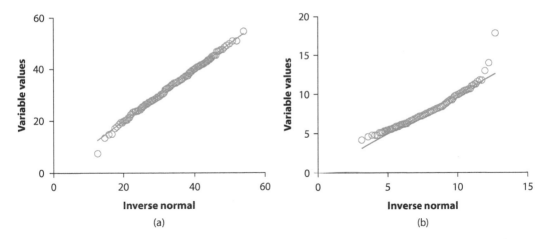

**Figures N.3a and N.3b** Normal plot: (a) variable with an approximately Normal distribution; (b) variable with a positively skewed distribution (drawn using Stata Statistical Software).

variables with a negative skew (note that if the variable itself is on the $x$-axis and the inverse normal is on the $y$-axis, the curvatures displayed by skewed distributions will be just the opposite: convex if positively skewed and concave if negatively skewed). The **Shapiro–Wilk** and **Shapiro–Francia tests** perform the formal testing of Normal plots. See also **skewness, kurtosis, goodness-of-fit (GoF)**.

## Normalizing transformation

A data **transformation** that results in a **Normal distribution** for a quantitative variable, as required by certain methods of analysis (see **assumptions**). Examples are the **logarithmic, square root** and **reciprocal** transformations, which are often employed as both normalizing and **variance-stabilizing** transformations for positively **skewed** variables. **Symmetry**, rather than normality of distribution, is sometimes all a transformation may achieve. See also **Box–Cox transformation, square** and **cubic power** transformations.

## NPV

Abbreviation for negative predictive value. See **predictive values**.

## Nuisance parameter

A **parameter** that is calculated to take some feature of the data into account and improve **inference**, although the parameter is not itself of interest. For example, the **variance** of the **random effects** in a **multilevel model** must be estimated, although the focus of the analysis is likely the **fixed effects** of exposures or treatments, and of additional risk and prognostic factors. The **baseline hazard function** in **Cox regression** is another example of a nuisance parameter, with values derived directly from the data at the specific time points at which the event of interest occurs. Its sole purpose is to give the model its proper structure, although the nuisance parameter is not of interest in itself and may not be used to compute the predicted outcome, the hazard or instantaneous rate. See also **ancillary statistic**.

## Null hypothesis

NH or $H_0$. A hypothesis put forward when carrying out **significance testing**, which states: (a) there are no differences between groups being compared (e.g. aspirin and placebo are equally effective in preventing death in patients following an acute myocardial infarction), or (b) there is no relationship or association between variables (e.g. caloric intake and body mass index), in the relevant **population**, i.e. the collective of people similar by some measure to those participating in a study. Under **frequentist inference**, significance tests are carried out on the assumption that $H_0$ is true. It is then necessary to decide whether the observed data deviates from what would be expected *if* $H_0$ were true. This is expressed as a probability or **P-value**. The smaller the *P*-value, the lower the probability of obtaining the result observed (or a more extreme result) in the **study sample** if $H_0$ were in fact true, in which case observed differences and associations are declared to be **statistically significant**, i.e. unlikely to be due to chance, and $H_0$ is rejected. If *P*-values are large, conventionally >0.05, there is said to be insufficient evidence to reject the NH (which is not the same as *accepting* the NH to be true). See also **alternative hypothesis**, **one-sided test**, **two-sided test**, **type I error**, **type II error**, **power**, **hypothesis testing**.

## Null model

A **regression model** that does not include any **predictor variables**. In a null model, the **predicted value** for each observation is given by the **intercept**, as an estimate of the overall group mean. An overall **significance test** for the predictors in a given model is a test against the corresponding null model. Similarly, **r-squared** and related measures evaluate the fit of a model against the null model. More generally, a model that excludes the variable or variables whose significance is being tested. See also **maximal model**, **saturated model**.

## Number at risk

The denominator in the formulae for the calculation of **risks**. It is usually taken to be the total number of individuals who are disease-free at the start of a **follow-up study** in which length of follow-up is uniform for the entire study group. This is in contrast with **person-time at risk** (**PTAR**), the denominator in the calculation of **rates**.

## Number needed to harm

Or its abbreviation, NNH. The reciprocal of the difference in risk of **adverse events**, i.e. 1/$ARD_{adverse\ events}$, where ARD is the abbreviation for **absolute risk difference**. See **number needed to treat** (**NNT**), **measures of impact**.

## Number needed to treat

Or its abbreviation, NNT. A **measure of the impact** of a treatment or intervention. The NNT gives the number of patients that must receive the treatment in question in order to prevent an event that would otherwise occur (COOK & SACKETT, 1995; SEDGWICK, 2013). The **risk** of the event in question, both in patients receiving the new treatment, and in patients receiving a standard treatment (or no treatment), needs to be known. From Table 2.b (p. 72), the NNT is calculated as:

$$NNT = \frac{1}{risk_0 - risk_1} = \frac{1}{ARD} = \frac{1}{\dfrac{c}{c+d} - \dfrac{a}{a+b}}$$

where $risk_0$ is the risk in the control group and $risk_1$ is the risk in the intervention group (both expressed as proportions). Because the NNT is based on the **absolute risk difference (ARD)**, it is possible for treatments of only moderate or little *relative* effect to have considerable *impact* when used to treat common diseases with a reasonably high incidence of adverse outcomes. An example is given in Box N.1. A critique of the number needed to treat is given by HUTTON (2000). Ebrahim, in EGGER, DAVEY SMITH & ALTMAN (eds., 2001), discusses issues and pitfalls around the calculation of NNTs from meta-analyses.

---

## BOX N.1

From **Box A.1**, p. 3.

The NNT is calculated as 1/ARD (i.e. if 2.4 deaths are prevented per 100 patients who would die otherwise, how many patients must be treated to prevent **1** death?). The calculation gives:

$$NNT - 1/0.24 = 42$$

This shows the intervention (aspirin, here) to have a reasonably high impact on vascular mortality at 5 weeks in patients with AMI.

If aspirin has any serious side-effects, the 'number needed to harm' should also be computed, and the trade-off between the two results, NNT and NNH, considered when making clinical and policy decisions (see **likelihood of being helped** vs. **harmed**).

---

## Numerical variable

See **quantitative variable**.

# O

### OAPR

Abbreviation for 'odds of being affected given a positive result' (synonymous with post-test odds). See **post-test probability**.

### O'Brien–Fleming approach

See **stopping rules**.

### Observation

A datum or piece of information or detail that is measured, counted or observed. The term is also used to refer to the row of information pertaining to a single individual or **study unit**, with respect to the different **variables** that are presented as columns in a **data set**.

### Observational study

A non-experimental investigation in which individuals are not assigned to actual treatments or interventions, but rather, information on relevant exposures and outcomes is collected, based on which inferences about **exposure effects** with regard to one or more specific diseases are made. Observational studies may be classified as **cross-sectional** or **longitudinal**, depending on whether the relevant information is collected at a single point in time, or study participants are followed up over a period of time, and information is collected either periodically or at the start and end of the study. Examples of the latter are **cohort** and **case–control studies**, although the case–control design does not involve actual follow-up, whereas the cohort design is usually, but not always, conducted prospectively. The information collected commonly includes disease and **exposure** status, and data on potential **confounding factors**. ROTHMAN, GREENLAND & LASH (eds., 2012), and ROTHMAN (2012) give a full discussion of issues relating to observational studies. See WALD (2004) and MACHIN & CAMPBELL (2005) for an overview, and Egger, Davey Smith & Schneider, in EGGER, DAVEY SMITH & ALTMAN (eds., 2001), for issues pertaining to systematic reviews of observational studies. See also **STROBE statement** for reporting guidelines.

### Observed frequency

The observed frequency ($O$) is the actual count or **frequency** in the different categories, classes or values of a **categorical** or **quantitative** (continuous or discrete) **variable**, or in the different cells of a **contingency table**, as opposed to the frequency that is **expected** ($E$) based on the parameters of a **theoretical distribution**, or on the **marginal totals** of a contingency table.

## Observed outcome

The actual **outcome** that is measured or observed to have occurred, as opposed to that which would be **expected** (or fitted/predicted) on the basis of a **regression model**.

## Observed value

The actual value of an observation with respect to a **continuous variable**, as opposed to the value that is **expected** based on the parameters of a **theoretical distribution**.

## Odds

The ratio of the number of times (or alternatively, the probability) an event occurs to the number of times (or probability) it does not occur, out of a given number of chances or trials. Odds convey the idea of **'risk'**, although the two are only approximately the same when considering rare events (e.g. probability of getting brain cancer). For a common event, such as a newborn baby being a boy or a girl, the probability or risk is roughly 0.5 or 50%, but the odds are 1 (50:50). Odds are always larger than the corresponding risk measure. When the risk or probability is 1, the odds are infinite. If the **probability** of the event of interest occurring is $p$, then the probability of it not occurring is $1 - p$. The odds of the event are given by:

$$\text{Odds} = p/(1 - p),$$

with

$$p = \text{odds}/(1 + \text{odds})$$

Unlike probabilities or proportions, odds may take any value from 0 to infinity. A transformation of the odds, the **logit**, may take any value from $-\infty$ to $+\infty$. For this reason, **logistic regression** is often used to model/predict **binary outcomes**. See also **odds ratio**.

## Odds of being affected if positive result

Or OAPR. Synonymous with post-test odds. See **post-test probability**.

## Odds ratio

A ratio of two **odds**, often used in epidemiological studies (in particular, **case–control studies**) and **clinical trials** as a **measure of association** between exposure and disease, or between treatment and outcome (Box L.1, **Logistic regression**, p. 198). If the odds are the same in the two groups, their ratio is 1. From Table 2.a (p. 72):

$$OR = \frac{odds\ in\ exposed}{odds\ in\ unexposed} = \frac{a}{b} \div \frac{c}{d} = \frac{ad}{bc}$$

For rare diseases, the odds ratio (OR) and the **risk ratio** (calculated using the actual **risks**, not the odds) are very similar. BLAND (2015) gives a derivation of the equivalence between these measures, showing that the OR is a good approximation to the risk ratio (RR) when prevalence of disease is low. When controls are selected from among the disease-free in a **cumulative case–control study** (at what would be the end of the follow-up or 'at-risk' period in a cohort study), the OR gives an estimate of the OR in the population, or, if the disease is rare, of the RR. If controls are selected as cases arise, as in a **density case–control study**, the OR estimates the **rate ratio** in the population. If controls are selected from among the initially disease-free population as in a **case–cohort study**, the OR gives an estimate of the **risk ratio** (KIRKWOOD & STERNE, 2003; ROTHMAN, 2012). MIETTINEN (1976) examines the 'rare disease' assumption and the estimability of various measures in case–control studies. Box O.1 gives a table from which ORs may be converted into a useful measure of impact in intervention studies, the **number needed to treat** (**NNT**). See also **diagnostic odds ratio**.

## BOX O.1

Reproduced from Straus SE *et al.* (2010). *Evidence-based Medicine: How to Practice and Teach It, 4th edition*. Churchill Livingstone (with permission).

**Translating ORs to NNTs:** Since results from clinical trials and meta-analyses are often presented as ORs, the table below can be used to convert these into a measure of treatment impact, the number needed to treat (NNT). Another quantity, the **patient expected event rate** (**PEER**), is also required. See STRAUS *et al.* (2010) for additional tables and formulae, and for calculations based on the **risk ratio** (**RR**).

|  |  | OR < 1 | | | | |
|---|---|---|---|---|---|---|
|  |  | 0.9 | 0.8 | 0.7 | 0.6 | 0.5 |
| Patient's | 0.05 | 209[a] | 104 | 69 | 52 | 41[b] |
| expected event | 0.10 | 110 | 54 | 36 | 27 | 21 |
| rate (PEER) | 0.20 | 61 | 30 | 20 | 14 | 11 |
|  | 0.30 | 46 | 22 | 14 | 10 | 8 |
|  | 0.40 | 40 | 19 | 12 | 9 | 7 |
|  | 0.50 | 38 | 18 | 11 | 9 | 6 |
|  | 0.70 | 44 | 20 | 13 | 9 | 6 |
|  | 0.90 | 101[c] | 46 | 27 | 18 | 12[d] |

The numbers in the body of the table are the NNTs for the corresponding odds ratios (for ORs <1) at that particular patient's expected event rate (PEER); [a]RRR = 10%, [b]RRR = 49%, [c]RRR = 1%, [d]RRR = 9% (RRR: **relative risk reduction**).

**To calculate the NNT for any OR <1 and PEER:**

$$NNT = \frac{1-\left[PEER\times\left(1-OR\right)\right]}{\left(1-PEER\right)\times PEER\times\left(1-OR\right)}$$

## Offset

In the context of **generalized linear models**, an offset is a regression term with **regression coefficient** fixed at one (1). An example is the regression term for **person-time at** risk (**PTAR**) – or more precisely, for the **logarithm** of PTAR or log($t$) – which is included as an explanatory variable in **Poisson regression** models to give the total person-time exposure for each group or for each individual (depending on whether data are individual- or aggregate-level), i.e. the number of person-time units over which a count is made or a frequency of occurrence registered. PTAR may be thought of as an index to the **count variable**, the expected value of the count being proportional to the index (AGRESTI, 2007). It may be thought of also as an adjustment [= -log($t$)] to the predicted log count, to give the model for the predicted **rate**. The larger the PTAR, the greater the **precision** with which regression coefficients for relevant predictors will be estimated. The extent of exposure may be given also by the total number of time or space units. See also **ancillary statistic**.

## Ogive

A **cumulative frequency polygon**, that is, a line graph in which the cumulative frequencies (on the vertical axis) are plotted against the corresponding upper **class limits** of a categorized quantitative variable (on the horizontal axis). See Figure C.4, p. 90.

## Oldham plot

In the context of the study of **change**, the Oldham plot is a plot of the *differences* between measurements obtained before and after a given treatment or intervention (on the $y$-axis), against the *average* of the same two measurements (on the $x$-axis) (OLDHAM, 1962). The average of the two measurements gives the best estimate of the true value of what is being measured. The technique enables an assessment to be made as to whether change scores correlate with magnitude of measurements. This is a more accurate assessment than would be obtained by plotting *differences vs. initial* or 'before' value, due to the problem of **regression to the mean**. Regression to the mean exaggerates the relationship or **correlation** between amount of change and initial value, as individuals with 'before' values in the extremes of what is being measured are bound to have less extreme measurements on second reading, regardless of whether or not a treatment is being administered concomitantly. A plot of 'differences' *vs.* 'initial value' shows a characteristic negative or positive slope that suggests a significant relationship between magnitude of initial measurement and amount of change experienced (note: the correlation between 'differences' and 'initial value' depends on the way the 'differences' variable is calculated: if calculated as 'after – before', the correlation is negative; if calculated as 'before – after', the correlation is positive). When initial measurement is replaced with 'average' measurement on the plot, it is often the case that a less steep slope is obtained, indicating a weaker relationship between magnitude of measurement and amount of change. This is shown in Figures O.1a and O.1b, in the study by SUMNER *et al.* (1988) on initial blood pressure as a predictor of the response to antihypertensive (AHT) therapy. A mixed group of 255 normotensive and hypertensive individuals were given either a placebo treatment or one of five types of AHT drug (ACE inhibitors, calcium antagonists, direct vasodilators, alpha-adrenoceptor blocker, beta-adrenoceptor blocker). Among those administered ACE inhibitors, the **correlation coefficient** between change in systolic blood pressure (SBP) (calculated as initial SBP *minus* minimum SBP reading in the 8 h period following administration of the drug) and initial SBP was 0.74. When initial SBP was replaced by the average of the two SBP measurements (BP1 and BP2), the correlation was attenuated to $r = 0.49$ ($P<0.001$):

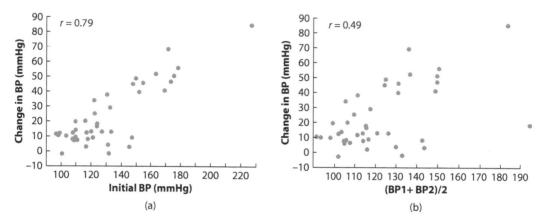

**Figures 0.1a and 0.1b** Oldham plot: the positive correlation between amount of *change* in systolic blood pressure (BP) (difference between initial BP and minimum reading in the 8 h period following the administration of single doses of ACE inhibitors; $n = 43$) and *initial* BP became more attenuated when the relationship was assessed against the *average* of the two BP measurements. (Reproduced from Sumner DJ *et al.* (1988). Initial blood pressure as a predictor of the response to antihypertensive therapy. *Br J Clin Pharmacol* **26**: 715–20 (with permission).)

BLOMQVIST (1977; 1987) suggests an alternative assessment of the relationship between change and initial value, where the assessment is made by adjusting for **measurement error** as opposed to calculating an average measurement. This approach is recommended by HAYES (1988), in particular where study participants have been selected on the basis of extreme initial values, and underlying treatment effect differs between individuals. CHIOLERO *et al.* (2013) compare a number of different methodologies for evaluating the relationship between change and baseline value. See additional discussion under **regression to the mean** (in comparative studies). See also **difference** *vs.* **average plots**.

## OLS

Abbreviation for **ordinary least squares**.

## Omega squared

A **standardized measure of effect**, which is considered a less **biased** population estimate than **eta squared** ($\eta^2$), especially with small **sample sizes**. Both may be calculated in the context of **analysis of variance (ANOVA)**. Similarly to the latter, omega squared ($\omega^2$) gives the proportion of total variance that is accounted for by an effect or factor under study. A *partial* measure may also be calculated for an effect where additional factors and/ or covariates add to the variability in the **outcome variable** (see **partial correlation coefficient**). This is not applicable where these factors and covariates reduce, rather, response variability. A *generalized* omega squared has been proposed for comparing results from different experimental designs (e.g. including just the **factor** of interest, a **covariate** and/or additional factors, **blocking** factors, and mixed fixed and random effects – see **linear mixed effects model**) (OLEJNIK & ALGINA, 2003). See also **effect size**.

## Omitted predictor variable

See **model selection**, **dependence**, **overdispersion**, **instrumental variable**.

## One-sided test

A **significance test** that only evaluates one of the two alternatives to the **null hypothesis** (**NH**). For example, under a one-sided test, as opposed to a **two-sided test**, the **alternative hypothesis** being tested could be that the risk of an adverse outcome is *lower* in the **intervention group** as compared to the **control group**. The possibility that the risk in the intervention group could be *higher* than in the control group is disregarded. A one-sided test should not be carried out unless one is certain only one alternative to the NH is possible. On the other hand, Sackett, in HAYNES *et al.* (eds., 2006), makes an argument for the use of one-sided tests, on the basis that "Clinicians ask one-sided questions of **superiority** and **non-inferiority**." (pp. 188, 190), and as a way of avoiding indeterminate non-inferiority and superiority conclusions. MOYÉ & TITA (2002) offer the opposite argument. MACHIN & CAMPBELL (2005) describe the calculation of one-sided **confidence intervals** in non-inferiority trials, which, just as one-sided tests are more powerful than two-sided tests (all other things being equal), are also less stringent than the corresponding $100(1 - \alpha)\%$ two-sided confidence interval. This is because the **alpha** ($\alpha$) level that was split equally between the lower and upper confidence limits ($100(\alpha/2)\%$ on each side) is now wholly shifted to the lower boundary. The result is a smaller difference at the lower boundary and a more 'determinate' conclusion of non-inferiority. See Box O.2.

---

### BOX O.2

Roberts M *et al.* (1984). The Edinburgh randomized trial of screening for breast cancer: description of method. *Br J Cancer* **50**: 1–6.

. . . . . . . . . . . . . . . . . . . . . . . . . . . . . . . . . . . . . . . . . . . . . . . . . . . . . . . . . . . . . . . . . . . . . . . . . . . . . . . . . . . . . . . . . . . .

The UK 7-year trial of breast cancer screening started in 1979. Edinburgh was one of the participating centres, with 65,000 women aged 45–65 years enrolled, in clusters defined by their general practices. The researchers in this trial based the required sample size calculations on the assumption that the outcome for women screened could not be worse than for women not screened (on the basis of a previous study, a 35% reduction in mortality was expected at the first analysis after 7 years of follow-up). Although this seems reasonable, there are also well-known harmful effects of screening that sometimes have to be taken into account in this type of investigation.

---

## One-tailed test

See **one-sided test**.

## One-way ANOVA

**Analysis of variance** of data classified according to a single factor or characteristic. For example, one may wish to compare **mean** birthweight among different ethnic groups (the classifying factor), or mean body mass index (BMI) among different groups that may be nutritionally vulnerable, as in the example in Box O.3 (VESPA & WATSON, 1995). As with the **independent** samples *t*-test that is carried out when there are just two groups, one-way ANOVA requires the **outcome variable** to have a **Normal distribution** and similar variances (**homoscedasticity**) in all the groups being compared. The **null hypothesis** of no differences between the groups is tested by the *F*-test. See also **two-way ANOVA**, **repeated measures ANOVA**, **multiple-comparison procedures**, **contrast**, **trend** (test for).

## BOX O.3

Reproduced from Vespa J, Watson F (1995). Who is nutritionally vulnerable in Bosnia-Hercegovina? *Br Med J* **311**: 652–4 (with permission).

Data collected as part of a nutrition and food security monitoring system set up by the WHO in three besieged cities in Bosnia-Hercegovina (Sarajevo, Tuzla, Zenica) between December 1993 and May 1994 were analysed in order to identify nutritionally vulnerable groups. The comparison between type of household with respect to mean body mass index (BMI) was as follows (for adults aged 18–59 years, excluding pregnant women):

Nutritional status of adults by household group in Bosnia-Hercegovina, February 1994

|  | | Displaced people | | |
|  | *Urban residents* | *In private accommodation* | *In collective centres* | *Rural residents* |
| --- | --- | --- | --- | --- |
| Sample size | 186 | 128 | 123 | 109 |
| Mean (SD) body mass index* | 22.5 (3.0) | 22.7 (2.9) | 23.0 (3.0) | 24.0 (3.7) |
| 95% confidence interval | 22.1 to 22.9 | 22.2 to 23.2 | 22.5 to 23.5 | 23.3 to 24.7 |
| % Undernutrition (body mass index <18.5) | 8.1 | 5.5 | 3.1 | 1.8 |
| % Low nutritional status | 18.3 | 18.0 | 13.8 | 6.4 |

\* ANOVA for mean body mass index: *F*-statistic = 5.417, *P*-value = 0.001.

*Interpretation:* The analysis of variance comparing adults in the different types of household with respect to mean BMI gives an *F*-statistic of 5.417, i.e. the between-groups variability ($MS_{between-groups}$) is more than five times greater than the within-groups variability ($MS_{within-groups}$), a strong indication that significant differences exist among the groups. Degrees of freedom (*df*) for the *F*-test are given by the number of groups (*k*) *minus* 1 (= 4 – 1 = 3), and the number of individuals *minus* the number of groups (= 546 – 4 = 542). It is possible a household or other **cluster** effect was not taken into account in this analysis.
　　See explanation of other quantities under the relevant entries (SD, **standard deviation**; MS, **mean squares**; SS, **sum of squares**; *df*, **degrees of freedom**; *P*-value).

## Open sequential design

See **sequential designs**.

## Ordered categorical variable

A **categorical variable** whose different levels or categories have an inherent ordering, although its values (or labels) cannot usually be interpreted in a strict numerical sense.

Nonetheless, successive categories represent an increment in the feature or characteristic being assessed. For example, the ordered categories may represent increasing levels of exposure to a risk factor, increasing intensity of experience of a subjective symptom such as pain or increasing stages of progression of an oncological disease. See also **chi-squared test for trend, ordered logistic regression**. Cf. **categorized continuous variable, ordinal variable**.

## Ordered logistic regression

Also termed proportional odds model. An extension of **logistic regression** that is carried out with **ordered categorical** outcome variables (for example, severity of pain categorized as no pain, minimal pain, moderate pain and severe pain). Cf. **chi-squared test for trend** for ordered *exposures* or *treatments*. See AGRESTI (2007), HOSMER, LEMESHOW & STURDIVANT (2013), HAMILTON (2012), and MITCHELL (2012b) for further details and illustrative examples. See also **polytomous logistic regression**.

## Ordinal variable

A *semi*-**quantitative variable** whose values are given by **ranks** and scores. Unlike **interval** or **ratio variables**, differences between any two consecutive values of an ordinal variable do not necessarily represent increments of the same magnitude. Ordinal data are often analysed using **non-parametric methods**, such as the **Mann–Whitney $U$ test**, the **Kruskal–Wallis test, Cuzick's test** and **rank correlation**. The **median, interquartile range** and other central ranges based on **centiles** of actual distribution are used as **descriptive measures**. See also **Likert scale, Guttman scale, visual analogue scale, composite score, measurement scale**.

## Ordinary least squares

Commonly referred to by its abbreviation, OLS. A term used to describe the standard method of estimating a **least squares regression** model (a **simple** or **multiple linear model**), in which no weighting or iteration is involved. **Assumptions** for OLS are **independence** of observations, a **linear relationship** between quantitative outcome and quantitative predictor variable, and **homoscedasticity**, with resulting errors (**residuals**) that are *Normal i.i.d.*, i.e. normally distributed with zero mean and identical variance for each value of the predictor variable, and independent of the value of the predictor and of the error of other observations (HAMILTON, 1992). Alternatives to OLS include **weighted least squares (WLS)** and **iteratively reweighted least squares (IRLS)** (which provide a robust alternative in the presence of outliers and non-Normal errors), models for **autocorrelated** errors and **multilevel models** (which are appropriate with dependence due to cluster effects), **logistic regression** (binary outcome and binomial errors), **Poisson** and **negative binomial regression** (non-negative count variable outcome and Poisson errors, or overdispersed counts) and **Cox regression** and other models for the analysis of survival times (non-Normal errors and censored outcomes). HUITEMA (2011) gives further details on the rationale for the various alternatives to OLS.

## Ordinate

The value on the vertical or $y$-axis for a datum point that is plotted on a two-dimensional graph. An individual or **study unit** is identified on such a graph by its coordinates, i.e. the point of intersection between the value of the **abscissa** and the value of the ordinate.

## Outcome variable

Also termed *y*, dependent or response variable. The endpoint event, measurement or characteristic (e.g. death or cholesterol levels) that is analysed to test the main hypothesis in an investigation. In the context of **regression analysis**, it is commonly referred to as the **y-variable**. A distinction is made between the *observed* values of *y*, and the **predicted values** of *y* or *ŷ* (read 'y hat') as those computed from the equation for any given regression **model**. The **measurement scale** of the outcome variable determines in large part the choice of statistical methods of data analysis. BLAND (2015) and KIRKWOOD & STERNE (2003) give comprehensive guides. See also **primary outcome**, **surrogate endpoint**, **multiple outcomes**. MACHIN & CAMPBELL (2005) discuss these various concepts. Cf. **predictor variable**.

## Outliers

Or extreme observations. Observations of a given variable whose values are significantly higher or lower than the 'average'. An important consequence of the presence of outliers is that the distribution of the variable in question will likely not be **Normal**. **Transformations** and **non-parametric methods** are often used to analyse variables whose distribution is **skewed** by the presence of outliers. In the context of **regression** and **correlation**, outliers tend to dominate (to varying degrees, see below), affecting the **strength**, and sometimes also the **direction**, of the association between the variables in question. Nonetheless, outlying observations should not be discarded without careful consideration. The identification of outliers can be accomplished with simple graphical methods such as **scatterplots**. Figure O.2 shows the relationship (without adjustment of food intake to 1 kg/day) between daily intakes of lecithin (in grams per day) and cholesterol (in mg per day) in the study by ISHINAGA *et al.* (2005), seeking to demonstrate that restriction of dietary cholesterol intake is associated with reduced intake of lecithin, a crucial nutrient for the production of choline, the precursor of the neurotransmitter acetylcholine (see also Figure P.1, p. 257). An outlier is circled on the scatterplot, and two *fictitious* ones are also shown. The likely effect of these outliers on the regression line is (would be) as follows:

1. Outlier in *y* (200:7, *fictitious*, black). Intercept: moderately increased; slope: slightly decreased; its own **residual** (vertical distance to solid line): large size; this is an observation not well explained by the model.
2. Outlier in *x* with *y* coordinate 5.6 (1150:5.6, circled). Although a high **leverage** point (high value for cholesterol intake), this outlier does not exert much influence on the regression line since its value for lecithin intake keeps it in line with the pattern of relationship in the main body of data. Intercept: slightly increased; slope: slightly decreased; its own residual: small size.
3. Outlier in *x* with *y* coordinate 1 (1150:1, *fictitious*, black). This is a high leverage point whose value for lecithin goes against the pattern of higher lecithin values with increasing cholesterol values, and it will affect the regression line possibly reversing the direction of relationship. Intercept: moderately increased; slope: moderately or greatly decreased; its own residual: moderate size. Outlier 3 is an **influential** observation.

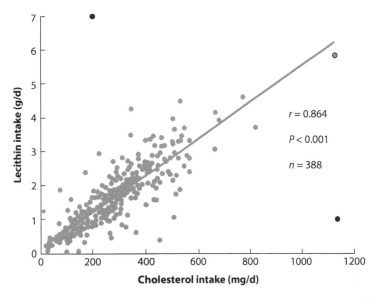

**Figure 0.2** Regression line with three outliers: relationship between daily lecithin (g/day) and cholesterol (mg/day) intakes (without adjustment of food intake to 1 kg/d) in 388 Japanese men, women and children 6–59 years old. The fitted regression model (without the fictitious outliers) is: lecithin intake (g/d) = 0.16 + 0.005 × cholesterol intake (mg/d) ($r^2$ = 0.747, $P$ < 0.001). (Reproduced from Ishinaga M *et al.* (2005). Cholesterol intake is associated with lecithin intake in Japanese people. *J Nutr* **135**: 1451–5 (with permission).)

'Good' outliers still affect statistical **inference**, if not the value of parameter estimates. See also **Normal plot, regression diagnostics**.

## Overall rate

The **rate** or frequency of occurrence of an event for all causes combined (e.g. all-cause mortality rate). Cf. **cause-specific rate**. See also **crude rate**, **age-specific rate**.

## Overdispersed Poisson model

See **overdispersion, Poisson regression**.

## Overdispersion

The characteristic of a **discrete variable** (a count or a grouped binary variable) that displays greater **variability** than would be expected under an assumed **probability distribution**, specifically, the **Poisson** and **binomial** distributions. Overdispersion may be due to the omission of important **predictor variables** from a **Poisson** or **logistic regression** model, or to unexplained between-subject **heterogeneity** and related within-subject **dependence**. For any given covariate pattern (e.g. different treatment groups), the **rate** of occurrence of an event, or the **probability** of a given outcome, may not then be assumed to be the same for all individuals, so that the distribution of the outcome variable within each covariate pattern (given same conditions such as extent of person-time exposure or number of 'trials') displays extra-Poisson or extra-binomial variability. An excess of zero counts may also cause overdispersion. In addition to between-subject heterogeneity, in **clustered designs**, within-cluster dependence or correlation with between-cluster heterogeneity, may result in, or add to, overdispersion in the variable of interest. In **survival analysis**, reference is made to *unshared* and *shared* **frailty models**, as accounting for heterogeneity at the individual and at the group level. In the presence of overdispersion, Poisson and logistic regression underestimate the magnitude of the **standard errors (SEs)** of the regression coefficients estimated for the different predictors, which leads to spurious precision and statistical significance. In the latter, overdispersion is reflected in larger than expected discrepancies between observed and predicted number of events. Generally, overdispersion is likely to be present if the **deviance** or **Pearson goodness-of-fit** statistics for a Poisson or logistic regression model are larger than the **residual degrees of freedom**. The ratio of a goodness-of-fit statistic (often, the Pearson $X^2$ statistic) to its number of degrees of freedom gives a **scale parameter**, the square root of which may be used to adjust (inflate) the value of standard errors. **Test statistics** and **residuals** should also be adjusted, by dividing by the scale parameter or by its square root, respectively (ARMITAGE, BERRY & MATTHEWS, 2002). A deviance statistic thus adjusted is referred to as 'scaled deviance' and has the same number of degrees of freedom as the unscaled deviance. A scale parameter should be estimated from a **maximal model**. Alternatively, different probability models may be considered for the data, commonly, the **negative binomial** and **zero-inflated Poisson** models for count data, the **beta-binomial** model for grouped binary data and models with additional **random effects** to account for between-cluster variability. See also **underdispersion**, **dispersion parameter**; GARDNER, MULVEY & SHAW (1995), AGRESTI (2007), DWIVEDI *et al.* (2010). Cf. **heteroscedasticity**.

## Overmatching

In the context of **case–control studies**, overmatching occurs when cases and controls are **matched** on variables that are *not* **confounding factors**. For example, if cases and controls were matched for parental alcohol consumption in a study investigating the relationship between parental smoking and asthma in their children, cases and controls would be 'made' to have very similar levels of **exposure** to parental smoking, since smoking is frequently associated with alcohol consumption. However, asthma in children is not related to parental drinking habits (at least not directly!), and, as a result, it may be wrongly concluded that parental smoking and asthma in children are unrelated. Matching on factors that are not confounders is not only unnecessary, as it also introduces **selection bias** into a case–control study. The need to control for the matching variable at the data analysis stage (through **stratification**) has the effect of reducing the **efficiency** of the study design.

## Overview

See **systematic review**.

# P

## p

See **proportion, probability, prevalence**.

## P-P plot

Or probability-probability plot. See **Normal plot**.

## P-value

In the context of **significance testing**, the $P$-value is the probability that a given difference (or one more extreme), with respect to means, proportions, rates, etc., is observed in a **study sample**, when in reality such a difference does not exist in the relevant **population**, i.e. is not a 'true effect'. Smaller $P$-values provide stronger evidence to reject the **null hypothesis (NH)** of no difference. For example, a $P$-value $= 0.004$ can be interpreted as a 4 in 1000 chance of observing a difference of a given magnitude (or a more extreme one), between, for instance, two groups of patients and with respect to a given mean measurement, when, in the population (i.e. if we could have carried out a study with *all* similar patients), the two groups being compared have similar means. Conventionally, a difference is said to be **statistically significant** if the corresponding $P$-value is less than 0.05. However, it is preferable to report exact $P$-values rather than the commonly used 'NS' (non-significant) or '$P < 0.05$': it is clear that the difference between $P = 0.049$ and $P = 0.051$ is too small to deserve such dichotomy. When carrying out **correlation** or **regression analyses**, the NH being tested is that the correlation or regression **coefficients** are equal to 0 (i.e. there is no relationship between the variables in question). For measures of **relative risk**, the NH is that RR = 1. The $P$-value may also be thought of as the probability that a **type I error** has occurred. A difficulty with $P$-values, as commented by ROTHMAN (2012, p. 152), is that "... [the $P$ value] confounds two important aspects of the data, the strength of the relation between exposure and disease and the precision with which that relation is measured. To have a clear interpretation of the data, it is important to be able to separate the information on strength of relation and precision, which is the job that estimation does for us." Thus, a $P$-value cannot be properly assessed in isolation, i.e. without reference to a **confidence interval**. This is the main issue with declaring studies to be **positive**, i.e. statistically significant, or **negative**, i.e. non-statistically significant. See Box P.1 for an example from the ISIS-2 study.

## BOX P.1

From **Box A.1**, p. 3.

The probability that an absolute risk difference (ARD) of 2.4% or greater could have been found in a study of this size, when, in fact, it is simply a chance finding, is less than 1 in 100,000 ($P < 0.00001$). The results of the comparison of aspirin *vs.* no aspirin (with respect to 5-week vascular mortality following an acute myocardial infarction) are therefore statistically significant, and likely to reflect a real effect. In other words, the data are not consistent with the null hypothesis, to use ROTHMAN's interpretation of $P$-values as not quite strict probabilities.

See also **negative study, positive study, frequentist inference, Bayesian inference (Bayes' factor), clinical significance, mid $P$-value**; GREENLAND *et al.* (2016).

## PACF

Abbreviation for partial **autocorrelation** function. See also **correlogram**.

## PAF

Abbreviation for **population attributable fraction** or $AF_{population}$.

## Paired data

Data that arise in the context of **before–after studies, matched pairs designs** and **crossover trials**. The lack of **independence** of paired observations requires the use of special tests and methods of analysis. The **paired $t$-test** and **Wilcoxon's matched pairs signed rank test** are used with quantitative data, while **McNemar's test** and methods for paired proportions are used with binary data. Regression models, such as obtained through **conditional logistic regression**, take the pairing into account. The assessment of measurement **repeatability** and categorical **agreement** are special applications of these methods. In contrast to the simple before–after design (i.e. without a **control group**), results from matched pairs and crossover designs do not typically suffer from lack of internal **validity** (HUITEMA, 2011).

## Paired $t$-test

A special form of the **$t$-test** that is carried out to compare the **means** of paired (i.e. not **independent**) quantitative variables. Examples of **paired data** are measurements taken in the same group of patients *before* and *after* some treatment or intervention, or after each treatment in a two-period crossover trial. To carry out the test, a new variable is computed as the *difference* between the paired variables, which will have mean equal to zero if there are no differences, on average, between paired measurements. The number of **degrees of freedom** ($df$) for the paired $t$-test is $n - 1$, where $n$ is the number of pairs. An **assumption** of the paired $t$-test is that these differences are **normally distributed**. The **Wilcoxon test for matched pairs** may be used as an alternative if this assumption does not hold, and the **sign test** with paired **ordinal data**. See also **two-way ANOVA**.

## Pairwise matching

Synonym for *individual* **matching** (as opposed to *frequency* matching) in **case–control studies**. See also **matched pairs design**.

## PAR

Abbreviation for **population attributable risk**.

## Parabolic curve

Synonym for **quadratic curve**.

## Parallel design

The most frequently used **study design** for a **clinical trial**. As opposed to the **crossover design** where participants act as their own controls, in a parallel design two (or more) separate groups of patients each receive just one of the treatments or treatment regimens being compared, one of the groups acting as the **control group**. Methods for **independent** samples are generally appropriate when analysing the results from parallel trials. See also **randomized controlled trial**, **factorial design**. See FLEISS (1999) and MACHIN & CAMPBELL (2005) for further details.

## Parameter

A measure pertaining to a **population**, and which summarizes information on demographic and socioeconomic indicators, and on pattern of disease distribution. Population parameters are almost invariably impossible to measure, except where the population is limited in size, well-defined and static (what is referred to as a 'closed population'). With large populations in constant flux, it is virtually impossible or highly costly to ascertain every member of the population. More commonly, the value of a parameter of interest is estimated or inferred from the value of **sample statistics**. Population parameters are conventionally denoted by Greek letters, such as $\mu$ (mu) for the population mean, whereas the sample mean is denoted by $\bar{x}$ (read, 'x bar'). A distinction is sometimes made between population parameters such as the **prevalence** of disease or of some other characteristic, the estimation of which requires unbiased **sampling**, and the 'true effects' of **treatments** and **exposures**, which are estimated from study samples more or less precisely and accurately, depending on whether the study sample is sufficiently large and the assessment of effect **unbiased**. See also **regression coefficient** (model parameter), **probability distribution** (defined by its parameters).

## Parametric methods

Statistical methods of data analysis that rely on one or more distributional **assumptions** for the data being analysed, commonly, normality (data follow an approximately **Normal distribution**) and **homoscedasticity** (or constant variance). *t*-tests and **Pearson's correlation** are examples of parametric methods. See also **non-parametric methods**, **robust method**, **bootstrapping**.

## Parametric survival models

Two main classes of models provide a **parametric** alternative to **Cox regression**: **proportional hazards models** and **accelerated failure time models**, depending on how the model is specified. Proportional hazards models provide estimates of relative hazard (**hazard ratios**), while accelerated failure time models provide a means to predict *time to* **failure**. However, these models are usually specified as predicting survival probability (i.e. the **survival function** or [$S(t)$]), which is computationally more straightforward. The parametric survival function is continuous, rather than a step function (cf. **Kaplan–Meier survival curve**).

Proportional hazards models make some **assumption** regarding the distribution of **survival times**, in contrast with models fitted through Cox regression, a semi-parametric method that does not require any such assumptions to be made. The **distribution** of survival times (and therefore, the distribution of regression errors or **residuals**) typically displays a *positive* **skew** (as is often the case when negative values are not allowed), for which reason **maximum likelihood estimation**, rather than ordinary least squares, is the usual approach to analysis. Unlike Cox regression, parametric hazards models give an estimate of the **baseline hazard function** and may be used to predict the hazard or instantaneous rate, $h(t)$, at any given time $t$. The difficulty these models present is that the particular functional form for the baseline hazard, $h_0(t)$, must be specified in order for a model to be correctly parameterized (CLEVES, GOULD & MARCHENKO, 2016). The choice of form for the baseline hazard function determines the distributional assumption for the regression errors. For example, the exponential model assumes a *constant* baseline hazard rate, which implies an **exponential distribution** for the 'time to event' variable conditional on the predictors.

## Parsimony

The balance one aims to achieve between fit and simplicity when selecting **predictor variables** to be included in a **regression model** (HAMILTON, 1992). The adjusted $R^2$, for example, "reflects parsimony, because it combines a measure of fit ($R^2$) with a measure of the difference in complexity between data ($n$, sample size) and model ($K$, number of parameters estimated). This difference, $n - K$, is called the *residual degrees of freedom*." (HAMILTON, 1992, p. 72). See also **goodness-of-fit**, **multiple correlation coefficient** squared (see *r-squared*), **Mallow's $C_p$**, **Akaike's information criterion (AIC)**, **Bayesian information criterion (BIC)**.

## Partial correlation coefficient

In the context of **multivariable** data analysis, a measure of the **correlation** between any two variables, while adjusting for a third variable. The partial correlation coefficient is calculated from the **correlation coefficients** for each pairing of the variables involved. Subscript notation is normally used to denote the variables in the analysis, as, for example, $r_{FH|A}$, which might be taken to represent the partial correlation coefficient between $FEV_1$ (forced expiratory volume at 1 minute) and height, conditional on (or 'while adjusting for') age. As in the case of bivariate relationships, partial correlation coefficients should only be calculated for data arising from **random samples**. ALTMAN (1991) gives an interpretation of the square of the partial correlation coefficient in the context or **multiple** (or multivariable) **linear regression**, as being equivalent to the proportion of the **residual sum of squares** (from a model excluding the third variable) that is explained by adding this variable to the model, i.e. the difference between the residual sums of squares from the two models (excluding and including the third variable), divided by the residual sum of squares from the model without the variable. See also *r-squared*, **multiple correlation coefficient**, **standardized measures of effect**, **eta squared**, **omega squared**.

## Partial *F*-test

See *F*-test.

## Patient expected event rate

An estimate of a particular patient's **risk** of an adverse outcome over a given period of time. STRAUS *et al.* (2010) discuss the various ways in which a patient expected event rate (PEER) may be obtained, which include using the overall event rate in the control group,

## BOX P.2

Reproduced from Chatellier G *et al.* (1996). The number needed to treat: a clinically useful nomogram in its proper context. *Br Med J* **312**: 426–9, 563 (with permission).

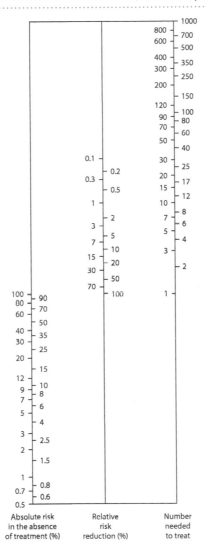

*Translating PEERs and RRRs into NNTs:*
To use the nomogram, a straight line is drawn through the value of the patient's PEER and the RRR estimate obtained from a relevant study, and the resulting NNT can be read off. CHATELLIER *et al.* (1996) discuss limitations of the method.

as given by a relevant research study, or, if available, using a subgroup-specific event rate. The PEER may be used in conjunction with the estimated **RRR** (**relative risk reduction**) to give a particularized estimate of the **NNT** (**number needed to treat**) for the same patient:

$$NNT = \frac{1}{(PEER \times RRR)}$$

Similarly, a particularized estimate of the **NNH (number needed to harm)** may be calculated on the basis of the PEER estimate for the adverse effect in question, and the corresponding **RRI (relative risk increase)** estimate. Box P.2 gives a **nomogram** that can be used to convert PEERs into NNTs, using RRRs. See also **likelihood of being helped** *vs.* **harmed (LHH)**.

## PCA

Abbreviation for **principal components analysis**.

## pdf

Abbreviation for **probability density function** or $f(x)$.

## Peaked curve

See **non-monotonic curve**. Cf. growth (**monotonic**) curve. See also **summary measures**.

## Pearson chi-squared statistic

A **test statistic** that is used to assess the overall **goodness-of-fit (GoF)** of **regression models** fitted by the method of **maximum likelihood**. The Pearson chi-squared statistic ($X^2$) is calculated as the sum of squared Pearson **residuals**, i.e. the square of the differences between **observed** and **fitted values** of the outcome variable (see AGRESTI, 2007). These are usually divided by the corresponding standard deviation, to be expressed as **standardized residuals**. This statistic plays a similar role (and is calculated in a similar way) to the **residual sum of squares** in least squares regression, in that the latter decreases as predictor variables are added to a model and the sum of squares due to regression increases, in the same way that the Pearson statistic decreases as variables are added to a model and the discrepancy between observed and fitted values decreases. Similarly to the **deviance statistic** ($D$), the Pearson $X^2$ statistic is based on a comparison between the current model and the corresponding **saturated model** (i.e. the observed data). (With zero count frequencies, Pearson residuals may still be calculated, but deviance residuals are undefined.) Under the **null hypothesis** of a similar fit, $X^2$ follows a **chi-squared ($\chi^2$) distribution** with **degrees of freedom** equal to the difference in number of **parameters** between the saturated model and the current model. With binary outcomes and data that are individual-level records (i.e. ungrouped), the validity of these assessments depends on the number of unique covariate patterns (see deviance statistic). A related statistic is $\Delta X^2$, which is the difference between the Pearson statistics of any two **nested models**, and is equivalent to the $G$ or **likelihood ratio test** statistic. See CLAYTON & HILLS (1993), HOSMER, LEMESHOW & STURDIVANT (2013) and Greenland, in ROTHMAN, GREENLAND & LASH (eds., 2012), for further details. When evaluating **overdispersion**, the *scale parameter* is estimated by the ratio of the Pearson $X^2$ statistic to the **residual degrees of freedom** (calculated as the number of observations *minus* the number of parameters in the model). Two additional applications are the assessment of goodness-of-fit of a **frequency distribution** or one-way table (see **chi-squared test for goodness-of-fit**) and the assessment of independence of the variables cross-tabulated in a $r \times c$ **contingency table** (see **chi-squared test**). Both applications involve the comparison of **observed** *vs.* **expected frequencies** in each cell of the table.

## Pearson's correlation coefficient

The product-moment **correlation coefficient**, *r*. A measure of the strength of the *linear* relationship between two **quantitative variables**. *r* may take any value between –1 and +1, where $r = -1$ represents a perfect negative correlation, $r = +1$ a perfect positive correlation, and $r = 0$ absence of a linear relationship (Figure C.2, p. 76). Thus, the absolute value of *r* indicates the **strength** of the linear relationship and its sign the **direction** of the relationship. It should be noted that $r = 0$ does not imply the absence of *any* relationship, but the absence of a *linear* one. An alternative way of assessing the strength of a relationship is to compute the square of *r*, i.e. **r-squared ($r^2$)**. The **statistical significance** of the correlation coefficient may be assessed by computing a *P*-value. It should be noted the latter cannot give information on the strength of the relationship itself: a small *P*-value is not synonymous with strong association, and may be an artefact of a very large sample size. An **assumption** of **parametric** correlation is that one or both variables (for significance testing or confidence interval estimation – see BLAND, 2015, for methodology) are **normally distributed**. When required assumptions cannot be met, **rank correlation** may be used instead. Figure P.1 shows a **scatterplot** of the positive association between daily intakes of lecithin (in grams per 1 kg of food intake) and cholesterol (in mg per 1 kg of food intake), in 388 Japanese men, women and children 6–59 years old (ISHINAGA *et al.*, 2005); the analysis is with adjustment of food intake to 1 kg/day. Pearson's correlation coefficient was 0.881, a strong positive correlation that replicates the results from the analysis without adjustment (see Figure O.2, p. 249). See also **Fisher's transformation**.

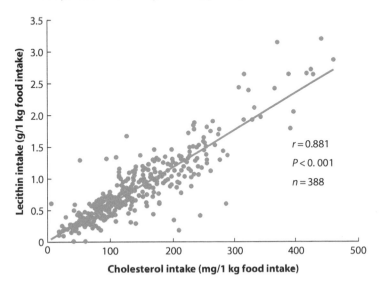

**Figure P.1** Pearson's correlation coefficient: scatterplot of daily lecithin intake (g/1 kg food intake) *vs.* cholesterol intake (mg/1 kg food intake) in 388 Japanese study participants. A strong positive correlation is obtained with and without adjustment of food intake to 1 kg per day (see Figure O.2, p. 249). (Reproduced from Ishinaga M *et al.* (2005). Cholesterol intake is associated with lecithin intake in Japanese people. *J Nutr* **135**: 1451–5 (with permission).)

## PEER

Abbreviation for **patient expected event rate**.

## Percentage

A ratio or **proportion** expressed as fraction in which the denominator is equal to 100. For example, $3/4 = 75/100$, i.e. 75%. See also **probability**, **percentage point.**

## Percentage change from baseline

See **change scores**.

## Percentage point

The difference between two **percentages** (which are each ratios) may be expressed as percentage points. Suppose the pass rate for a postgraduate medical examination used to be 30% 5 years ago, but is now 36%. The increase in the pass rate for this examination over the last 5 years is *not* 6%, but rather '6 percentage points'. In terms of percentage increase, the increase is $100 \times (36 - 30)/30 = 20\%$. The term 'percentage point' is also used to refer to threshold values in a **theoretical probability distribution** that correspond to given **probabilities** in the tails of the distribution (one- or two-sided). As the sampling distribution of **test statistics** is often approximated by such a distribution under the assumption that the **null hypothesis** is true, these threshold values coincide with the **critical values** for statistical significance at different levels of significance.

## Percentiles

See **centiles**.

## Perinatal mortality rate

The number of perinatal deaths occurring during a given time-period, in a given geographical region (such as a country), divided by the total number of births in the same region during the same time-period. The perinatal mortality rate is often multiplied by 1000 to be given as a rate per 1000 births (births = stillbirths and live births), and the time-period chosen is usually 1 year. A perinatal death is the death of a fetus or neonate (28 weeks of gestation to 1 week postpartum). See also **stillbirth rate, neonatal mortality rate, infant mortality rate.**

## Period effect

In the context of two-period and multiperiod **crossover trials**, this term refers to the effect of time on disease, as measured by relevant outcomes. This acknowledges the fact that both disease and patients' responses may vary from one period to the next, regardless of whether treatments are being administered concomitantly. Period effects are sometimes due to learning effects, as, for example, when patients learn to cope with pain. The presence of a period effect is not as much cause for concern as the presence of a **treatment–period interaction**, since treatment order is **randomly allocated** in crossover trials. A simple period effect should therefore affect all study treatments equally.

## Period prevalence

See **prevalence**.

## Permutation tests

Statistical **significance tests** that make an assessment of statistical significance by carrying out repeated permutations of the data between two groups that are being compared, to find out the proportion of permutations that gives rise to a **test statistic** that is at least as large as the test statistic first obtained by carrying out the relevant significance test on the data as actually observed. This proportion is the significance level or **P-value** for the given permutation test. Permutation tests do not make an assumption regarding the **sampling distribution** of the test statistic, and no other assumptions are made apart from assuming the observations to be **independent**. An example of a permutation test is **Fisher's exact test**. With fast computers readily available, permutation tests for significance testing may be carried out with relative speed; however, calculation of the corresponding **confidence intervals** using the same methodology can still sometimes prove too computationally expensive for some problems.

## Perprotocol analysis

In the context of **randomized controlled trials**, an approach to data analysis that only includes the data from patients or individuals who have adhered to the trial **protocol**. Those who, for some reason, **crossed-over** to the alternative treatment, or were not in **compliance** with their allocated treatment, are not included. This approach is more commonly adopted in the analysis of **explanatory** rather than **pragmatic trials**, but nonetheless can open the results to **bias** (specifically, selection bias). See also **Phase III trial**. Cf. **intention-to-treat analysis**.

## Person-time at risk

Or its abbreviation, PTAR. The sum of the lengths of time each individual is under observation in a **follow-up study** (**observational study** or **clinical trial**). It may be estimated as the average number at risk of the event of interest (for example, contracting a disease or dying) multiplied by the length of the study period. Person-time is often expressed as person-years – person-years at risk (PYAR) – but it may also be expressed as person-days, person-weeks, etc. Person-time at risk is the denominator in the computation of **rates**. Box P.3 gives a worked example of a PYAR calculation.

---

**BOX P.3**

**Worked example:**
Follow-up study with five patients (not really a good idea!) over a 3-year period. Two deaths (event of interest) are observed during the follow-up period. The length of follow-up for each patient is:

| Patient | Duration of follow-up | |
| --- | --- | --- |
| 1 | 3 years | **Total PYAR =** |
| 2 | 2 years and 7 months | 12 person-years and 4 person-months |

*continued...*

*continued...*

| Patient | Duration of follow-up | |
|---------|----------------------|---|
| 3 | 1 year and 9 months | = 12.333 person-years |
| 4 | 3 years | **Mortality rate** = 2 per 12.333 PYAR |
| 5 | 2 years | = 0.16 per PYAR = 16 per 100 PYAR |

*Interpretation:* With a constant death rate of 16 per 100 per year (year⁻¹), the average time to the event (or the average **life expectancy**) among a cohort with similar characteristics to the patients above, is given by the inverse of the rate, i.e. 1/(16/100) = 1/0.16 = 6.25 years. Over 100 person-years of observation, 16 deaths are expected to occur.

Where length of follow-up varies among study participants, **risks** may not be calculated. **Survival analysis** and **Poisson regression** are often used to analyse these data (see also **offset**). See KIRKWOOD & STERNE (2003) for alternative approaches to defining 'time at risk' in a follow-up study.

## Peto's method

A statistical method for **pooling** or combining **odds ratios (OR)** in a **meta-analysis**, to produce a single summary or overall measure of **treatment** or **exposure effect**. The method, also known as Yusuf and Peto's method, is particularly useful with rare events, provided treatment groups have similar sizes, and the effect in question is not too large, i.e. provided the estimated OR is not too far from 1, the null value (BRADBURN *et al.*, 2007). A **two-by-two table** summarizes the results in each **primary study** and the estimated OR in each of these studies is based on the comparison between **observed** and **expected frequency** for cell *a* (see Table 2.b, p. 72; cell *a* is treatment YES/outcome YES). The estimated overall odds ratio is a **weighted average** of the odds ratios obtained for each individual study. This parallels the computations for the **logrank test** (the Mantel–Haenszel $\chi^2$ test variation), and provides an alternative method of pooling **hazard ratios** (*HR*), by first pooling across time strata within each individual study and then across all studies ($HR_{Peto}$). See also **inverse variance method**, **Mantel–Haenszel method**. See Deeks, Altman & Bradburn, in EGGER, DAVEY SMITH & ALTMAN (eds., 2001), for formulae and illustrative examples.

## Pharmacovigilance

The study of risks with regard to **adverse drug reactions**. Methods can include observational studies and clinical trials. Spontaneous (and *ad hoc*) reports of adverse reactions to drugs can be very difficult to interpret but still also fall within the scope of pharmacovigilance. See also **Phase IV study**. See WALLER & EVANS (2003), and COLEMAN, FERRER & EVANS (2006) for a comprehensive discussion of issues around pharmacovigilance.

## Phase I trial

In the context of pharmacological research, a **clinical trial** that is conducted early on with a relatively small number of patients in order to evaluate the safety of a new drug or compound. The aim is to determine the maximum tolerable dose or MTD, i.e. the dose just below that at which dose-limiting toxicity (DLT) occurs. Phase I trials are usually preceded by preclinical and pharmacokinetic (or **bioequivalence**) studies. POCOCK (1983), MACHIN & CAMPBELL (2005), Sackett, in HAYNES *et al.* (eds., 2006), and SENN (2008) give details. See also **crossover design**, **Phase II trial**, **Phase III trial**, **Phase IV study**; $C_{max}$, $T_{max}$, **AUC**.

## Phase II trial

A **clinical trial** that is conducted with a small number of patients with the target disease, to find the dose and dose schedule that appear to have the most **efficacy**, as *preliminarily* assessed by comparing the activity level or pharmacodynamics of several doses and schedules, based on the maximum tolerable dose evaluation of a preceding **Phase I trial**. Phase II trials may be subdivided into non-comparative Phase IIA trials, which are primarily concerned with confirming dose requirements for the desired pharmacodynamic effect (i.e. the effect on the structure and function of tissues and organs), and comparative Phase IIB trials (or randomized selection designs), which are primarily concerned with comparing the activity level of different compounds. MACHIN & CAMPBELL (2005) discuss **study designs** for Phase II trials, which include single-stage (**Fleming–A'Hern**) and two-stage designs (**Gehan**, **Simon-optimal**, **Simon-minimax**, **Tan–Machin** single- and dual-threshold designs, and **Bryant–Day**). Two-stage designs are **sequential**, for which reason they incorporate an **interim analysis**. See also POCOCK (1983), Sackett, in HAYNES *et al.* (eds., 2006), and SENN (2008); **Case–Morgan design**, **drop-the-losers design**, **adaptive seamless Phase II/III design**, **crossover design**, **Phase III trial**.

## Phase III trial

A **clinical trial** that is conducted to evaluate the **efficacy** of new (or existing) drugs against standard treatments or placebos, or the **effectiveness** of the same once their safety and efficacy have been provisionally established. Phase III trials are normally conducted in the typical settings where patients and clinicians interface. Efficacy or explanatory trials are conducted under a stricter **protocol** than effectiveness trials, including more restrictive **eligibility criteria**. The latter require a larger number of patients, in order to account for **protocol breaches** and greater between-patient **variability** of response, and to allow small **treatment effects** to be detected when evaluating treatments for common diseases. In the latter situation, while the treatment effects may be modest the net impact may nonetheless be considerable. See **superiority trial**, **equivalence trial** and **non-inferiority trial**; **crossover design**, **parallel design** and **factorial design** for types of study and study designs for Phase III trials. See also **explanatory trial**, **perprotocol analysis**, **pragmatic trial**, **intention-to-treat analysis**, **Phase II trial**, **Phase IV study**; POCOCK (1983), MACHIN & CAMPBELL (2005), Sackett, in HAYNES *et al.* (eds., 2006), and SENN (2008).

## Phase IV study

Also termed postmarketing surveillance or monitoring, Phase IV studies (not trials, usually) are conducted after a new drug has been introduced in the market, in order to monitor acceptability, **compliance** and the occurrence of **adverse events**. WALLER & EVANS

(2003) and COLEMAN, FERRER & EVANS (2006) provide in-depth discussion of issues around **pharmacovigilance**. See also Sackett, in HAYNES *et al.* (eds., 2006), SENN (2008) and ROTHMAN (2012).

## PI

Abbreviation for **prognostic index**.

## Pick-the-winners design

See **drop-the-losers design**.

## Pictograph

A **graphical** representation of **treatment** or **exposure effect**, which may be used as a communication tool to convey both *absolute* and *relative* effect. The example in Figure P.2 (TAIT *et al.*, 2012) shows **incidence risk** in each treatment group as the number of individuals out of 100 in which the event of interest has occurred. 'Individuals' with the event of interest in each group are shown in highlighted colouring so that an immediate comparison between groups is possible (relative effect). The contrast with the

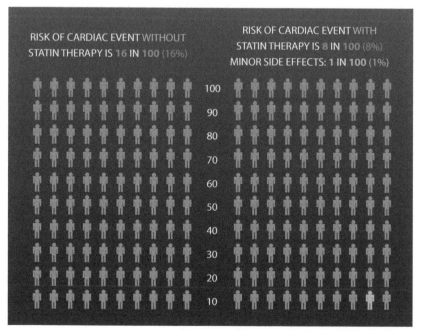

**Figure P.2** A pictograph comparing the risk of a cardiac event in patients with hypercholesterolemia and receiving statins *vs.* not receiving statins. Relative and absolute treatment effect are readily communicated. (Reproduced from Tait R *et al.* (2012). Using animated computer-generated text and graphics to depict the risks and benefits of medical treatments. *Am J Med* **125**: 1103–10 (with permission).)

number of individuals within each group without the event enables an assessment to be made as to how common or rare the event in question is, and the difference between these assessments gives a representation of absolute effect. This type of information, when communicated to a patient, allows **relative** and **absolute effects** to be put in perspective. For example, a large **relative risk** may look less dramatic when overall risks are very low, but a small one may result in large **risk differences** when risks are moderate or high. See also MUSCATELLO *et al.* (2006).

## Pie chart

A **graphical display** that is used to depict the **relative frequencies** of the different groups or categories within a **categorical variable**, with each sector ('slice') of a circular disc (the 'pie') being proportional to the corresponding relative frequency or percentage. If a group within the categorical variable has an observed frequency of $x$, and if the total frequency for the variable is $N$, then the relative frequency in that group is $x/N$, and the angle of the corresponding slice of the pie chart is $2\pi N/x$, or $360N/x$ in degrees. Figure P.3 shows the estimated distribution of causes of 4 million neonatal deaths for the year 2000, in the study by LAWN, COUSENS & ZUPAN (2005), with the corresponding percentages given next to the sectors.

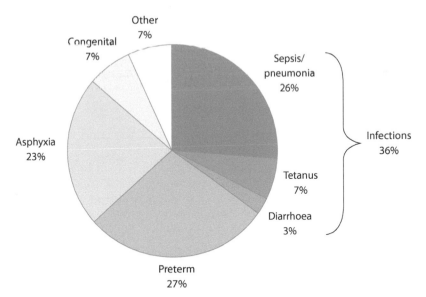

**Figure P.3** Pie chart: distribution of direct causes of 4 million neonatal deaths for the year 2000 based on vital registration data (45 countries) and modelled estimates (147 countries). (Reproduced from Lawn JE *et al.* (2005). Neonatal survival 1: 4 million neonatal deaths: When? Where? Why? *Lancet* **365**: 891–900 (with permission).)

## Piecewise regression

Synonym for **spline regression**.

## Pilot study

A small-scale study that is carried out in order to obtain information with which to design and plan the logistical needs of a larger study. As an example, a pilot study may be carried out to obtain an estimate of **variability** for a given measurement (the outcome variable), in order for **sample size** requirements to be calculated more accurately. Data collected during a pilot study may or not be incorporated as part of the main study. See also **sensitivity analyses**.

## Placebo

An inactive or dummy treatment that is given to the **control group** in a **clinical trial** in order to prevent **information biases**, as it enables both patients and researchers to remain **blind** to treatments given. Placebos must be similar to active treatments (colour, taste, mode of administration) if they are going to have the desired effect. The administration of placebos is widely regarded as unethical (ROTHMAN & MICHELS, 1994; MICHELS & ROTHMAN, 2003) if standard treatments are available that, albeit with drawbacks, are indicated and effective for the condition or disease in question. In these situations, experimental treatments should be evaluated against existing treatments and not against a placebo, especially where the target disease is likely to have an unfavourable outcome in absence of any treatment. See POCOCK (1983) for further discussion. See also **placebo effect**, **placebo group**.

## Placebo-controlled trial

A **clinical trial** in which the **control group** is administered a **placebo** treatment. Cf. a clinical trial in which the control group is administered an **active treatment**.

## Placebo effect

A component of **treatment effect** that may be mediated by the brain, through neurophysiological processes unrelated to the biological **efficacy** of the treatment itself. These appear to derive from the mere fact that one is undergoing some form of treatment. Thus, whenever possible, the **control group** in a **clinical trial** should be administered either an **active treatment** or a **placebo**, and trial participants should remain **blind** (as should researchers) as to which treatment, new active *vs.* standard active, or active *vs.* placebo, is being administered. Although observed effects in the placebo treatment group (for example, a reduction in average blood pressure measurements) are often ascribed to a placebo effect, SENN (2011) points out that it is in fact not possible in most instances to distinguish between a placebo effect and **regression to the mean**. Whereas clinical trials usually include just two treatment arms, a third treatment arm comprising individuals not subjected to any treatments or placebos would be needed to accomplish this goal. BLAND (2015) discusses a number of factors affecting response to placebo treatments, including the colour and appearance of inert tablets and the nature of the target disease. A discussion of ethical issues and constraints is given by BLAND (2015) and POCOCK (1983).

## Placebo group

In the context of **clinical trials**, a **control group** to whom a dummy or **placebo** treatment is administered. See also **placebo effect**. Cf. **active control group**.

## Platykurtic

The quality of a **distribution** that has a negative **kurtosis**, i.e. is flatter (higher tail densities) than the corresponding **Normal distribution**. At the extreme, this may be a peakless **uniform** or rectangular distribution that is bounded by a lower and upper value. See also **mesokurtic**, **leptokurtic**.

## Plunger plot

Synonym for **error bar chart**.

## PMC

Abbreviation for probability of misclassification. See **classification table**.

## PMR

Abbreviation for **proportional mortality ratio**.

## Pocock's approach

See **stopping rules**.

## Point estimate

See **estimate**.

## Point prevalence

See **prevalence**.

## Poisson distribution

The **probability distribution** that is followed by **independent** processes or events that may be counted over time or space. It is assumed these events occur **randomly**, and at a constant **rate**, $\lambda$ (lambda). The Poisson distribution is defined by one **parameter** alone, the **mean** ($\mu$ or mu), which is estimated by the mean number of occurrences of the event in question over time intervals of equal length. When the mean number of events is calculated in reference to unit of time, area or volume, the mean, $\mu$, is given by the rate itself, $\lambda$. The **exact probability** of the occurrence of $r$ events per unit of time, area or volume is given by the Poisson **probability mass function**:

$$\text{Prob}(X = r) = \frac{e^{-\mu}\mu^r}{r!}$$

where $X$ is a Poisson **random variable**, $\mu$ is the mean, $r!$ is **factorial** $r$, and $e$ is the mathematical constant 2.718.... As an example, suppose admissions to a medical ward average a mean number of three per day. To work out the probability of there being no more than two admissions on any one day, we proceed as follows:

Required probability = probability of 0, 1 or 2 daily admissions

= (probability of 0 daily admissions) + (probability of 1 daily admission) + (probability of 2 daily admissions)

= $e^{-3}3^0/0! + e^{-3}3^1/1! + e^{-3}3^2/2!$

= $e^{-3}(1/1 + 3/1 + 9/2)$

= $8.5\ e^{-3}$

= 0.423 (to 3 significant figures) or 42.3%

As the mean increases, the positively skewed shape of the distribution increasingly resembles a **Normal distribution** (as the probability of zero or low occurrences decreases) and the Poisson distribution may be approximated by the Normal. For the purposes of **estimation** and **significance testing**, the **variance** is also equal to the mean, from which the standard error (SE) of the mean is calculated as $\sqrt{\mu}$ (square root of mu). A distinguishing factor between the Poisson and **binomial** distributions is the fact that for the former the number of 'trials' does not need to be known. The Poisson distribution may be used to approximate the binomial when $p$ (the probability of a trial being a success) is small (for example, <0.05) and sample size is large. In addition to describing the **sampling distribution** of the number of events (or alternatively, the sampling distribution of the **rate**) that may arise in a given time interval, surface area or capacity volume, the Poisson distribution may also appropriately describe the **frequency distribution** of *individual* **counts** (or individual rates). When the null hypothesis is true, the Poisson distribution is the sampling distribution of the observed frequencies in each cell of a **contingency table**. The link between Poisson and **chi-squared distribution** is explained under **approximation**. See also **count variable, overdispersion, negative binomial distribution, Poisson regression**.

## Poisson heterogeneity test

Synonym for **chi-squared test for goodness-of-fit**.

## Poisson regression

A **regression** method that is used to model **counts** and **rates**. It may be used, for example, to compare two **exposure groups** with regard to the number of occurrences of a disease of interest. The **outcome variable** in a Poisson model is the count or number of occurrences in each group (the numerator of the rate; at the individual level, the outcome is a 'occurred/did not occur' binary variable). The denominator (**person-time at risk** or **PTAR**) is included as an **offset** explanatory variable, on a log scale. Poisson models are usually reported as predicting the log of the rate (not the log of the count), and take the following form, with a **logarithmic transformation** of the predicted outcome as a linear function of the log baseline rate (in this example, the log rate in the unexposed) and the **predictor variable(s)** in the model:

$$\ln(rate) = b_0 + b_1x_1$$

where 'rate' is the predicted number of events per person-time at risk, $b_0$ is the log of the estimated baseline rate, and $b_1$ is the estimated **regression coefficient** for the predictor variable, $x_1$ (for example, a binary exposure coded '0' if absent or '1' if present). Anti-logging this coefficient gives the **rate ratio**, i.e. the relative effect of the exposure (or the factor by which the predicted rate increases for each unit increase in a quantitative predictor variable). As is the case with all **generalized linear models**, additional predictors (for example, confounding variables and interaction terms) may be added to the model. See KIRKWOOD & STERNE (2003) and HAMILTON (2012) for illustrative examples. Another example of group- or population-level count data is illustrated by BLAND (2015) with the analysis of an interrupted **time series**. The offset variable gives the number of time units over which counts were recorded. Poisson regression may be used also to model *individual* counts, provided the **assumption** of a **Poisson distribution** is met. Here, and for each observation, the offset gives the number of time, space or person-time units over which counts were recorded. Overdispersed Poisson and **negative binomial regression** are alternative methods that may be employed when the count variable shows **overdispersion** (GARDNER, MULVEY & SHAW, 1995; AGRESTI, 2007; ALEXANDER, 2012). **Zero-inflated** regression (Poisson or negative binomial) may be used when overdispersion is due (or due in part) to an excess of zero counts (DWIVEDI *et al.*, 2010), and **random effects** models may be employed when overdispersed counts arise in the context of **clustered designs**. Poisson regression with categorical predictors is equivalent to **log-linear modelling** for contingency tables. An example of the type of outcome that may be modelled using Poisson regression is shown in Figure P.4, from the randomized placebo-controlled trial by ERMERS *et al.* (2009) of the effects of high-dose inhaled corticosteroids on wheeze in infants after respiratory syncytial virus infection (RSVI). The primary outcome is the number of days with wheeze in the year after the 3-month intervention period that followed a hospital admission for 243 infants. **Back-transformation** of the **regression coefficient** from the fitted Poisson model gives treatment effect as a **rate ratio**. From the results obtained, the authors conclude that "Early

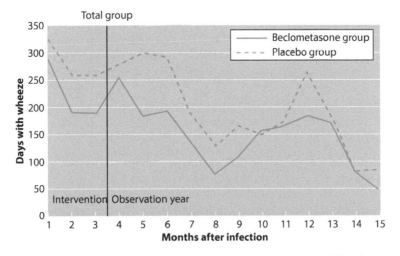

**Figure P.4** Poisson regression: comparison of days with wheeze between 119 infants administered beclometasone (1761 out of 33,568 total days of observation) and 124 infants administered a placebo inhaler (2301 out of 36,556 total days of observation) in the year after a 3-month intervention following hospital admission due to RSVI (*P*-value = 0.31). (Reproduced from Ermers M *et al.* (2009). The effect of high dose inhaled corticosteroids on wheeze in infants after respiratory syncytial virus infection: randomised double blind placebo controlled trial. *Br Med J* **338**: b897 (with permission).)

initiated high-dose extra fine HFA beclometasone to infants during the first 3 months after hospital admission for respiratory syncytial virus infection has no major effect on recurrent wheeze. The general use of such treatment during lower respiratory tract infection with respiratory syncytial virus should not be advocated."

## Polychotomous variable

Synonym for **nominal variable**.

## Polynomial regression

A method of **regression analysis** in which a continuous variable and its square, cubic or quartic power **transformations** are included as **predictors** in order to accommodate a non-linear relationship between outcome and continuous predictor. Reference is made to lower and higher order polynomials, depending on the number of 'turn points' in the relationship that is being modelled. As an example, the equation for the **quadratic curve** (a second order polynomial with one turn point – see Figure Q.1, p. 292) may be written as follows:

$$\hat{y} = a + b_1 x_1 + b_2 x_1^2$$

where $\hat{y}$ (read 'y hat') is the predicted value of the **outcome variable**; $x_1$ are the observed values of the continuous predictor or independent variable; $b_1$ is the **regression coefficient** associated with the *untransformed* or linear predictor; $b_2$ is the regression coefficient associated with the *square* power transformed predictor; and $a$ is the **intercept** or constant ($b_2 x_1^2$ is the **quadratic term**). This corresponds to a **fractional polynomial** with powers from the set {1, 2} (polynomial powers are integers, fractional polynomial powers are a mix of integers and fractions). A test of significance for the quadratic term may be carried out to test for a departure from a **linear relationship**. In addition, higher power terms (cubic, $x^3$; quartic, $x^4$, etc.) may be included for the same predictor variable to test for departures from a quadratic or parabolic curve. Additional predictor variables may be added to this **model**, where, for each predictor, a differently shaped relationship with the outcome variable may be specified. **Collinearity** may be present in polynomial models as linear predictors and their power transformations may be highly correlated. BLAND (2015) gives a simple method for reducing, if not eliminating, the correlation between these variables. See also **non-linear relationship, curvilinear regression**; MITCHELL (2012b).

## Polytomous logistic regression

A **logistic regression** method for **categorical outcomes** with more than two unordered categories (e.g. different conditions associated with chest pain – angina, acute myocardial infarction, acid reflux, pneumonia, etc., or different categories of cause of death). Also termed multinomial logistic regression. See AGRESTI (2007), HOSMER, LEMESHOW & STURDIVANT (2013), HAMILTON (2012) and MITCHELL (2012b) for further details and illustrative examples. See also **ordered logistic regression**.

## Pooled estimate

An estimate of **exposure** or **treatment effect** that is obtained in the context of **meta-analysis**, and also when evaluating these same effects across categories or strata of a

**confounding variable**. The pooled estimate is a **weighted average** across individual studies or across the categories of the confounder. Weights are commonly based on the **inverse variance** method, the **Mantel–Haenszel** method or **Peto's** method. Where there is marked **heterogeneity** of effect, the **fixed effect** assumption is no longer valid, and the pooled estimate of effect is calculated as an estimate of the mean or 'average effect' rather than an estimate of the 'true effect'. Modified weights are used in these calculations to accommodate the **variance** of the **random effects**. See also pooled **diagnostic odds ratio**.

## Pooling

See **pooled estimate**.

## Population

In statistical terms, a population is the collective of persons or items that is the subject of an investigation, and from which **study samples** are taken so that **inferences** regarding population **parameters** and 'true effects' may be made. A population may be finite (e.g. the human population of a country at a specific time point) or infinite (e.g. the result of rolling a couple of dice repeatedly). As it may not be practical (or indeed possible, in the case of an infinite population) to sample the whole population to determine the values of its parameters, sample **statistics** or **estimates** are calculated instead, which, if based on unbiased **sampling** and sufficiently large **sample sizes**, can give an accurate representation of the distribution of the features of interest in the population. Likewise, the true, underlying effects of treatments and exposures are estimated from study samples in comparative studies, and aim to provide **unbiased** and **precise** assessments of **treatment** and **exposure effect**. See also **study population, source population, target population**.

## Population at risk

The population that, at a given point in time, is disease-free or has not yet experienced some event to which it is susceptible, and thus is at risk for the occurrence of this same disease or outcome. In research studies, the population at risk may be expressed as **number of people at risk** (leading to the calculation of incidence and mortality **risks**), or as person-contributed time units or **person-time at risk** (leading to the calculation of incidence and mortality **rates**).

## Population attributable fraction

The **population attributable risk** (**PAR**) may be expressed as a fraction of the incidence of disease in the **study population**, the population *proportional* attributable risk or attributable fraction (PAF or AF$_{population}$), which is a **measure of the impact** of an **exposure** on a population, with regard to a specific disease (see illustrative example in Box P.4, p. 270):

$$Population\ attributable\ fraction = \frac{incidence\ in\ population - incidence\ in\ unexposed}{incidence\ in\ population}$$

i.e. PAF = PAR/(incidence in population). The population attributable fraction is sometimes referred to as population risk proportion, or population attributable risk percent when expressed as a **percentage**. Box P.4 gives an alternative formula for calculating the PAF based on **relative risk** measures and on an estimate of **prevalence** of exposure. Yet an alternative calculation is by multiplying the **attributable fraction** among the exposed (**AF**$_{exposed}$) by the *proportion of cases* in the population that are exposed (ROTHMAN, 2012). The last two formulae may also be used to calculate the PAF for a population that is broader than the actual study population. In case–control studies, in which risks and risk differences may not usually be obtained, the equation in Box P.4 allows the computation of the population attributable fraction, using the **odds ratio** as the measure of association (HENNEKENS, BURING & MAYRENT (eds.), 1987). See also Greenland, in ROTHMAN, GREENLAND & LASH (eds., 2012), for formulae and additional discussion and interpretation. Both Greenland, and KIRKWOOD & STERNE (2003) discuss the more realistic concept of *impact fraction* or *percentage impact*, in connection with the more likely scenario of partial, not total, removal of exposure.

## Population attributable risk

A **measure of the impact** an **exposure** or risk factor has on a **study population**, in terms of excess risk of disease (i.e. in *net* terms). The population attributable risk (PAR) depends not only on how strongly associated the exposure in question is with a particular disease, but, more importantly, on the **prevalence** of the exposure. It is calculated as follows:

*Population attributable risk = incidence in population – incidence in unexposed*

where incidence in population = (incidence in exposed) + (incidence in unexposed). Alternatively, it may be calculated as (**attributable risk**) × (prevalence of exposure); see HENNEKENS, BURING & MAYRENT (eds., 1987). A valid estimate of exposure prevalence is particularly important in calculating the PAR for a broader population than the actual study population. The example given in Box P.4 (WALD, 2004, pp.12–14) illustrates the concepts discussed in this entry and under **population attributable fraction (PAF)**.

---

**BOX P.4**

Adapted from Wald NJ (2004). *The Epidemiological Approach: An Introduction to Epidemiology in Medicine, 4th edition.* Wolfson Institute of Preventive Medicine & The Royal Society of Medicine Press (with permission).

. . . . . . . . . . . . . . . . . . . . . . . . . . . . . . . . . . . . . . . . . . . . . . . . . . . . . . . . . . . . . . . . .

The study by DOLL *et al.* (1994) has become a classic example to demonstrate the concepts of relative and absolute effect. It considers the association between smoking and mortality to lung cancer and ischaemic heart disease (IHD). In the first case, the association is rather strong (RR = 14.9), and in the second case, it is weak (RR = 1.6) (RR stands for risk ratio, or, as in this example, for rate ratio). However, the *impact* of the exposure (cigarette smoke) is greater for ischaemic heart disease than for lung cancer (as judged by the absolute excess risk, i.e. the attributable risk or absolute risk increase), due to the fact that the former is a more common condition and makes a greater contribution to overall mortality than the latter. PAR = absolute excess risk × prevalence of exposure.

*continued...*

*continued...*

| Cause of death | Age-standardized annual death rate per 100,000 | | | Absolute excess risk (death rate per 100,000 per year) |
| | Non-smokers | Current smokers | RR | |
| --- | --- | --- | --- | --- |
| **Lung cancer** | 14 | 209 | 14.9 | 209 – 14 = 195 |
| **IHD** | 542 | 892 | 1.6 | 892 – 542 = 350 |

*Source:* Doll R *et al.* (1994). Mortality in relation to smoking: 40 years' observations on male British doctors. *Br Med J* **309**: 901–11.

WALD gives a hypothetical but realistic example of how RRs may be translated into number (or rather, proportion) of premature deaths prevented in a particular population, with a given prevalence (*p*) of exposure to cigarette smoke. It assumes approximately 30% of men in the age group 45–54 (the population) to be smokers, and the risk of dying from ischaemic heart disease to be 3 per 1000 per year among smokers and 1 per 1000 per year among non-smokers (RR = 3). The PAF may be calculated using this alternative formula:

$$PAF = \frac{p(RR-1)}{p(RR-1)+1} = \frac{0.3(3-1)}{0.3(3-1)+1} = \frac{0.6}{1.6} = 0.38 \text{ or } 38\%$$

*Interpretation:* 38% of IHD deaths in this population of 45–54-year-old males may be attributed to cigarette smoking, i.e. could be prevented (in principle) by removal of the exposure.

## Population attributable risk percent

Synonym for **population attributable fraction** (expressed as a **percentage**).

## Population-averaged model

See **marginal model, generalized estimating equations (GEEs)**.

## Population-based case–control study

See **case–control study, control group**. Cf. hospital-based case–control study.

## Population parameter

See **parameter**.

## Population pyramid

A **graphical display** of the age/gender **distribution** of a given **population**, where the **absolute** or **relative frequency** in the different age groups is presented in the form of horizontally stacked bars, the length of each bar being proportional to the frequency in the corresponding age group; basically, a sideways **histogram**. The age distribution of each gender group may be presented side by side on the same graph, as shown in Figures P.5a and P.5b. The same display may be used to compare the age distributions of any two populations. The pyramid in Figure P.5a (age/sex population structure of Cuba in 2015) may be described as a *stable* population pyramid (BLAND, 2015), with a relative frequency in the older age groups that is higher than would be seen on an *expanding* population pyramid (Figure P.5b, age/sex population structure of Guatemala in 1990 and 2015). The former reflects a population with lower birth and fertility rates, lower infant and child death rates and, to some extent, lower mortality in the older age groups. On the other hand, expanding

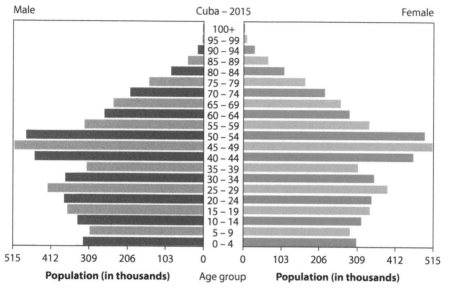

Figure P.5a Stable population pyramid: age structure of the male and female populations of Cuba (2015) as absolute frequency (in thousands) in each age group. (Reproduced from US Census Bureau.)

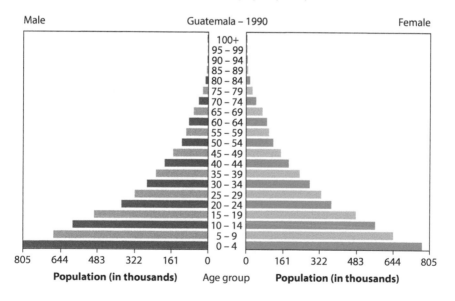

Figure P.5b Expanding population pyramid: age structure of the male and female populations of Guatemala (1990 and 2015) as absolute frequency (in thousands) in each age group. (Reproduced from US Census Bureau.)

*(Continued)*

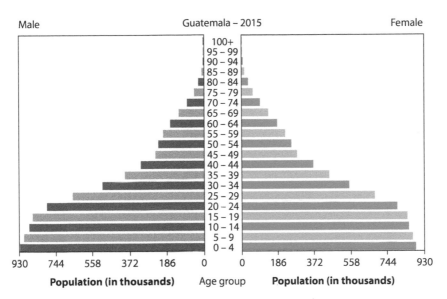

Figure P.5b *(Continued)*

population pyramids have a characteristic triangular shape, with a wide base reflecting higher birth and fertility rates, higher infant and child mortality and, to some extent, lower life expectancy. The population pyramids for Guatemala give an indication that infant and child mortality rates have decreased between 1990 and 2015. See also **demographic indicators, standardization**.

## Positive correlation

See **correlation**.

## Positive predictive value

See **predictive values**.

## Positive skew

See **skewness**.

## Positive study

A study that yields **statistically significant** results. This, however, does not necessarily imply **clinical significance**, especially in large studies where statistical tests will have greater **power** to detect small or negligible effects as statistically significant. This illustrates the difficulties with drawing inferences based solely on statistical significance. The **confidence interval** for the same statistically significant result would need to be evaluated for an assessment of clinical significance and potential impact. See also **negative study,** ***P*-value**.

## Post-test odds

Or 'odds of being affected if positive test result' (OAPR). See **post-test probability**.

## Post-test probability

In the context of **diagnostic testing**, the post-test probability of disease is the probability that an individual actually has the disease or condition of interest, given a particular test result. The post-test probability depends not only on the **prevalence** of the condition in question, but also on the **likelihood ratio (LR)** for the particular test result. It is calculated as follows:

$$Post\text{-}test\ probability = \frac{post\text{-}test\ odds}{post\text{-}test\ odds + 1}$$

where post-test odds = LR × pretest odds (see **pretest probability**). For dichotomous test results, the post-test probability of disease given a positive test result is the *positive* **predictive value** (or PPV) of the test, and the post-test probability of disease given a negative test result is given by 1 − NPV (*negative* predictive value). See Guyatt, Sackett & Haynes, in HAYNES *et al.* (eds., 2006), for further discussion. Box P.5 shows a **nomogram** that may be used to convert pretest probabilities into post-test probabilities given the likelihood ratio for a particular test result (or alternatively, and for a dichotomous test result, given the sensitivity and specificity of the test). WALD (2004) points out the greater usefulness of post-test odds (or OAPR) *vs.* post-test probability (or PPV), as it lends itself to the numerical calculations in sequential testing: the post-test odds for a given test result may be used as the pretest odds for the subsequent test, provided the tests are independent. It also better reflects differences in performance or detection rate between tests. See also FAGAN (1975); **SnNout, SpPin**.

### BOX P.5

Reproduced from Caraguel CGB, Vanderstichel R (2013). The two-step Fagan's nomogram: *ad hoc* interpretation of a diagnostic test result without calculation. *Evid Based Med* **18**: 125–8 (with permission).

**The two-step Fagan's nomogram:** This nomogram is used in two steps: in step I, the LR for the particular test result is obtained (LR⁺ if positive test result, LR⁻ if negative test result), by drawing a straight line that connects the values for sensitivity and specificity on the respective scales (light green for positive test result, dark green for negative test result). In step II, the value for post-test probability is read off by drawing a straight line that connects the value for pretest probability and the LR from step I, and intersects the post-test probability scale. If the LR value is known, the procedure simplifies to step II.

*— continued...*

continued...

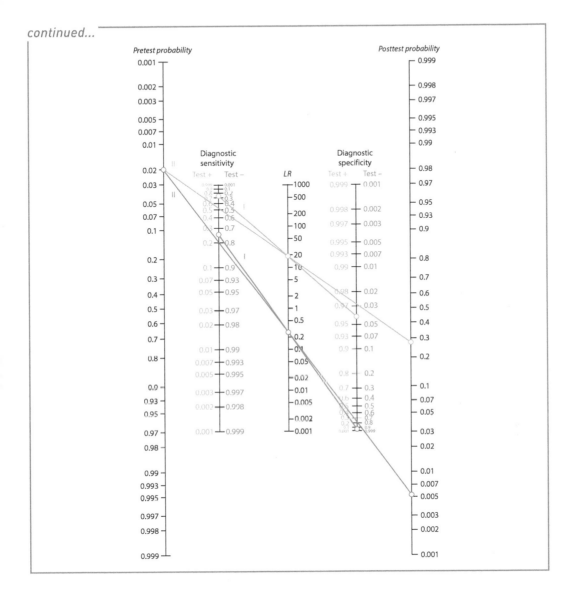

## Post-treatment measurement

See **outcome variable, before–after comparison, change** (study of), **analysis of covariance (ANCOVA)**. Cf. pretreatment or **baseline measurement, change scores**.

## Posterior distribution

The **probability distribution** of a **parameter** given the observed data, which derives from its **prior distribution** and **likelihood**, i.e. probability of the data given the model parameter. The posterior distribution is used to obtain the range of likely values or **credible interval (CrI)** for the parameter of interest. See **Bayesian inference, Bayes' factor**.

# Power

In the context of **significance testing**, the probability of detecting a true effect of a given magnitude as **statistically significant**. Also, the probability of meeting a stipulated level of statistical significance for a study result when the **null hypothesis** is false, or the probability of avoiding a **type II error**. For example, in a clinical trial of size N, 80% power means an 80% chance that a specified **minimally important difference** (**MID**), if a true effect,

## BOX P.6

Reproduced from Altman D (1991). *Practical Statistics for Medical Research*. CRC Press (with permission).
.................................................................................................................................

**Nomogram for sample size or power calculations:**
To use this nomogram, differences are standardized by dividing the MID by the **standard deviation** of the measurements. A straight line going through the value of the **standardized difference** and the desired level of power gives the required total **sample size** (N) for a **significance level** (alpha or α) of 0.01 or 0.05 (1% and 5%). Alternatively, the level of power for specific sample sizes and α levels may also be read off. Calculations for binary outcomes are given under 'standardized difference'.

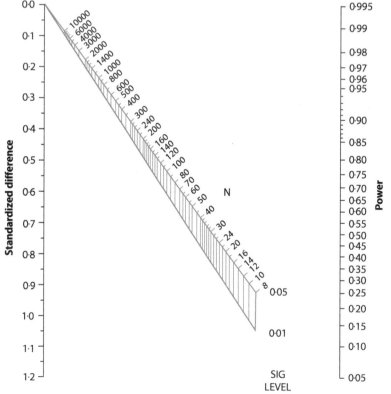

Reproduced from Altman D (1982). How large a sample? In: *Statistics in Practice*. Gore S, Altman D (eds.), p. 7, Figure 2. British Medical Association.

will be found to be statistically significant at the stipulated level of significance or **alpha**. The larger the difference or effect to be detected, the greater the power of the relevant statistical test. Power may be increased by increasing a study's **sample size** and/or decreasing the level of significance required for the results (i.e. by increasing the tolerance for a **type I error**). In addition, with quantitative outcomes, the greater the **variability** of individual measurements, the lower the power of a statistical test. The complement of power is the **type II error** ($\beta$) (power = $1 - \beta$). ALTMAN (1991) gives a **nomogram** for power and sample size calculations (Box P.6). KIRKWOOD & STERNE (2003) and BLAND (2015) give formulae for calculating sample size requirements for a number of **summary measures**, for both power and **precision** calculations. See also GREENLAND *et al.* (2016).

## Power transformation

See **transformations**.

## PPV

Abbreviation for positive predictive value. See **predictive values**.

## Pragmatic trial

As opposed to **explanatory trial**. A **clinical trial** that evaluates the **effectiveness** of treatments and interventions. Sackett, in HAYNES *et al.* (eds., 2006), describes pragmatic trials as being on a continuum with explanatory trials, in that explanatory trials are able to rule out "**minimally important improvements**", but pragmatic (or 'management') trials are necessary for evidence of clear benefit in 'real world' settings and circumstances. Larger pragmatic trials would then ideally follow smaller, more restrictive explanatory trials whenever the latter are able to demonstrate a minimally important improvement with benefit clearly greater than harm. See also **Phase III trial, intention-to-treat analysis**.

## Precision

The number of **significant figures** obtained for a measurement. For example, the height of an individual recorded as 1.734 m is more precise than if recorded as 1.7 m. It is important to note that a precise measurement is not necessarily an **accurate** or correct one. Care should be taken to avoid an unnecessary degree of precision (such as a person's height as 1.734 m). In the context of **estimation**, the term 'precision' refers to the inverse of the **standard error** (**SE**) of an estimate, i.e. 1/SE. The magnitude of the precision statistic is in inverse proportion to the magnitude of the standard error. The greater the precision of an estimate, the narrower the width of the corresponding **confidence interval** (**CI**) at any given level of confidence. A precise estimate is only useful if also **unbiased**. See also **inverse variance method, Egger's test, funnel plot, Galbraith plot**.

## Predicted outcome

Or $\hat{y}_i$ (read 'y hat'), as opposed to **observed outcome** (or $y_i$). For any given observation $i$ in a data set, the value of the **outcome variable** as predicted by a **regression model**, based on the actual values of the independent or **predictor variables** and on the estimated values of the **regression coefficients**, including the **intercept** or baseline coefficient. In **linear regression models**, the predicted outcome is on the same **measurement scale** as the observed outcome (which may be a transformed or untransformed measurement). With **generalized linear models** (fitted to counts, rates and binary outcomes), the predicted outcome is usually a **logarithmic transformation** of predicted rates and odds. See also **prediction**.

## Predicted value

As opposed to **observed value** or outcome. The value predicted for a particular quantile of a continuous distribution, given the set of parameters of a continuous **probability distribution**, or the value predicted by a **regression model**, given the observed values of the predictors and the estimated values of the regression coefficients. See also **predicted outcome**, **expected value**.

## Prediction

For an individual or **study unit**, the computation of the value of a variable, based on knowledge of the value of at least one other variable, and a **model** that links the former (**outcome** or *y* **variable**) to the latter (**predictor** or *x* **variable**). Prediction may be of the *average* value of *y* for any given value of *x*, or it may be a prediction of the value of *y* for an *individual* with a given value of *x*. In the first instance, interval **estimation** around the **regression line** is given by a **confidence interval**, and in the second instance by a **prediction interval**. Prediction intervals are wider than the corresponding confidence intervals (Figure P.6). See also **predicted outcome**, **predictive model**, **extrapolation**, **goodness-of-fit (GoF)**. Cf. **forecast**.

## Prediction interval

The *x*% (often 95%) prediction interval around a **regression line** is the interval for which there is an *x*% probability that the **predicted value** for an individual will lie. It is therefore wider than the corresponding *x*% **confidence interval** for the same regression line, owing to greater uncertainty when making an *individual* prediction *vs.* an *on average* prediction, for any given value of the **predictor variable(s)**. Both intervals (confidence and prediction) are narrowest at the average values for both the *x* and *y* variables. Figure P.6 shows a regression line with 95% confidence (CI) and prediction (PI) interval, for the relationship between serum concentrations of sulfoconjugated steroids (DHEAS and E1S) in 989 Hungarian women with primary postmenopausal IDC (invasive ductal carcinoma) breast cancer prior to surgical intervention (VINCZE *et al.*, 2015). 'On average' predictions should be fairly precise given the narrow 95% CI. However, the 95% PI is rather wide, and too much uncertainty would be attached to any given individual prediction. See also **prediction**. See RILEY, HIGGINS & DEEKS (2011) for PI estimation in the context of random effects meta-analyses, based on a concept developed by HIGGINS, THOMPSON & SPIGELHALTER (2009).

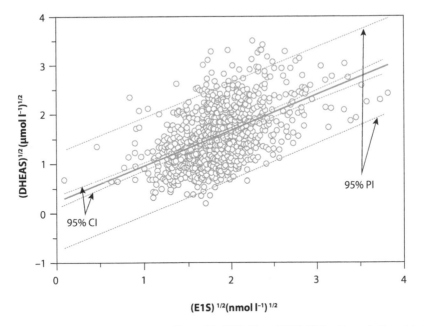

Figure P.6 Prediction interval: regression line with 95% CI and 95% PI for the relationship between serum concentrations of DHEAS (dehydroepiandrosterone sulfate) and E1S (estrone sulfate) in 989 Hungarian women with primary post-menopausal IDC breast cancer. (Reproduced from Vincze B *et al.* (2015). Serum estrone concentration, estrone sulphate/estrone ratio and BMI are associated with human epidermal growth factor receptor 2 and progesterone receptor status in primary post-menopausal breast cancer patients suffering invasive ductal carcinoma. *SpringerPlus* **4**: 387–97.)

## Predictive model

A **regression model** that is used for the purpose of **prediction**, as opposed to **causal inference**. Predictive models are often developed from large data sets, and may be used in clinical settings to predict a patient's prognosis based on a number of patient and disease characteristics (**prognostic factors**), or to derive the risk of a given diagnosis based on a number of **risk factors**. These need not be causal factors in order to be included in a predictive model. Variables are added to the model on the basis of their predictive ability, i.e. their ability to improve the **fit** of the model and therefore decrease prediction error, and also on the basis of the **classifying** accuracy of the resulting model. The **APACHE III** prognostic system is one such example. Cf. **causal inference model**. See also **prognostic index, risk score, validation, calibration, discrimination**. See **TRIPOD statement** for reporting guidelines. See **categorized continuous variable** for a discussion of the treatment of continuous variables in multiple regression models.

## Predictive values

In the context of **diagnostic testing** using dichotomous test results, predictive values measure a test's usefulness in practice. Thus, they help interpret test results outside of the research settings where diagnostic tests are compared against **gold standards** to determine their accuracy or diagnostic ability, as expressed by the **sensitivity** and **specificity** of a test. The positive predictive value (PPV) of a test is the probability of actually *having* a condition, *given* that the test result is positive. The negative predictive value (NPV) is the probability of *not* having the disease, *given* that the test is negative. From Table 4 (**Likelihood ratios**, p. 191):

$$PPV = \frac{all\ testing\ positive\ and\ diseased}{all\ testing\ positive} = \frac{a}{a+b}$$

$$NPV = \frac{all\ testing\ negative\ and\ non\text{-}diseased}{all\ testing\ negative} = \frac{d}{c+d}$$

Predictive values are affected by changes in the **prevalence** of a condition. Lower prevalence decreases the PPV, and higher prevalence increases the PPV. The opposite is true for the NPV. Thus, a diagnostic tool with a high **detection rate** may nonetheless produce a large number of **false-positive** diagnoses (low PPV) when used in settings with low disease prevalence. The PPV is also known as the **post-test probability** of disease given a positive test result. The post-test probability of disease given a negative test result is given by $(1 - NPV) \times 100\%$ if expressed as a percentage. See also **conditional probability**, **SnNout**, **SpPin**.

## Predictor variable

Also termed $x$, explanatory or independent variable. In the context of **regression analysis**, a variable that is used to determine or **predict** the values of the response or **outcome variable**. Predictor variables are typically exposures or risk factors, confounding variables, treatments and other prognostic factors, baseline measurements, etc. The type and number of predictor variables determines to a large extent how simple or complex data analyses may be. Although the terms 'predictor' and 'explanatory' are usually employed interchangeably, a distinction could be made between the role and purpose of independent variables in **predictive models** and in **causal inference models**. In the latter, the term 'explanatory' may be more appropriate as the aim is not as much prediction, but **estimation** of effects of putative causal factors.

## Pretest odds

See **pretest probability**.

## Pretest probability

In the context of **diagnostic testing**, the probability that an individual patient has a disease or condition *prior* to the undertaking of relevant diagnostic procedures. The pretest probability of having a disease is usually estimated by the **prevalence** of the disease. The following formula is used to convert pretest probabilities ($p$) into pretest odds:

$$Pretest\ odds = \frac{p}{1-p} \qquad \left(and\ p = \frac{odds}{1+odds}\right)$$

**Likelihood ratios** are then used to convert pretest odds into post-test odds, which in turn go into the calculation of the **post-test probability** of disease. See Box P.5 (p. 274) for a **nomogram** that bypasses these calculations.

## Pretreatment measurement

Synonym for **baseline measurement**. See **before–after comparison**, **change** (study of), **analysis of covariance** (**ANCOVA**). Cf. post-treatment measurement or **outcome variable**, **change scores**.

## Prevalence

A measure of the burden of disease in a given population and at a given time. As opposed to **incidence**, it is the total number of *existing* cases of a disease or condition at a particular point in time (*point* prevalence) or in a specified period of time (*period* prevalence), divided by the total population or by the total population at mid-point of the specified time interval. Usually expressed as a percentage or per 1000, 10,000 or 100,000 if very small. Period prevalence reflects both point prevalence at the start of the specified period, and incidence over its duration (HENNEKENS, BURING & MAYRENT (eds.), 1987). ROTHMAN (2012) discusses factors that affect prevalence of disease, in particular its incidence rate and average length or duration. With regard to the interplay between these factors, and although higher disease incidence will normally result in higher prevalence, with diseases of short duration, high incidence may nonetheless result in low prevalence of disease at any given time. The opposite is true for chronic diseases of longer duration. The following equivalence between prevalence, $P$ (or, more precisely, **odds** of disease), and incidence rate ($I$) is given:

$$\frac{P}{1-P} = I\overline{D} \quad [or\ P \approx I\overline{D},\ for\ small\ prevalences]$$

which may be rewritten as:

$$P = \frac{I\overline{D}}{1+I\overline{D}}$$

where $\overline{D}$ is the average duration of disease (or the average time spent in a given age group while diseased if the prevalence in question is age-specific). Although prevalence, unlike incidence, gives no indication of 'risk' of disease and has limited usefulness in studying disease causation, there are instances (such as when studying birth defects and diseases with insidious onset, and also in health services research – ROTHMAN, 2012) where prevalence is the measure of choice due to the impracticality of estimating incidence, or simply due to its greater usefulness. When studying **cause–effect relationships**, the prevalence of a given **exposure** (relative to the prevalence of other exposures participating in different **causal mechanisms** for the same disease) is an important determinant of the strength of its relationship with the disease in question. In the context of **diagnostic testing**, the overall prevalence of a given disease is often taken as the estimate of **pretest probability** of disease.

## Preventable fraction

Synonym for **relative risk reduction (RRR)** and efficacy. Cf. **attributable fraction (AF)**, **excess relative risk (ERR)**. See **measures of impact**.

## Preventive factor

A protective **exposure** such as dietary and lifestyle habits, genetic traits or interventions that decreases an individual's probability of experiencing a given disease or outcome, when compared to individuals in whom the factor in question is absent. See also **absolute benefit increase (ABI)**, **relative benefit increase (RBI)**. Cf. **risk factor, prognostic factor**.

## Primary outcome

Or primary endpoint. In a research study, the response or **outcome variable** that tests the main study hypothesis. POCOCK (1983) gives details on the various aspects of the evaluation of patient response, and a summary of descriptive and analytic methods pertinent to the analysis of results from clinical trials. Tugwell & Guyatt, in HAYNES *et al.* (eds., 2006), highlight **responsiveness** as a necessary feature for an outcome measure, i.e. the ability to reflect even small changes in 'exposure', which allows detection of **minimally important differences**. On the issue of interpretability of results with **continuous outcomes** such as blood pressure measurements, fasting blood glucose, etc., Guyatt, Haynes & Sackett, in HAYNES *et al.* (eds., 2006), suggest analysing the uncategorized continuous outcome for an assessment of statistical significance, while deriving a *dichotomized* outcome based on a prespecified threshold value, for a presentation of results that are more readily interpretable and more meaningful to clinicians. See also **multiple outcomes, surrogate endpoint**.

## Primary study

Each of the individual studies included in a **systematic review** or a **meta-analysis**, which provide the estimates of effect and of sampling variation that are used in the quantitative evaluation of heterogeneity of effect, and in the estimation of overall measures of effect.

## Principal components analysis

Also referred to by its abbreviation, PCA. A **multivariate method** of data reduction in which the original measurements on several variables are combined to produce an equal number of composite variables that are uncorrelated with each other. The new 'variables' are termed first, second, etc., principal components, in order of the amount of variability in the data they are able to explain (the first principal component is the one which maximizes differences between individuals or observations). The *eigenvalue* is a measure of the proportion of **variance** explained by each principal component. A plot of eigenvalues *vs.* component order (a **scree plot** – see Figure S.1, p. 325) helps in deciding on the number of principal components to retain. The analysis may provide a single index that uses information contained in all the variables considered. Principal components are equivalent to postulated factors (or latent variables) in **factor analysis**. In distinguishing between the two types of analysis, HAMILTON (1992) states that "Principal components [analysis] attempts to explain the observed variables' variance, whereas factor analysis attempts to explain their intercorrelations." (p. 252). Each principal component ascribes a **composite score** to each individual or observation in the data, and plots of these scores may be used to detect multivariate **outliers**, and to aid the detection of clusters when carrying out **cluster analysis**. PCA may also be employed to deal with **collinearity** in regression analysis. See HAMILTON (1992; 2012) and BLAND (2015) for further details and illustrative examples.

## Prior distribution

The **probability distribution** for the parameter of interest, prior to incorporating additional information that will modify the prior belief about the parameter to produce a **posterior** belief, also expressed as a probability distribution. See **Bayesian inference**.

## PRISMA statement

Formerly known as the QUOROM (Quality of Reporting of Meta-analyses) statement (MOHER *et al.*/QUOROM group, 1999), PRISMA (Preferred Reporting Items for Systematic Reviews and Meta-analyses – MOHER *et al.*/PRISMA group, 2009) is a collaborative statement that sets out standards and checklists for reporting the rationale, methodology, results and conclusions of systematic reviews, in order to facilitate the proper appraisal of the same. The PRISMA statement consists of a 27-item checklist and a four-phase flow diagram. See Shea, Dubé & Moher, in EGGER, DAVEY SMITH & ALTMAN (eds., 2001), LIBERATI *et al.* (2009), and www.prisma-statement.org for further discussion and details, including proposed revisions and extensions. See also **systematic review**, **meta-analysis**, **CONSORT statement**, **STROBE statement**, **EQUATOR Network**, **critical appraisal**.

## Probabilistic model

A model that contains probabilistic or **random** elements. Most **regression** models encountered in medical research are probabilistic, where the effect of predictor or explanatory variables is estimated by **regression coefficients** or parameters. Unless a **saturated model** is fitted, probabilistic models typically produce an error or **residual** for each observation in a data set, as a proportion of the observed variability in the outcome variable will remain unexplained. Cf. **deterministic model**.

## Probability

The number of times an event will occur out of a large number of trials, as estimated by the **proportion** of trials that give rise to the event. This is equivalent to the **risk** of developing a given outcome or disease, which is also a proportion, calculated as the number of individuals who develop the outcome of interest out of the total number who were at risk at the beginning of a given time-period. This interpretation of probability, as observation based on repetition, underlies the **frequentist** approach to statistical **inference**. The probability of an event taking place is 0 if that event can never take place. The probability of an event taking place is 1 if that event is certain to take place. The probability that two **independent events** will both occur is calculated by *multiplying* their respective probabilities.

Where the events in question are not independent, their joint probability of occurrence is given by multiplying the 'probability of the first event' by the 'probability of the second event, *conditional* on the first event having occurred'. This is known as a **conditional probability** and is a central concept to **Bayesian inference** and to methods based on **likelihood**. The probability of one of two events occurring, where the events are **mutually exclusive**, is calculated by *adding* up their respective probabilities. Where the events in question are not mutually exclusive, i.e. can both occur concurrently, the probability of at least one event occurring is calculated as the 'sum of their respective probabilities' *minus* the 'probability that both will occur'. These are known as the *multiplicative* (both events) and *additive* (either or both) *rules* of probability. See also **odds**, the ratio of the 'probability of an event occurring' to the 'probability of event not occurring'.

## Probability density function

Also, pdf or f(*x*). A mathematical equation that gives the probability densities for a **continuous probability distribution**. Plotting f(*x*) on the *y*-axis against *x* (the values of the distribution) on the *x*-axis produces a theoretical curve, as, for example, a **Normal distribution curve** (Figure N.1, p. 235) or an **exponential distribution curve** (Figure E.3, p. 126). The probability density gives the height of the curve at any given point on the continuous *x*-axis, which cannot however be interpreted as the probability of that value. Rather, the **area under the curve** between any two points on the *x*-axis is the *density* or **probability** that an observation from the distribution is between those two values. The total area under a probability curve is 1 (or 100%). See also **histogram, frequency density, cumulative distribution** (or density) **function (CDF)**. Cf. **probability mass function**.

## Probability distribution

The set of theoretical probabilities (adding up to 1 or 100%) for each of the **mutually exclusive** outcome values of a **discrete random variable** (as in **binomial** and **Poisson distribution**), or, in the case of a **continuous random variable**, a curve (as in **Normal curve**) that is used to calculate the theoretical probability *below* any given value, or, indirectly, between any two values (since, for continuous variables, the probability of any single value is essentially zero), where the total area under the curve equals 1. A mathematical equation (a **probability mass function** or a **probability density function**) gives these theoretical probabilities (for continuous distributions, the probability density or height of the curve) for a number of known probability distributions. Probability distributions are defined by one or more **parameters**, as, for example, the **mean** and **standard deviation**, which give the location and scale (or dispersion) of the **Normal distribution**. See ARMITAGE, BERRY & MATHEWS (2002) for details and illustration of a number of theoretical probability distributions. See also **theoretical distribution**.

## Probability mass function

A mathematical equation that gives the probabilities for each of the values of a **discrete probability distribution**. It is usually denoted by Prob($X = x$), where $X$ is a discrete **random variable**, and $x$ is the specific value from a set of possible outcomes. The probability mass function for the **binomial** and **Poisson distributions** is given under the respective entries. The sum of the probabilities for any given set of outcome values is 1 (or 100%). See also relative **frequency distribution**. Cf. **probability density function**.

## Probability of misclassification

Or PMC. See **classification table**.

## Probability-probability plot

Or P-P plot. See **Normal plot**.

## Probability sampling

A method of **random sampling** from a **population** of finite size, whereby each member of the population is enumerated and ascribed a probability of being sampled or selected. This probability may be the same for all members of the population, or it may be such that certain individuals, or certain groupings within the population, have greater probability of being selected.

## Probit analysis

The analysis of **proportions** (which range in value from 0 to 1) that have been transformed into an unconstrained scale (from $-\infty$ to $+\infty$) through the **probit transformation**. This type of analysis is often carried out to model **dose–response relationships**, where different doses of a given drug or toxic substance are administered to different groups, and the proportion in each group with the outcome of interest is calculated. The relationship between dose and response (transformed proportion) may then be expressed through a linear model. See AGRESTI (2007) for further details. ARMITAGE, BERRY & MATHEWS (2002) discuss statistical methods for laboratory assays. See also **logistic regression**, **generalized linear model**.

## Probit transformation

A **transformation** that is used to **linearize** the **sigmoid** (or S-shaped) **curve** of a **dose-response relationship**, where the response is the **proportion**, $p$, with a given outcome of interest. The transformation is usually obtained by adding a constant to the 'probit', i.e. for each proportion or probability, the corresponding **quantile** of the **standard Normal distribution**. The addition of the constant avoids getting negative values for the transformed variable; otherwise, its range of values is unconstrained. See also **cumulative distribution function** or **CDF** (which gives the probabilities for the values or quantiles of a theoretical distribution), **arcsine square root** transformation, **complementary log-log** transformation, **logit** transformation, **probit analysis**.

## Product-limit estimate

An estimate of **survival probability** that is obtained with the **Kaplan–Meier method**.

## Product term

A term in a regression model that represents the **statistical interaction** between two or more predictor variables. See also **higher-order interaction**.

## Prognostic factor

A patient or disease characteristic that influences the course of a particular condition or disease and can determine its outcome. Common examples are age, immune competency, duration of symptoms, comorbidities, etc. See also **clinical trial**, **survival analysis**, **prognostic index**. POCOCK (1983) discusses a number of related issues, from assessment of **comparability**, to **subgroup analyses**. See also Guyatt, in HAYNES *et al.* (eds., 2006), for an overview of the study of prognosis, and Altman, in EGGER, DAVEY SMITH & ALTMAN (eds., 2001), for issues pertaining to systematic reviews of evaluations of prognostic variables.

## Prognostic imbalance

See **comparability**, **baseline characteristics**.

## Prognostic index

A **classification** tool derived from the **fitted values** of a **predictive regression model** (for example, a multivariable linear or logistic model), or from the linear predictor or 'prognostic index' of a **Cox regression** model (i.e. the regression equation minus the baseline hazard component), which is used to assign predictive scores to patients with a variety of clinical diagnoses. In the case of Cox models, the relationship between **survival** and **cumulative hazard function** results in the following equation, which relates the survival function, $S(t)$, to the Cox regression model:

$$S(t) = \exp[-H_0(t) \times \exp(\eta)], \text{ which may also be expressed as } S(t) = S_0(t)^{\exp(\eta)}$$

where $H_0(t)$ is the baseline cumulative hazard function, $S_0(t)$ is the baseline survival function, and $\eta$ (eta), the exponent of the constant $e$, is the prognostic index (all of which are given by the Cox model). $\eta$ or eta may also be written as $b_1 x_1 + b_2 x_2 + b_3 x_3 + ... + b_p x_p$, where the $x$s represent the **predictor variables** in the model, and the $b$s represent the corresponding **regression coefficients**. The range of values provided by a prognostic index (PI) is further analysed to determine its accuracy of prediction (**calibration**) and classification (**discrimination**). **Validation**, using an independent data sample, is an important additional step when evaluating prognostic indices and **risk scores**. The information conveyed by a prognostic index may be presented as **post-test probabilities** to facilitate its use in clinical settings (Guyatt, in HAYNES *et al.* [eds., 2006]). See ALTMAN (1991), MOONS *et al.* (2009) and ROYSTON *et al.* (2009) for additional details. MACHIN & CAMPBELL (2005) give details of the design of studies developing and validating prognostic indices. See also **APACHE score**, **severity of illness index**. See **TRIPOD statement** for reporting guidelines.

## Propensity scores

A type of confounder summary score that is used in the analysis of **observational studies** in order to prevent the problem of overfitting (ROTHMAN, 2012). This is a situation that occurs when too large a number of **confounding variables** must be taken into account in a **regression model** with a limited number of **observations**. Propensity scores are calculated as **exposure** summary scores (as opposed to disease risk scores), by reducing the information on all potential confounders to a single summary variable (in respect of the exposure of interest), usually by means of regression analysis. Variables thus included in a propensity score must fully meet the criteria for being a confounder, otherwise their inclusion will be likely to affect the **precision** of estimates of **exposure effect**. ROTHMAN (2012) points out a useful application of propensity scores in carrying out **restriction** efficiently, when this must be accomplished in respect of more than one potential confounder. The distribution of a set of propensity scores facilitates the identification and subsequent exclusion (trimming) of outlying observations from the study sample. HUITEMA (2011) gives additional details.

## Proportion

The ratio of the number of individuals in a group with a given characteristic or experiencing a certain event to the total number of people in the same group. The incidence risk, or simply, **risk**, a frequently used measure of disease occurrence, is a proportion, more specifically termed 'incidence proportion'. *Differences* between risks or proportions give estimates of *absolute* treatment or exposure effect, and their *ratios* give estimates of *relative* effect. A related statistic is the **odds**, which is the ratio between two complementary proportions or **probabilities** (i.e. the ratio of the probability that an event will happen to the probability that it will not happen). Proportions are commonly analysed with methods suitable for **binary** and **binomial outcomes** and **contingency tables**.

## Proportion-of-variance-explained measures

In the context of **correlation** and **regression analysis**, measures that give an estimate of the proportion of total **variance** or variability observed in a given variable that is explained or accounted for by one or more other variables. These measures include the square of **Pearson's correlation coefficient**, *r*-squared or $r^2$, the square of the **multiple correlation coefficient**, $R^2$, eta squared ($\eta^2$) and **omega squared** ($\omega^2$). The square of a **partial correlation coefficient** estimates the proportion of residual variability that may be explained by considering the effect of an additional variable. See also **standardized measures of effect**.

## Proportional attributable risk

Synonym for **attributable fraction** (**AF**).

## Proportional hazards assumption

In the context of **survival analysis**, and in particular the **Cox regression** model, this term refers to the assumption of a constant **hazard ratio** (*HR*), at any point in time, and between any two groups that are being followed up. Where *HR* changes with time, it suggests the existence of a 'time-exposure' **interaction**. KIRKWOOD & STERNE (2003) discuss strategies for dealing with non-proportionality with regard to the main exposure under study, and also in reference to a confounder. See also **proportional hazards models**.

## Proportional hazards models

A class of **parametric survival models** (exponential, Weibull, Gompertz), which assumes a *proportional* **hazard** over time for one of the treatment or exposure groups as compared to another, such that at any given time the hazard in one group is a constant proportion of the hazard in the other group, i.e. the **hazard ratio** between any two groups is assumed to remain constant over time. Unlike **accelerated failure time models**, acceleration and deceleration of effects cannot be accounted for. See also **Cox regression**, a semi-parametric proportional hazards model that provides estimates of relative hazard for the predictor variables in the model, i.e. it allows a comparative assessment to be made, without, however, making any assumptions with regard to the functional form of the **baseline hazard function**, $h_0(t)$, and the distribution of **survival times**. It also does not provide a parameterization of the baseline hazard. Whereas Cox regression does not have an **intercept** that is distinct from the baseline hazard, the intercept in an exponential model, for example, is $h_0(t)$. See CLEVES, GOULD & MARCHENKO (2016) for further details. See also **proportional hazards assumption**.

## Proportional mortality ratio

Or its abbreviation, PMR. A measure of the impact of a disease on a given exposed population, that may be calculated when the structure of the population (i.e. its size and age distribution, for example) is not known (HENNEKENS, BURING & MAYRENT (eds.), 1987). It is calculated as the ratio of the proportion of deaths from all causes, among the exposed, that is due to a particular cause to the same proportion among the comparison population (unexposed or general population). Alternatively, it may be calculated as $PMR = O/E$, where $O$ is the observed number of cause-specific deaths in the population, and $E$ is the expected number were the proportion in the comparison population applied to the total number of deaths in the exposed population (i.e. $E = O \times PM$[comparison population]). Rothman & Sanderland, in ROTHMAN, GREENALND & LASH (eds., 2012), also point out the limitations of proportional mortality studies (mainly, the difficulty in determining whether excess deaths due to a specific cause represent increased risk, or simply a decrease in the number of deaths due to competing causes), and draw a parallel between these and **case–control studies**. Cf. **standardized mortality ratio (SMR)**.

## Proportional odds model

Synonym for **ordered logistic regression** model.

## Prospective study

A study in which **exposure** status is established at the beginning of the investigation, with participants then **followed up** for the development of a given disease or **outcome**. **Cohort studies** and **clinical trials** are in this category. The term is also used to refer to a study that uses newly collected data, as opposed to existing information. In this sense, **case–control studies** can sometimes be carried out prospectively, in particular case–control studies that are **nested** in cohort studies.

## Protective factor

See **preventive factor**.

## Protocol

A blueprint that details all aspects of the design, conduct, monitoring and evaluation of a **clinical trial**. Background information and stated goals and objectives give the necessary rationale for the conduct of the trial. **Minimally important differences** should be hypothesized. **Eligibility** and **exclusion criteria**, and mode of obtaining **informed consent**, are also detailed, and **safety** concerns addressed. Aspects of design include the specific **study design** to be employed, **sample size** requirements and method of treatment **allocation**. **Concealment** of allocation, **blinding** of study participants and researchers and details on treatment regimens and schedules are all important aspects in conducting a trial. Monitoring and evaluation encompasses assessment of **compliance**, ascertainment or measurement of **outcomes** and planned approaches to data analysis. The latter include not only the specific steps and methodology to be employed, but also the timing and frequency of **interim analyses** (if any), and intended **subgroup analyses**. The approach to **protocol breaches**, with the view to minimize potential bias and attrition, should also be stated. POCOCK (1983) gives additional details. ALTMAN (1991) recommends the use of formal protocols in all research studies. See also CHAN *et al.* (2013) – SPIRIT statement.

## Protocol breach

Non-compliance with the **protocol** specifications for a **clinical trial**. For example, in a randomized, double-blind, placebo-controlled trial of omega-3 fatty acids, study participants may be instructed not to take omega-3 supplements obtained privately (e.g. from a health store). A person who is taking part in the trial while also self-administering the treatment under study is in breach of protocol, as is an investigator who does not follow treatment and evaluation schedules and procedures. Protocol breaches may be intentional, or simply due to mistakes or poor understanding. POCOCK (1983) discusses a number of pertinent issues, the "underlying objective [...] to try and avoid protocol deviations from [occurring and] biasing any therapeutic comparisons." (p. 176). See also **eligibility, compliance, concomitant treatment, withdrawal, loss to follow-up, selection bias, information bias, pragmatic trial, intention-to-treat analysis**.

## PTAR

Abbreviation for **person-time at risk**.

## Publication bias

A type of **bias** that is due to selective publication in medical journals of articles that report **statistically significant** results ('**positive study**'). Given that statistical significance is not synonymous with quality or **validity**, this practice may cause studies of poor quality and misleading results to have much greater impact on clinical and policy decisions than they merit, as their results are often biased in the direction of greater magnitude of effect.

In addition, studies that conclusively demonstrate a lack of treatment effect or a lack of association may be considered less consequential and withheld from publication. The importance of such studies is often underestimated: if a study is well designed and properly conducted so that it may provide reliable answers to pertinent questions, the results it produces are important, regardless of their magnitude or statistical significance. The issue of publication bias is central to **systematic reviews**, as reviewers must make an effort to obtain and evaluate all published and unpublished studies on the particular question of interest. Publication bias may be assessed using graphical methods (**funnel plot**), formal tests (**Begg and Mazumdar, Egger's**) and **meta-regression**. The assessment of publication bias is part of the larger assessment of statistical **heterogeneity**. See Sterne, Egger & Davey Smith, in EGGER, DAVEY SMITH & ALTMAN (eds., 2001), and BORENSTEIN *et al.* (2009) for a fuller discussion. See also de BRÚN & PEARCE-SMITH (2014) for a comprehensive discussion on search strategies.

## PYAR

Acronym for person-years at risk. See **person-time at risk (PTAR)**.

# Q

## Q-Q plot

Or quantile-quantile plot. See **Normal plot**.

## Q test

Also known as Cochran's $Q$ test. A test that is used in the context of **meta-analysis**, to test for **heterogeneity** of treatment or exposure effect across the different **primary studies** included in a meta-analysis. This test is similar to the **chi-squared test for heterogeneity** that is used with **Mantel–Haenszel** stratification methods. The two tests differ in the way the stratum- or study-level components of the test statistic are weighted, using either Mantel–Haenszel or **inverse variance** weights. **Degrees of freedom** for the test are calculated as the number of studies *minus* 1. The larger the test statistic, the smaller the $P$-value and the greater the evidence against the **null hypothesis** that the underlying exposure or treatment effect is the same across the different studies. Due to the test's lack of **power**, in particular where a meta-analysis encompasses only a small number of studies, less stringent levels of significance are often suggested. The **index of heterogeneity** ($I^2$) may offer a better assessment in these situations. See also **forest plot**, **Galbraith plot**, **L'Abbé plot**, **meta-regression**.

## QALYs

Acronym for **quality-adjusted life-years**.

## Quadratic curve

See **quadratic term**.

## Quadratic term

A power term that is included in a **polynomial regression model** to account for a curvature in the relationship between an outcome or response variable and a continuous predictor or explanatory variable. A quadratic term is computed by taking the square (power 2) **transformation** of the **explanatory variable**, as shown in the following equation:

$$\text{Predicted response variable} = \text{constant} + \text{coefficient}_1 \times (\text{explanatory variable}_1)$$
$$+ \text{coefficient}_2 \times (\text{explanatory variable}_1)^2$$

where the last term of the equation, $\text{coefficient}_2 \times (\text{explanatory variable}_1)^2$, is the quadratic term. ALTMAN (1991) describes the quadratic or parabolic curve as one "which rises and then falls (or vice-versa) in a symmetric manner about its maximum (or minimum) value" (p. 310). As always, **scatterplots** are invaluable for understanding the pattern of association between the variables involved. See BLAND (2015) for another illustrative example. Methodology for dealing with the potential **collinearity** or high correlation between the untransformed explanatory variable and its power transformation is also discussed. See also **non-linear relationship** (also, linear relationship), **fractional polynomials**. Figure Q.1 shows the quadratic or U-shaped relationship between vitamin D levels and thickness of inner vascular layers in children undergoing dialysis for chronic kidney disease, in the study by SHROFF *et al.* (2008). The authors concluded "both low and high $1,25(OH)_2D$ levels are associated with adverse morphologic changes in large arteries, [...]. For optimization of strategies to protect the vasculature of dialysis patients, careful monitoring of $1,25(OH)_2D$ levels may be required."

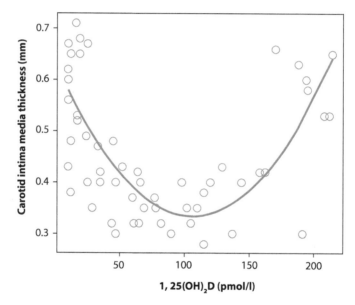

**Figure Q.1** Quadratic curve: relationship between $1,25(OH)_2D$ (vitamin D3) levels and carotid intima-media thickness (cIMT) in children undergoing dialysis for chronic kidney disease. (Reproduced from Shroff R et al. (2008). A bimodal association of vitamin D levels and vascular disease in children on dialysis. *J Am Soc Nephrol* **19**: 1239–46 (with permission).)

## Qualitative study

A study that explores a research question that cannot be answered through objective measurements and assessments, with the aim of providing an in-depth and multidimensional description or explanation of the attitudes, beliefs and behaviours of a group with regard to issues such as perceptions of specific health risks, responses to health-promoting messages and initiatives and provision and access to health care services. See AJETUNMOBI (2002) for a comprehensive overview of research methodology and guidelines for **critical appraisal**. HIGGINS & GREEN (eds., 2008) give guidance for undertaking **systematic reviews** of qualitative studies.

## Qualitative variable

See **categorical variable**.

## Quality-adjusted life-years

Usually abbreviated to the acronym QALYs, an adjustment of **life expectancy** that takes into account quality as well as quantity of life. For example, if it is estimated a given intervention would result in $x$ years of prolonged life, in a 'perfectly healthy' state, then it can be said to be able to add $x$ QALYs. On the other hand, if it is estimated a given intervention would result in $x$ years of prolonged life, in a far from healthy state, then the intervention can be said to have the potential to add only $y$ QALYs, where $0 < y < x$. (Tables are available that estimate $y$ under different circumstances.) Also, if it is estimated that a given intervention would result in immediate death, then it would add zero QALYs to a patient undergoing this same intervention. (Some argue that certain outcomes may actually be 'worse than death' and should be assigned negative-value QALYs.) QALYs are widely used in health economics, where they play a role in determining how financial and other resources are allocated to different services and programmes (see **cost-utility analysis**), and in **decision analysis** as a measure of utility. AJETUNMOBI (2002) gives additional details. Tugwell & Guyatt, in HAYNES *et al.* (eds., 2006), offer some discussion of issues around the selection of health-related quality of life outcomes.

## Quantile-quantile plot

Or Q-Q plot. See **Normal plot**.

## Quantiles

The values of an empirical or theoretical **distribution** below which a given **proportion** of the observations if found, when these are sorted according to the magnitude of their values. Some quantiles also divide the total number of observations into equal-sized groups, such that each group holds the same number (or the same proportion) of observations. Thus, **quartiles** divide the data into four equal-sized groups, each holding one quarter, or 25%, of the observations, and **deciles** into ten, each holding one tenth or 10% of the observations. Other commonly used quantiles are **tertiles** and **quintiles**, each division encompassing respectively 1/3 and 1/5 of the observations. See also **centiles**, **cumulative frequency distribution**, quantile-quantile plot (**Normal plot**).

## Quantitative variable

A count (**discrete variable**, e.g. number of children, number of practice visits) or a measurement (**continuous variable**, e.g. height, HDL cholesterol). For such variables, there is usually a true zero representing the absence of a quantity or a zero count, and, in addition, most measurements and counts may be doubled or halved in a meaningful way. Quantitative variables are usually summarized by the **mean** and **standard deviation**, or by resistant measures such as the **median** and **interquartile range**. Statistical methods for this type of data include, among others, *t*-tests, **analysis of variance**, **linear regression**,

Poisson regression, Pearson's correlation, calculation of reference intervals, method comparison studies and also non-parametric methods. Graphical methods include, among others, histograms, scatterplots, dotplots, Normal plots and regression lines. A quantitative variable may sometimes be categorized into classes or levels. Ordinal variables are considered to be semi-quantitative. See also interval and ratio variables. Cf. categorical variable.

## Quartic power transformation

See transformations, polynomial regression.

## Quartiles

For a given ordinal or quantitative variable with values or observations sorted in ascending order, the 25th centile or lower quartile is the value below which 25% of all observations fall, and the 75th centile or upper quartile is the value below which 75% of the observations fall. The range of values falling between the two quartiles is the interquartile range, which is further divided into two equal-sized halves by the median, the second quartile (Figure B.6, Box-&-whiskers plot, p. 40). See also quantiles, tertiles, quintiles, deciles.

## Quintiles

The 20th, 40th, 60th and 80th centiles. Quintiles divide the total number of observations in a given variable into five equal-sized groups. The first quintile (i.e. the 20th centile), for example, is the observation value below which we find 20% or 1/5 of all observations, when these are sorted in ascending order. See also quantiles, tertiles, quartiles, deciles.

## QUOROM statement

See PRISMA statement.

# R

## r

See **Pearson's correlation coefficient**.

## R

See index of **reliability**. Also, **multiple correlation coefficient**.

## $r^2$

The coefficient of determination, i.e. the square of **Pearson's correlation coefficient**, $r$. See **r-squared**.

## $R^2$

The coefficient of multiple determination, i.e. the square of the **multiple correlation coefficient**, $R$. See **r-squared**.

## $r \times c$ table

A **contingency table** resulting from the cross-tabulation of two categorical variables, with $r$ and $c$ number of categories respectively. See also **two-by-two (2 × 2) table**, **chi-squared test**, **log-linear model**.

## r-squared

Also termed 'coefficient of determination'. The square of **Pearson's correlation coefficient**, $r$-squared ($r^2$) ranges in value between 0 and 1, i.e. between 0 and 100%. This measure is used in the context of **correlation** and **simple linear regression**, and estimates the proportion of the total **variance** of a variable (the **outcome**, in regression) that is explained by the other variable (the **predictor**, in regression). In other words, $r^2$ gives a measure of how much of the value of one of the variables can be accounted for *solely* by the value of the other variable, and provides a way of assessing the **clinical** (or public health) **significance** of an association. The corresponding measure for **multiple linear regression** is $R^2$, the square of the **multiple correlation coefficient**. In linear regression (simple or multiple), the coefficient of determination may be calculated as $SS_{regression}/SS_{total}$ (see **sum of squares**). A more useful measure is the *adjusted $r^2$* (or adjusted $R^2$), which is corrected for chance predictions, thus enabling regression **models** with a different number of predictor variables to be compared (ALTMAN, 1991; HUITEMA, 2011). The adjusted $R^2$ statistic reflects **parsimony**, as it combines a measure of **fit** with a measure of the relative complexity of the model with regard to the data (HAMILTON, 1992). The former is given by the unadjusted coefficient of multiple determination, and the latter by the **residual degrees of freedom**. See also **partial correlation coefficient** (squared), **standardized measures of effect, eta squared, omega squared**. Cf. **Mallow's $C_p$**.

## Random

The quality of something that has no defined pattern. This term is commonly used in the context of **survey sampling** to refer to a sample that is **unbiased**, and therefore does not display any patterns or trends that are systematically different from those displayed by its **source population**. It is also used in the context of **comparative intervention studies** to describe a method of treatment **allocation** that is unbiased. The entries that follow describe a number of terms all of which involve an interpretation or application of the concept of randomness.

## Random allocation

See **randomization**.

## Random effects

In the context of **analysis of variance (ANOVA)** and **regression analysis**, a term that is used to refer to **factors** whose categories are not **fixed**, but rather, are taken as a random sample of all possible 'values'. For example, a 'subject' factor may have as 'values' each of the patients undergoing **repeated measurements** in a longitudinal study. If, however, a different set of patients is selected, the 'categories' or 'values' of the variable 'subject' will be different. Likewise, the categories of a 'cluster' factor are the different clusters sampled or selected, but a different set of clusters might have been chosen. Inclusion of random effects allows **dependence** in the data to be taken into account, or, in other words, accounts for unexplained between-subject or between-cluster heterogeneity. Often, these effects are not the primary focus of the analysis. In addition to estimating regression coefficients for **fixed effects** predictor variables (which are *cluster-specific* given the random effects), one or more random terms are also estimated, with baseline values (random **intercept** model) and rate of change associated with any given predictor (random **slope** model) allowed to vary randomly between **study units**. The **distribution** of these random effects is assumed to follow a given **probability distribution** (whose variance must be estimated), which induces a **correlation** pattern among within-cluster observations, given the predictors. Examples are **linear mixed effects models, negative binomial models** and generalized linear mixed models (GLMMs) for count variables, and GLMMs for binary outcomes, in which random effects are assumed to follow, respectively, a Normal, gamma and Normal, and Normal distribution, while the **outcome variable** is described by a Normal, Poisson and binomial distribution. The analysis of **longitudinal studies** and other **clustered designs** are common applications. An important **assumption** is that of independence between random effects and predictor variables. **Missing data** are assumed to be 'missing at random' or MAR (cf. **generalized estimating equations**). The terms 'random effects model', **'multilevel model'** and **'latent variable** model' are used interchangeably. See BLAND (2015), KIRKWOOD & STERNE (2003), AGRESTI (2007) and HAMILTON (2012) for an overview. See also **maximum likelihood estimation**; DIGGLE *et al.* (2002), RABE-HESKETH & SKRONDAL (2012). Random effects models are **conditional models**. Cf. **marginal model, transition model; beta-binomial regression**.

## Random effects model

As opposed to **fixed effect model**. In the context of **meta-analysis**, a **pooling** method that does *not* assume an underlying 'true' effect that is the same for all **primary studies** included. The **DerSimonian and Laird random effects model** is widely used in this application. The term 'random effects model' is also employed in the context of **analysis of variance (ANOVA)** and **regression analysis** to refer to a **model** that accounts for **random effects**.

## Random error

The component of **variability** in a given variable that is not explained by known factors. In **regression analysis**, this is the **residual** variation that remains after accounting for the effect of the predictor variables in the model. The term is also used to refer to fluctuations or errors of **measurement** and **classification** that occur without a pattern, and with equal probability in all treatment or exposure groups (**non-differential**). Lastly, the term may be employed to refer to variation in sample **estimates** that is due to **sampling error** and not to biased estimation. See also **measurement error**, non-differential **misclassification**.

## Random intercept model

See **multilevel model, random effects** model, **correlation structure**.

## Random numbers

A sequence of numbers that displays no underlying pattern from which the numbers can be guessed or predicted. In practice, to provide a short run of random numbers, one may throw a (fair) die, use a (fair) roulette wheel or toss a (fair) coin. The concept of random numbers finds its application with **random sampling** and **random allocation**, so that representative study samples may be generated (for example, in surveys), and unbiased comparisons of treatments and interventions may be made (for example, in clinical trials). See also **sampling frame, randomization list, random permutations**.

## Random permutations

Random rearrangements of an ordering or sequence, usually in reference to an array of numbers that may be used for **random allocations**. See also **block, Latin square**. FLEISS (1999) gives a table of random permutations of the first 100 integers, which may be used in **simple** and **restricted randomization**. See also POCOCK (1983).

## Random sample

A **study sample** that is selected at random and does not display any systematic differences from its **source population**, although there will likely be differences due to sampling variation or **sampling error**, especially with small study samples. The concept of random sampling is particularly relevant in **surveys** and **cross-sectional studies**, and in the selection of **controls** in **case–control studies**. Random samples are not usually employed in **clinical trials**, which are more commonly carried out using a sample of available patients who fulfil the **eligibility criteria** for inclusion in a trial. Here, a biased assessment of treatment effect is prevented by randomly **allocating** patients to the different treatments under study. See **sampling**. Cf. **systematic sampling**.

## Random slope model

See **multilevel model, random effects** model.

## Random variable

A quantity whose values are determined by a chance or random event. A value sampled from a **population distribution** is a random variable, as is a value sampled from a **sampling distribution**. In the latter case, the random variable is a sample estimate as opposed to an individual value. The values of a random variable occur with probability determined by its **probability distribution**, which often can be approximated by a given **theoretical distribution**. See also **discrete variable, continuous variable**.

## Random variation

Synonym for **random error**. See also **measurement error, sampling error**.

## Randomization

A method for allocating **study units** (patients, practices, communities) to the alternative treatments and interventions in **clinical trials** and other **experimental studies**. The purpose of randomization is to produce comparable treatment groups with respect to important **prognostic factors** (known and unknown), and thus avoid **confounding** effects. To this aim, **randomization lists** are produced using computer-generated random numbers, random number tables or random permutations. Sackett, in HAYNES *et al.* (eds., 2006), highlights the use of randomization as a strategy (or rather, a 'tactic') for ensuring **concealment** of treatment allocation, and notes that simple random allocation does not always produce the desired effects in terms of prognostic balance, especially when **sample sizes** are small. Modifications of the simple procedure are sometimes necessary. **Minimization** is a quasi-random allocation procedure that ensures a similar distribution of important prognostic factors in the treatment groups. **Stratified randomization** (within groups of patients with similar characteristics) may be used to the same effect, especially with larger samples. Random allocation will sometimes produce treatment groups with unequal sample sizes. This may be prevented with use of block or **restricted randomization** or the **biased coin method**. Sackett discusses the need to 'derandomize' *post hoc* patients found to be ineligible for participation. POCOCK (1983) discusses this and other issues relating to **protocol breaches**, in addition to the various methods for treatment allocation. A comprehensive discussion of the rationale and methodology for generating allocation sequences in clinical trials is given by SCHULZ & GRIMES (2002). FLEISS (1999) gives details of randomization procedures for experimental designs making use of **blocking**. MACHIN &

CAMPBELL (2005) give an overview of the various methods of randomization (including the use of blocks and Latin squares) in preclinical studies and clinical trials. See also **baseline characteristics**, **comparability**, **restriction**, **randomized controlled trial**, **cluster randomization**.

## Randomization list

In the context of **clinical trials** and other types of **intervention studies**, a randomization list is the blueprint for carrying out random treatment allocations or **randomization**. For example, when carrying out a randomized, placebo-controlled trial, the randomization list details the sequence of assignments, i.e. which group to allocate each successive patient, such as:

Patient #1 – Placebo
Patient #2 – Placebo
Patient #3 – Active
Patient #4 – Placebo
Patient #5 – Active

and so on, which also means the sequence of assignments is determined prior to any knowledge of who the patients will be. **Concealment** of treatment allocation is an important additional feature. Randomization lists are usually created from tabulated or computed-generated **random numbers** or **random permutations**. See POCOCK (1983) for further details and illustrative examples of randomization lists for different methods of allocation, random and quasi-random.

## Randomized block design

A **study design** for an **experimental study** in which treatment **allocation** is carried out within **blocks**, with allocations randomly permuted between blocks. This design (also referred to by its abbreviation, RBD) may be used to provide greater control for **prognostic variables**, but in clinical trials it is mostly used to provide a **matching** for time of entry into a study, as conditions and criteria for inclusion can sometimes vary throughout the length of a trial (FLEISS, 1999). Analysis of RBDs takes account of the blocking factor, which makes the design more **efficient** than one which utilizes **simple randomization** (HUITEMA, 2011). In addition to studies in which randomization is carried out within blocks comprised of different subjects, this method of analysis may be extended to studies in which **repeated measurements** are recorded for each individual in a group under different treatment conditions, "So long as treatments may be assigned randomly to the ultimate experimental units [in the example given, the ultimate units are blood samples, four per each subject] and so long as the response to one treatment is not affected by the other treatments […]" (FLEISS, 1999, p. 125). This is in contrast with **longitudinal** repeated measurements, which are analysed using repeated measures ANOVA and related methods (see also **split-plot design**). The RBD may be used also to ensure that treatment groups in randomized controlled trials have equal or similar size. See block or **restricted randomization**. Cf. **completely randomized design**. See also POCOCK (1983).

## Randomized controlled trial

A **clinical trial** in which two or more treatment groups are compared, one being the **control group**, and treatment **allocation** is carried out using a **random**, **unbiased** method. Often, simply referred to by its abbreviation, RCT. **Concealment** of allocation and **blinding** (to the extent that it is feasible) are also important features of properly conducted trials. Further details are given by ALTMAN (1991), POCOCK (1983) and HAYNES *et al.* (eds., 2006). JÜNI, ALTMAN & EGGER (2001) focus on the issue of study quality, and in particular the evaluation of internal and external **validity**. HIGGINS *et al.* (2011) report on the Cochrane Collaboration's tool for assessing risk of bias in randomized trials. See also **study design**.

## Range

The interval that goes from the minimum to the maximum value in a set of **ordinal** or **quantitative measurements**. Sometimes reported as a single figure (e.g. '6'), but preferably, both the minimum and maximum should be quoted (e.g. '11 to 17'). The range is not usually the preferred **measure of variability** or spread as it may be more representative of extreme observations than of the observations in the main body of data, and it also becomes wider with increasing **sample size**. In addition, the range does not generally lend itself to statistical calculations, as does the **standard deviation**. See also **interquartile range**, **central range**, **reference interval**, **limits of agreement**, **high–low graph**.

## Rank

The relative position taken by the values of a variable, as determined by the magnitude of the same. For example, if one had five observations in a variable, such as 'age', with values 65, 49, 31, 57 and 49 (sorted in ascending order: 31, 49, 49, 57, 65), these would be given the ranks 1, 2.5, 2.5, 4 and 5. When values are ordered according to magnitude into a 'league table', the rank of a given value represents its position in the table. Rank data are on the **ordinal scale**, and **non-parametric methods** are usually appropriate for their analysis. The **median** and **interquartile range** are often used as descriptive measures.

## Rank correlation

A **non-parametric** alternative to **Pearson's correlation**, which may be employed with **ordinal data**, or with quantitative measurements where the **assumptions** for parametric correlation cannot be met. **Spearman's** and **Kendall's rank correlation** are the methods commonly employed. The resulting coefficients ($\rho$ and $\tau$) are usually interpreted in the same way as **Pearson's correlation coefficient** (see comment on interpretation of $\rho$ or rho). However, in rank correlation, the **linear relationship** that is being evaluated is that between the **ranks** given to the values of each variable, not the values themselves.

## Rate

Commonly denoted by the lower case Greek letter $\lambda$, or lambda. A **summary measure** that conveys the idea of incidence of disease (**incidence rates**) or occurrence of death (**mortality rates**) per person and per unit of time, as estimated by risk/$t$ measured over a very small time interval, $t$ (see KIRKWOOD & STERNE, 2003, p.233, for an illustration). In the formulae for the calculation of rates, the numerator is the number of new occurrences of a particular event over the entire **follow-up period**, and the denominator is the total **person-time at risk** (**PTAR**). KIRKWOOD & STERNE (2003) discuss the relationship between rates and **risks**, which depends on the magnitude of the rate estimate, and on the length of the time-period over which risk, also known as *cumulative incidence*, is accumulating. With small rates, risk up to time $t$ may be estimated by the rate multiplied by time ($t$), i.e. risk ≈ $\lambda t$. To follow the example given, if the rate is estimated at 0.03 per person per year (this is equivalent, for example, to 30 per 1000 person-years at risk, where 1000 PYAR could have been 100 people followed for 10 years each, giving rise to one thousand person-years of observation), the risk over 1 year will be equal to 0.03 × 1, i.e. the same value as the rate. Over 2 years of follow-up, the risk would be 0.03 × 2, i.e. twice the risk at 1 year. This simple relationship does not hold with larger rates. For a rate of 0.3 per person per year, the risk at 1 year would be slightly lower than the value for the rate, and at 2 years it would be less than twice its value at 1 year. As the authors explain, this has to do with the rate (assumed to be constant) being applied on an increasingly smaller at-risk population, as those experiencing the event of interest, by reason of the force of incidence, also leave the at-risk pool so that the constant incidence rate now produces fewer cases. Thus, with larger rates, the relationship between risk and rate is as follows,

$$Risk = 1 - e^{-\lambda t}$$

which reflects the decaying **exponential curve** of the decrease in the **proportion** of the at-risk population over time as this population experiences the stated incidence rate. With smaller rates, this decay takes on a less steep, negatively sloped linear form. Regardless of the magnitude of the rate, the shorter the length of follow-up, the closer the rate will be to the risk estimate divided by length of follow-up; in other words, the closer the risk is to the rate multiplied by length of follow-up. See also **rate difference**, **rate ratio**, **hazard rate**.

## Rate difference

The absolute difference in **incidence** or **mortality rate** between the exposed and unexposed, or between the control and treatment groups, in a **comparative study**. The rate difference is a **measure of impact**, and may sometimes be calculated when the **absolute risk difference** or **attributable risk** may not. See KIRKWOOD & STERNE (2003) for an illustrative example of **confidence interval** estimation based on the Normal approximation to the **Poisson distribution**. See also **measures of effect**.

## Rate ratio

The ratio of two **incidence** or **mortality rates**, which is a **measure of association** between exposure and disease or between treatment and outcome in a **comparative study**. The rate ratio is one of a few measures of **relative risk** commonly used in research studies, and is often calculated in **follow-up studies** where length of follow-up is variable and outcomes may be censored. Where no difference exists between the rates in the two groups being compared (exposed *vs.* unexposed; treatment *vs.* control), the rate ratio is 1. A rate ratio greater than 1 suggests a higher rate of the event in the exposure group. The opposite is true if the rate ratio is less than 1. From Table 2.a (p. 72):

$$Rate\ ratio = \frac{a/PTAR\ in\ the\ exposed}{c/PTAR\ in\ the\ unexposed}$$

where PTAR is the **person-time at risk** in each group. Cf. **risk ratio, odds ratio, hazard ratio**. See KIRKWOOD & STERNE (2003) for an illustrative example of confidence interval estimation and significance testing based on the **delta method** (in which standard errors are calculated for the log of the rate ratio), and application of the **Mantel–Haenszel method** for control of **confounding**. See also ROTHMAN (2012); **measures of effect**.

## Ratio variable

A **quantitative variable** that has a true zero, representing the absence of the quantity or measurement in question. Unlike **interval variables**, the ratio of any two values retains its magnitude regardless of the scale on which measurements are made. An example of this type of variable is weight: a 10% increase in weight from 30 to 33 pounds still corresponds to the same 10% increase when measurements are expressed in kilograms (approximately from 13.6 to 15.0 kg). Another example is temperature measured in kelvins, or K. Unlike temperature measured in degrees Celsius and Fahrenheit, temperature in K has an absolute zero, 0 K (corresponding to –273.15 °C), and a measurement of 40 K is twice a measurement of 20 K. See also **measurement scale**.

## Raw data

Data in their 'long form' state (i.e. 'as collected'), that have not been summarized or analysed.

## RBD

Abbreviation for **randomized block design**.

## RBI

Abbreviation for **relative benefit increase**.

## RCT

Abbreviation for **randomized controlled trial**.

## Recall bias

See **information bias**.

## Receiver operating characteristic curve

See **ROC curve**.

## Reciprocal

The inverse of a quantity or measurement $x$, calculated as $1/x$. The notation $x^{-1}$ may also be used. For example, **rates** are measured in units of the reciprocal of time (e.g. year$^{-1}$ or per year). See also **reciprocal transformation**, **harmonic mean**.

## Reciprocal transformation

A **transformation** that may be applied to **quantitative variables** displaying a moderate to severe positive **skew**. The transformation is achieved by calculating the **reciprocal** of the values of the variable in question, which has a **normalizing** and **variance-stabilizing** effect. It is usually indicated in the analysis of **rates** and speeds. **Back-transforming** the mean of a set of reciprocals gives the **harmonic mean**. See FLEISS (1999) for an illustrative example. See also **logarithmic transformation**, **square root transformation** (all transformations for positively skewed variables).

## Reference interval

A range of values that reflects the **variability** of a given measurement among 'normal' individuals (thus, sometimes referred to as 'normal range'). 'Normal' usually refers to non-diseased individuals, but the definition of 'normal' may vary with the context in which it is used. Thus, a clear description of the characteristics of the **sample** used to construct a reference interval should be provided. Within a 95% reference interval we find 95% of all individual observations for a given measurement, 2.5% lying outside of either limit of the interval. To be sure this range is calculated with a fair degree of certainty, it is important to have a large enough **sample size** (some authors suggest at least 200, especially if based on centiles of distribution – see below). If measurements follow an approximately **Normal distribution**, their **mean** and **standard deviation** may be used to construct the reference interval:

$$95\% \text{ Reference interval} = mean \pm 1.96 \times SD$$

Reference intervals may also be constructed using the relevant **centiles** of the distribution of the variable in question (e.g. the 2.5th and 97.5th centiles for a 95% reference interval). This does not require that the data be normally distributed. See also **central range**; ALTMAN (1991), BLAND (2015). ARMITAGE, BERRY & MATHEWS (2002) and MACHIN & CAMPBELL (2005) give details of the design of studies to establish reference intervals. Cf. **confidence interval**, which reflects *uncertainty*, not spread or variability, about an estimated mean.

## Regression analysis

A statistical method that is used for **prediction** of outcomes or responses, and **estimation** of treatment and exposure effects. In **simple linear regression**, the relationship between the **outcome variable** ($y$) and the **predictor variable** ($x$), both **quantitative**, is summarized by means of a **linear model** (see Figures O.2 and P.6, pp. 249 and 279). The model specifies by how much the value of $y$ will increase (or decrease) for each unit increase in the value of $x$. 'By how much' is given by the **regression coefficient** or slope of the line of best fit.

Another parameter of this line is the **intercept**, i.e. the predicted value of $y$ when $x$ is equal to zero. The line of best fit is found using **least squares estimation**, which seeks to minimize the sum of the squared differences (i.e. vertical distances or **residuals**) between each observation and any given straight line going through the data points. Residuals are analysed to evaluate the **goodness-of-fit** of regression models, and to run **regression diagnostics**. **Categorical** predictors may also be included in regression models, either on their own (equivalent to **analysis of variance**) or with **covariates** (equivalent to **analysis of covariance**; see Figure A.1, p. 11). **Multiple** or **multivariable regression** allows for the inclusion of several predictor variables. See also **generalized linear models**, in particular, **logistic regression** (**binary** outcomes), **Cox regression** (**survival times**) and **Poisson regression** (**counts** and **rates**); **curvilinear** and **non-linear regression**; **non-parametric** and **robust regression**. See HAMILTON (1992; 2012) and MITCHELL (2012b) for further discussion with a focus on graphical methods and techniques. See also ARMITAGE, BERRY & MATHEWS (2002).

## Regression coefficient

Or slope of the line of best fit. In **simple linear regression** (see Figure O.2, p. 249), the regression coefficient represents the amount of change predicted in the **outcome variable** for each unit increase in the **predictor variable**. When the predictor is a **categorical variable**, the regression coefficient represents the average difference between any given level of the variable and the level taken as the baseline (e.g. smokers *vs.* non-smokers; active treatment *vs.* placebo treatment – see Figure A.1, p. 11; Box M.1, p. 219). As with **Pearson's correlation coefficient** ($r$), a slope of 0 indicates absence of a relationship between the variables. However, regression coefficients are not constrained between –1 and +1. In theory, they can take any value from $-\infty$ to $+\infty$: unlike $r$, which has no units, regression coefficients are expressed in the same units as the predicted outcome. In the context of **logistic**, **Poisson** and **Cox regression**, regression coefficients are usually interpreted as the **logarithm** of the measure of **relative risk**, i.e. when converted back to the original scale, the factor by which the 'risk' of the event in question is increased for each unit increase in the predictor variable. The term 'risk' is used here in its widest sense, to mean risk, odds, rate or hazard.

## Regression diagnostics

Graphical and other techniques that are used to assess the adequacy and consistency of fit of **regression models**, as part of the process of **model checking**. Diagnostic techniques are often based on the analysis of **residuals**, i.e. regression errors: their **distribution** and pattern of relationship with **predicted outcome** and/or **predictor variables** is often able to uncover problems with **misspecification** and **fit**. In addition, measures expressing **leverage** and **influence** may be computed for each observation in a data set. These measures give additional information as to which observations have exerted unusual or undue influence on a regression model. In **linear regression**, the outcome variable is assumed to have a **Normal distribution** and constant variability across all values of a predictor variable. A **linear relationship** is also assumed between the outcome variable and quantitative predictors. Plots of the residuals may be used to verify these **assumptions**. Specifically, the **Normal plot** is used to assess the assumption of normality, plots of residuals *vs.* fitted outcome can detect any departure from an assumption of **homoscedasticity**, and plots of residuals *vs.* each predictor can detect **non-linear relationships**. When assumptions do not hold in any significant way, a model will likely need to be respecified. A **scatterplot** of the observed outcome *vs.* each predictor variable in turn can be more helpful in detecting influential observations, as these typically have small to moderate residuals that may not stand out as **outliers** in plots of residuals – unless points are plotted with size in proportion to the magnitude of influence statistics. Commonly, regression methods assume **independence** of observations, and therefore uncorrelated residuals (see **autocorrelation**). See ALTMAN (1991), HAMILTON (1990; 1992; 2012) and KIRKWOOD & STERNE (2003) for further details and illustrative examples. HOSMER, LEMESHOW & STURDIVANT (2013) and HAMILTON (1992; 2012) discuss regression diagnostics in the context of logistic regression. This is generally based on **deviance** and **Pearson** residuals. CLEVES, GOULD & MARCHENKO (2016) give diagnostics for survival models. See also **collinearity**, **goodness-of-fit** (**GoF**).

## Regression dilution bias

A type of bias that results from **random errors** of measurement and classification, with respect to exposure and disease status (for quantitative *outcomes*, however, random errors of measurement lead to lack of **precision** of estimates of effect). The effect of **measurement error** and non-differential **misclassification** is the attenuation of any differences that might exist between **exposure groups**, thus leading to underestimation of **exposure** (or treatment) **effects**. For a quantitative exposure variable, the extent of bias or deviation from an accurate estimate of effect depends on the magnitude of the **intraclass correlation coefficient** or **ICC** (between replicate measurements of the variable in question – KIRKWOOD & STERNE, 2003). The closer this is to 1, the lesser the bias. BARNETT, van der POLS & DOBSON (2005; 2015) illustrate the occurrence of regression dilution bias in the context of **regression analysis**, as resulting from the wider range of **variability** of a quantitative predictor that is affected by measurement error, as compared to the narrower range of variability of the 'true' measurements (i.e. the mean or average for each individual). Here, the bias is reflected in a less steep relationship between predictor and outcome variable. See also FROST & THOMPSON (2000) for strategies for correcting for regression dilution bias.

## Regression through the origin

A **linear regression** analysis in which the value of the **intercept** or alpha-coefficient is set to zero. A regression line can be made to start at, or to pass through, the origin if the predicted value of the **outcome variable** is known to be zero when the value of the **predictor variable** is also zero. Thus, only the beta regression coefficient or **slope** is estimated. Interpretation of the **F-statistic** and $r^2$ (see **r-squared**), resulting from fitting the regression model, should take into account that these will be inflated due to the shift in what constitutes a **null model**, from one that predicts all observations as sharing the same mean or average value to one that predicts all observation values to be equal to zero (HAMILTON, 1992). See also **Galbraith plot**, **Egger's test**. Cf. **centering**.

## Regression to the mean

A phenomenon that occurs when taking measurements which are subject to **measurement error** or fluctuation (such as measurements on physiological and biochemical variables, for example), whereby a **repeated measurement** yields a less extreme value than previously measured. For example, a very high blood pressure measurement is usually lower at a second reading, as it likely represents one extreme of an individual's range of variability. At a second reading, the pendulum is likely to swing back to lower values. The importance of regression to the mean (RTM) in both clinical and research settings cannot be overstated. In both contexts, the usual focus of attention are individuals with the highest or lowest values for some marker of risk or disease severity. On a second evaluation, their values for the measurement in question are expected to be less extreme, due to regression to the mean. If treatments are being administered concomitantly, it will be difficult to separate a beneficial **treatment effect** from the effect of RTM, or, as noted by SENN (2011), to distinguish between "consequence and subsequence". A number of study design and data analysis strategies may be employed to improve the **reliability** of **baseline measurements**, and the assessment of treatment effect (BARNETT, van der POLS & DOBSON, 2005; 2015). These include repeated baseline measurements for a more accurate estimate of true baseline value, and inclusion of a **control group** to allow discrimination between RTM and treatment effect. Baseline values thus estimated lead to a more accurate assessment of who should be followed up, or who is eligible for trial participation. Data analysis strategies include estimation of the 'RTM effect' (which may then be subtracted from the estimate of 'change' for a treatment group), and **analysis of covariance** (**ANCOVA**), which gives more **precise** estimates of treatment effect. The higher the **correlation** between repeated measurements, and the smaller the **variability** of the measurement in the population, the lesser the effect of RTM. BLAND & ALTMAN (1994a) have noted that as long as the correlation is less than perfect ($r<1$), RTM is certain to occur. On the other hand, the more extreme the **cut-off** for selection, the greater the RTM effect. BLAND & ALTMAN (1994b) describe a number of instances in which an assessment or evaluation may be belied by the occurrence of RTM. Included are the evaluation of treatment effects, as discussed above, and the issue of whether magnitude of before–after differences correlates with magnitude of initial value (see **Oldham plot**, Figures O.1a and O.1b, p. 244). See also BLAND (2015) and KIRKWOOD & STERNE (2003); **differences** *vs.* **average plots**, **Bland–Altman plot**, **regression to the mean** (in comparative studies), **placebo effect**, **regression dilution bias**.

## Regression to the mean (in comparative studies)

In **comparative studies**, **change** from **baseline** is sometimes of special interest when estimating **treatment effect**. Due to **regression to the mean**, individuals with the highest values for a measurement (for example, blood pressure) which one intends to reduce will likely experience the largest changes (and those with the lowest values, the smallest changes or even an increase). Likewise, individuals with the lowest values for a measurement (for example, HDL cholesterol) that one intends to raise will likely experience the largest changes (and those with the highest values, the smallest changes or even a decrease). Thus, in the first instance, if 'before' or baseline measurements are higher (worse) on average in the **treatment group** than in the **control group**, the analysis of 'change score' *overestimates* treatment effect and the analysis of 'post score' *underestimates* it. In the second instance, if baseline measurements are lower (worse) on average in the treatment group, the analysis of 'change score' also *overestimates* treatment effect and the analysis of 'post score' *underestimates* it. For this reason, **analysis of covariance** (**ANCOVA**) should be used to carry out the data analysis if baseline imbalances between treatment groups are observed. See also **before–after comparison**, **differences** *vs.* **average plots**, **Oldham plot**.

## Relationship

See **association**, **linear relationship**, **non-linear relationship**.

## Relative benefit

Or benefit ratio. The relative benefit or RB is the ratio between the **probability** of a favourable or 'good' outcome in the **treatment** or protective exposure **group**, and the same probability in the **control group**. This parallels the calculation of **risk ratios**, as the ratio between the probabilities of a 'bad' or detrimental outcome. Cf. **absolute benefit increase (ABI)**. See also **relative benefit increase (RBI)**, **measures of association**, **measures of effect**.

## Relative benefit increase

Or its abbreviation, RBI. An alternative way of expressing **treatment effect** when the outcome of interest is a favourable ('good') rather than an adverse outcome. As a **relative difference**, it is calculated as the ratio between the **absolute benefit increase (ABI)** and the probability of a good outcome in the control group (assumed to have experienced a smaller proportion of good outcomes). Alternatively, it may be calculated as RB − 1, where **RB** is the **relative benefit** measure. For example, a relative benefit of 2.3 means the probability of a good outcome has increased by 130% (i.e. RBI = 2.3 − 1 = 1.3 × 100%, where 1 is the null value for the RB). The **relative risk reduction (RRR)** conveys a similar idea when analysing adverse outcomes. Cf. **relative risk increase (RRI)** (synonymous with **excess relative risk** or **ERR**). See also **measures of impact**, **measures of effect**.

## Relative change

Or percentage change from baseline. See **change scores**.

## Relative difference

A relative excess/increase or a relative reduction (depending on context). Synonym for **relative risk reduction (RRR)** and **excess relative risk (ERR)**, also termed **relative risk increase (RRI)**, and also for **relative benefit increase (RBI)**, all **measures of** relative **impact**. Cf. **absolute difference**, as in **absolute risk reduction (ARR)** and **absolute risk increase (ARI)**, and also **absolute benefit increase (ABI)**.

## Relative dispersion

As opposed to **absolute dispersion**, the extent of variability or dispersion in a quantitative variable, expressed as a fraction of its mean or average value. For example, a **standard deviation (SD)** of 100 g for weight measurements that average to 1000 g (1 kg) has different implications than a standard deviation of the same value, 100 g, for weight measurements with a mean of 10 kg (10,000 g); the relative dispersion gives a measure of this by taking the **measure of central tendency** (in this case, the **mean**) into account. Thus, by relating absolute dispersion (in this example, an SD of 100 g) to the mean through a measure such as the **coefficient of variation** or dispersion, we obtain 100 g/1000 g = 0.1 or 10%, in the first instance, and 100 g/10,000 g = 0.01 or 1% in the second instance. See **measures of dispersion**.

## Relative effect

The **magnitude** and **direction** of a **measure of effect**, which expresses in *relative* or *proportional* terms the estimated effect of a given treatment or exposure. Measures of relative effect are calculated as **relative differences** and simple *ratios*. The relative risk reduction and the relative risk increase are examples of measures of relative effect, as is the relative benefit increase. Examples of simple ratios are the risk and rate ratio. This is in contrast to measures of **absolute effect** such as the absolute risk increase, which give *net* effects. See also **measures of impact, measures of association, standardized measures of effect, effect size**.

## Relative frequency

See **frequency, cumulative frequency**.

## Relative risk

A **measure of effect** that is calculated as the ratio of the risk experienced by each of two comparison groups, where risk broadly represents **risk, rate, odds** and **hazard**. The term is often used as a synonym for **risk ratio**, but, in its broad sense, it also refers to **odds ratios, rate ratios** and **hazard ratios** (ROTHMAN, GREENLAND & LASH (eds., 2012) discourage the use in reference to odds ratios). When the 'risk' of the event of interest is the same in the two exposure or treatment groups, the relative risk (RR) is 1. It is less than 1 if the group represented in the numerator is at a lower 'risk' of the event, and greater than 1 if the opposite is true. **Confidence intervals** for ratio measures are asymmetrical around the estimated measure (see **delta method**). The relative risk is a **measure of association** and may be used to derive **measures of impact** (the **relative risk reduction** or **RRR**, for example, and the **attributable fraction, AF**). Cf. **absolute risk difference (ARD)**.

## Relative risk increase

Or its abbreviation, RRI. An alternative terminology for the **excess relative risk (ERR)**. Cf. **relative benefit increase (RBI), relative risk reduction (RRR), absolute risk increase (ARI)**.

## Relative risk reduction

An alternative way of expressing the **relative risk (RR)**, this time as a **measure of impact** (or, more specifically, a measure of *relative* impact, as opposed to the absolute risk reduction or ARR, which is a measure of *net* impact). The relative risk reduction or RRR is calculated as follows:

$$RRR = (1 - RR) \times 100\%$$

and is interpreted as the percentage of the baseline 'risk' that is prevented by a given treatment or intervention (or by avoidance of exposure to a risk factor) (Box R.1), as given by the alternative calculation, $RRR = ARR/risk_{control\ group}$, where ARR is the **absolute risk reduction**, calculated as $risk_{control\ group}$ minus $risk_{treatment\ group}$. When the RR estimate is greater than 1 (often the case with harmful exposures), what is calculated is the **excess relative risk** (**ERR**). The term 'relative risk' is being used to mean risk or rate ratio.

---

**BOX R.1**

From **Box A.1**, p. 3.

. . . . . . . . . . . . . . . . . . . . . . . . . . . . . . . . . . . . . . . . . . . . . . . . . . . . . . . . . . . . . . . . . . . . . . . . . . . . . . . .

The RR for the effect of aspirin relative to no aspirin is 0.80 and the RRR is 20%.

*Interpretation:* The risk of vascular death in the aspirin group, at 5 weeks, is 80% that in the control group, and therefore, aspirin appears to reduce the risk of vascular death at 5 weeks by 20%, following an acute myocardial infarction.

---

The terms **efficacy** and **preventable fraction** are synonymous with relative risk reduction. The **relative benefit increase** (**RBI**) conveys a similar idea when analysing 'favourable' outcomes. Cf. **attributable fraction** (**AF**).

## Reliability

In the context of **clinical measurement**, the quality of a measurement method or tool that consistently gives the same result. Reliability requires **repeatability** (of measurements repeated under the same conditions) and **reproducibility** (of measurements repeated under different conditions). An index of reliability (R) may be calculated from the **variability** of the repeated (or paired) measurements (see repeatability):

$$R = 1 - \frac{observed\ disagreement}{chance\text{-}expected\ disagreement}$$

where observed disagreement = 'variance of errors' and chance-expected disagreement = **variance** of all measurements, ignoring the pairing (DUNN & EVERITT, 1995). R takes values from 0 (no reliability) to 1 (perfect reliability). There is a parallel between this measure of agreement for **quantitative** measurements and the **kappa statistic** that is used to evaluate agreement between assessments on a **categorical** scale: R measures the proportion of the observed variability in the measurements that is over and above that due to **measurement error** (i.e. the proportion that is due to true variability). R (like kappa) is population-dependent; for the same measuring device or method, the value of R will vary according to the variance of the measurements in different populations. Greater variability has the effect of increasing the value of R, which puts repeatability in context. The reliability of a measuring method gives information on how well it distinguishes between individuals in the relevant population. Another measure of reliability is the **intraclass correlation coefficient** (**ICC**). Further details are given by BLAND (2015) and FLEISS (1999).

## Repeatability

In the context of **clinical measurement**, the quality of a measurement that shows little **variability** when replicate measurements are taken under similar conditions. Repeatability is given by the **standard deviation (SD)** of the measurement errors (also termed 'standard error of measurement' or SEM):

$$SD \ of \ errors = \sqrt{variance \ of \ errors}$$

$$Variance \ of \ errors = \frac{\Sigma(differences)^2}{2n}$$

where the sigma notation, $\Sigma$, represents summation, difference = measurement$_1$ – measurement$_2$ and $n$ is the number of measurement pairs (DUNN & EVERITT, 1995). The SD of errors may be used to calculate, for example, 95% **limits of agreement** for the repeatability of a given measurement, the interpretation of which is similar to that of **reference intervals** (i.e. an expression of variability, not of uncertainty). The SD of errors, with regard to a given measurement of interest, should therefore be estimated from a large, unbiased sample of individuals. BLAND (2015) gives an alternative computation of the SEM, as the square root of the **residual variance** or mean square from a one-way analysis of variance with 'subject' as the factor variable. Repeatability is also relevant to the assessment of **reliability** (in the formula for $R$, observed disagreement = variance of errors). When **measurement error** is proportional to the average measurement for each individual, the **coefficient of variation** is used preferably as a measure of within-subject variability. See also **reproducibility**.

## Repeated measurements analysis

The analysis of **measurements** taken on one or more groups of individuals, where more than one measurement per person is taken, usually over a period of time (**serial measurements**) in a **longitudinal study**. The main issue here is the lack of **independence** of observations pertaining to the same individual or **study unit**. Data of this sort are sometimes analysed using inappropriate methods, such as **multiple significance testing** (multiple comparisons at different time points); ordinary **analysis of variance**, in which the lack of independence of the observations is not taken into account; and somewhat uninformative **graphical displays**, with graphs only showing the average for each group at the different time points, thus 'hiding' individual response patterns. Also relevant to choosing a correct method of analysis, is whether or not measurements are taken with equal spacing over time (i.e. whether data are *time-structured* or *time-unstructured*), and whether or not the same number of measurements is taken on each study participant (i.e. whether data are *balanced* or *unbalanced*). Although **repeated measures ANOVA** and **multilevel modelling** (linear mixed effects models) may be used, which deal with the problems mentioned above, other straightforward and effective methods may also be used, requiring solely the choice of sensible **summary measures** (MATTHEWS *et al.*, 1990). These summaries reduce the multiplicity of data to fewer 'observations' (the chosen summaries), which in turn may be analysed using standard methods for independent data. An example of a graphical display may be found in Figure A.2 (p. 16), and also Figures S.2a–S.2d (p. 330), where the pattern of response over time is presented separately for each individual. Repeated measurements over time allow the **analytical** and **descriptive** study of **change**, i.e. the estimation of the effect of one or more predictors (**fixed effects**) on the individual patterns of change (**random effects**). SINGER & WILLETT (2003) describe a 'multilevel model for change', a composite two-stage analysis subsumed into one model, where the first stage describes the individual growth model and the second stage models the effects of relevant predictors on individual change trajectories. See also **longitudinal data**; DIGGLE *et al.* (2002). One- and two-factor **experimental designs** may also include repeated measurements under different experimental conditions. **Two-way ANOVA** and extensions are usually employed in the analysis of these data (see **randomized block design** with repeated measurements; **split-plot design**). See MACHIN & CAMPBELL (2005) for details on calculating sample size requirements.

## Repeated measures ANOVA

An extension of **analysis of variance (ANOVA)** and **linear regression** to the analysis of **longitudinal data**. As in **two-way ANOVA**, the data are often classified according to two factors, with the factors in this case being 'treatment' and 'time' ('subject' being the **blocking** factor – see **split-plot design** with repeated measurements over time). An important **assumption** for repeated measures ANOVA is that a complete data record is available for each individual or **study unit**, i.e. that the data are **balanced**. The analysis implies a uniform or exchangeable correlation pattern between measurements pertaining to the same individual, which is also the same for all individuals. The **null hypotheses** to be tested are that (a) treatment means are the same, and (b) the pattern of change over time is the same in all treatment groups, i.e. mean response profiles are parallel (DIGGLE *et al.*, 2002). **Linear mixed effects models** (**multilevel** linear models) allow for incomplete data, and **autocorrelation models**, for a different choice of error **correlation structure**. See also **serial measurements**, **repeated measurements analysis**, **hierarchical model**; FLEISS (1999). KIRKWOOD & STERNE (2003) give details on partitioning the sum of squares (more specifically, the **mean square**), when testing different effects where **fixed** and **random effects** may be present.

## Reporting guidelines

See **EQUATOR Network**, **critical appraisal**.

## Reproducibility

In the context of **clinical measurement**, the quality of a measurement that shows little **variability** when replicate measurements are taken under different methods or conditions. **Repeatability** within *each* method is an important determinant of reproducibility, and should always be assessed. See BLAND & ALTMAN (1986) and ALTMAN (1991) for illustrative examples. See also **method comparison studies**, **reliability**.

## Residual confounding

A **confounding** effect that may remain after procedures such as **restriction** and **stratification** have been employed, due to eligibility not being sufficiently restrictive, or strata, i.e. categories of the confounding variable, being too broad. It may also result from non-differential **misclassification** of study participants with regard to the potential confounder, with a resulting **bias** that may underestimate or overestimate **exposure effect**, depending on whether the confounding effect is negative (weakens the association), or positive (exaggerates the association). This confounding effect may be difficult to control by employing the standard methodology (e.g. stratification). See ROTHMAN (2012) and Rothman, Greenland & Lash, in ROTHMAN, GREENLAND & LASH (eds., 2012), for further discussion.

## Residual degrees of freedom

The **degrees of freedom** for the residual component in **analysis of variance (ANOVA)** and **regression analysis**. It is calculated as the total sample size *minus* the number of groups in one-way ANOVA, and as the number of observations *minus* the number of parameters in regression analysis. The **residual variance** (the denominator of the *F* statistic) is calculated as the ratio of the **residual sum of squares** to the residual degrees of freedom. Residual degrees of freedom are also used to compute a scale parameter where data are **overdispersed**, and to compute a measure of **parsimony**.

## Residual deviance test

See **deviance statistic, likelihood ratio test**.

## Residual *F*-test

A **goodness-of-fit (GoF)** test for regression models fitted by the method of **least squares**. It is assumed the data contain at least two observations (i.e. replicates) for each unique covariate pattern among predictor variables. The test is based on the decomposing of the **residual sum of squares** into a lack-of-fit (LoF) component and a true or random error (TE) component. Each of these components is then divided by the corresponding number of **degrees of freedom**, $m - p$, and $n - m$ (where $m$ is the number of unique covariate patterns, $n$ is the number of observations, and $p$ is the number of parameters in the model), to give a LoF and a TE **mean square**. The **test statistic**, $F$, is the ratio of these two mean squares, and is referred to tables of the $F$ distribution with $m - p$ and $n - m$ degrees of freedom for an assessment of statistical significance. Large test statistics and small **P-values** are indicative of poor fit. See also **F-test, residual variance**; ARMITAGE, BERRY & MATHEWS (2002).

## Residual mean square

Or residual variance. It is calculated as the ratio of the **residual sum of squares** to the **residual degrees of freedom**. In **analysis of variance**, the residual mean square is the estimate of common variance in the comparison groups, under the assumption of **homoscedasticity**. The residual variance and the residual standard deviation (**root mean square error** or RMS error) may both be used as overall measures of **goodness-of-fit (GoF)**. See also **mean squares, residual F-test, standardized residual**.

## Residual sum of squares

The within-groups **sum of squares** in an **analysis of variance**. In **linear regression** analysis, the sum of the squared **residuals**, i.e. the component of the total sum of squares for the **outcome variable** that is not explained by the predictors in the model. As with the **deviance statistic** in generalized linear models, the closer the fit of the model, the smaller the residual sum of squares (and the larger the sum of squares due to regression). The **residual variance** may be used as an overall measure of **goodness-of-fit (GoF)**. A test of significance for the fit of a model may be carried out using the lack-of-fit or **residual F-test**. See also **Pearson statistic**.

## Residual variance

Synonym for **residual mean square**.

## Residuals

In the context of **regression analysis**, residuals ($e_i$) are the numerical differences between **observed** and **predicted values** for the **outcome variable**. Summary measures calculated from the residuals are used in evaluating a **model**'s overall **goodness-of-fit (GoF)**. The analysis of the pattern of residuals is also useful in determining the adequacy of a particular model over the entire range of values of the **predictor variables** (or, equivalently, over the entire range of the predicted outcome), and plays a central role in a set of procedures known as **regression diagnostics**. For example, **Normal plots** of residuals help in making a visual assessment of the assumption that the errors (the residuals) resulting from **least squares estimation** have an approximate Normal distribution. A plot of residuals *vs.* fitted values (or *vs.* a quantitative predictor) should display a lack of pattern, with points randomly scattered around a mean residual value of zero. A curved pattern suggests the need to consider a **nonlinear relationship**. Increased variability of the residuals with increased magnitude of the fitted values (**heteroscedasticity**) suggests the need for a **logarithmic transformation** of the outcome variable. The **residual variance** is an overall measure of GoF for linear regression models. For models fitted through **maximum likelihood estimation**, these assessments are carried out by analysing **deviance** and other types of residuals. Regression models commonly assume their errors to be **independent**, i.e. uncorrelated (see **autocorrelation**). See HAMILTON (1992; 2012), HOSMER, LEMESHOW & STURDIVANT (2013), CLEVES, GOULD & MARCHENKO (2016). See also **standardized residual**.

## Resistant estimate

A statistical summary or **estimate** whose value is not much affected by small changes in sample data, with 'small changes' referring to either large changes in a small fraction of cases, or small changes in a large fraction of cases (HAMILTON, 1992). The **median**, **interquartile range (IQR)** and other ranges based on **centiles** of actual distribution are common examples, as they are not sensitive to **outlying** observations. A related concept is that of **robustness**, and applies to methods of statistical analysis that still give valid results even when distributional and other **assumptions** about the data are not met.

## Response bias

See **assessment bias**, **information bias**.

## Response rate

In the context of **analytical observational studies**, the proportion of individuals for whom there is information on **disease outcome** (cohort studies) and **exposure status** (case–control studies). In comparative studies, low response rates open study results to the possibility of **selection bias** if 'low response' is *informative*, i.e. likely to be associated with a given outcome or with a given exposure, and in particular if *differential*, i.e. affecting the comparison groups differently. ROTHMAN (2012) makes a distinction between low response and low participation (in the context of cohort and case–control studies), arguing the latter need not be a source of bias but is in fact preferable to the later withdrawal of reluctant participants. Cf. **volunteer bias** in the context of cross-sectional studies and surveys.

## Response variable

Synonym for **outcome variable**.

## Responsiveness

The quality of a response or **outcome variable** that reliably reflects the effects and actions of the treatments and exposures under evaluation, so that sufficient discrimination may be achieved between comparison groups to enable **minimally important differences** to be detected where they exist. The ability to measure an effect with sufficient sensitivity depends to an extent on the **measurement scale** of the outcome variable. A continuous response variable that is dichotomized will likely show less sensitivity than if measured on its original scale. Tugwell & Guyatt, in HAYNES *et al.* (eds., 2006), illustrate the approach to evaluating the responsiveness of outcome measures with an example from OMERACT (Outcome Measures in RheumAtology Clinical Trials).

## Restricted randomization

Also termed block randomization. A treatment **allocation** method that aims to pro-duce treatment groups with an equal (or predetermined differential) number of patients. CAMPBELL, MACHIN & WALTERS (2007) give an example of a trial where two treat-ments, A and B, are compared. **Blocks** of four patients are generated (i.e. a multiple of the number of treatments), to include all possible permutations of the two treatments that give equal allocation. In this case, six possible sequences are generated:

| | | | |
|---|------|---|------|
| 1 | AABB | 4 | BABA |
| 2 | ABAB | 5 | BAAB |
| 3 | ABBA | 6 | BBAA |

A sequence of **random digits** is then generated (e.g. 225, 673, 451), to represent the com-binations that will be used. The random digit sequence above gives the following order of assignment for the first 12 patients:

ABAB ABAB BAAB ... (combination 2 + combination 2 + combination 5 + ...),

resulting in treatment groups with equal **sample sizes**. A **randomized block design** is a **parallel trial** in which restricted randomization, rather than **simple randomization**, is employed. **Biased coin allocation** is used to the same aim as block randomization. See also **complete block design, incomplete block design**. Further details are given by ALTMAN (1991), POCOCK (1983) and FLEISS (1999), and also under randomized block design.

## Restriction

An approach to selection of study participants whereby **eligibility** is restricted, so that the resulting study group will be fairly **homogeneous** with regard to one or more potential **confounders** or to relevant **prognostic factors**. Restriction results in a study sample that is not representative of the **target population**, or of all patients with a given condition or disease. However, the ability to make an **unbiased** comparison, and ensure *internal* **validity**, is the paramount issue in **comparative studies** seeking to test research hypotheses. As noted by Rothman & Greenland, in ROTHMAN, GREENLAND & LASH (eds., 2012), a better approach to representativeness and ability to generalize study results is to conduct separate studies that focus on specific subgroups that are thought to respond differently to treatments and exposures, rather than to rely on 'representative' samples that are likely not to have sufficient numbers in the different subgroups to allow for an evaluation of **interaction** effects. HENNEKENS, BURING & MAYRENT (eds., 1987) point out as limitations of this approach the possibility of **residual confounding**, and the inability to assess interactions involving the restricting factor. See also **propensity scores**; ROTHMAN (2012).

## Retrospective study

An **observational study** in which disease status is ascertained at the beginning of the study, and information on past **exposure** to a **risk factor** of interest is subsequently collected (usually through interviews or by looking at employment or other records). **Cumulative case–control studies** are in this category. The term is also used to refer to a study that uses existing data, as opposed to data that is collected from newly occurring cases of disease. In this sense, **cohort studies** may sometimes be carried out retrospectively.

## Reverse J-shaped curve

See **J-shaped curve**.

## Reverse J-shaped distribution

See **J-shaped distribution**.

## Reverse U-shaped curve

See **U-shaped curve**.

## Reversibility

See **cause–effect relationship**.

## Rho

See **Spearman's rho ($\rho$)**.

## Risk

The **probability** of the occurrence of a given event among a group of people at risk. It is alternatively termed 'incidence proportion', 'cumulative incidence' and 'incidence risk', or 'mortality risk' when the event of interest is death. As is the case with probabilities and proportions, risks may only take values in the range 0 to 1 (or 0 to 100%):

$$Risk = \frac{number\ of\ people\ who\ experienced\ the\ event\ over\ a\ given\ time\text{-}period}{number\ of\ people\ at\ risk}$$

Risks may be calculated only from study designs that allow for **follow-up** over a period of time (prospectively or retrospectively), and where 'number of people at risk' can be ascertained. This is generally the case with **clinical trials** and other **intervention studies**, and also **cohort studies**. In some instances, the case–control design allows the estimation of risk in each of the exposure groups, or, at a minimum, the estimated odds ratio provides a good approximation to the **risk ratio** (see **case–cohort study**). See also **incidence risk, risk difference (absolute risk difference, attributable risk)**. Cf. **rate, odds, hazard**. Additional discussion is provided under **rate**, where the relationship between risks and rates is explored.

## Risk difference

Depending on context, synonym for **absolute effect, absolute risk difference, absolute risk increase** or **attributable risk, absolute risk reduction**. See also **absolute benefit increase; measures of effect, measures of impact**.

## Risk factor

A factor, for example an individual characteristic, a positive family history, an occupational exposure, socioeconomic and demographic factors, or a particular dietary or lifestyle habit, which increases an individual's probability of experiencing a given disease when compared to individuals in whom the factor in question is absent. WALD, HACKSHAW & FROST (1999) discuss the quantitative relation between risk factors and **screening tests**, and how strongly a risk factor needs to be associated with a disease before it is likely to be a useful screening test. See also **exposure**. Cf. **preventive factor, prognostic factor**.

## Risk ratio

The ratio of the **risk** of a given event among individuals in the **exposure** or intervention group to that in the **control group**. The term **relative risk** is often used as a synonym for risk ratio. The risk ratio (RR) is 1 when the risk is the same in the two comparison groups. A risk ratio greater than 1 suggests a greater risk of the event in the exposure group. The opposite is true if the risk ratio is less than 1, which is indicative of a protective effect by the exposure or intervention. The range of possible values for the risk ratio, a unitless measure, is 0 to +∞. From Table 2 (p. 72):

$$Risk\ ratio = \frac{risk\ in\ exposed\ or\ treatment\ group}{risk\ in\ unexposed\ or\ control\ group} = \frac{a/(a+b)}{c/(c+d)}$$

The magnitude of the risk ratio speaks to the **strength of the association** between disease and exposure, or treatment and outcome (the statistical significance, however, does not). It will, however, depend on **length of follow-up**, so that if measured at the end of a long period of follow-up for an outcome such as 'death' it will tend toward the null value of 1 (HENNEKENS, BURING & MAYRENT (eds.), 1987). Rate or hazard ratios may give a better estimate of relative risk in these situations. Also, RR cannot be larger than 1/'risk among the unexposed' (or smaller than 'risk among the treated'/1), so that if the risk in these groups is high (common events) the risk and rate ratios will differ more so (ROTHMAN, 2012). For rare diseases, risk, rate and **odds ratio (OR)** will be approximately equal (KIRKWOOD & STERNE, 2003). In **cumulative case–control studies** (if the disease is rare) and **case–cohort studies**, the odds ratio gives an estimate of the risk ratio. The **attributable fraction** and the **relative risk reduction** (depending on whether the exposure is harmful or protective) are **measures of *relative* impact** that may be calculated from the risk ratio (or from the **absolute risk difference**, which is a measure of *net* impact). See also **measures of effect, measures of association**.

## Risk score

A score derived from a risk assessment tool, which ascribes individual risk or **probability** estimates for a given disease or condition based on information on relevant **risk factors**. The risk assessment tool is often derived through **regression modelling**. CHD (coronary heart disease) and CVD (cardiovascular disease) risk calculators are commonly used examples. Among these, the Framingham Risk Score is widely employed to predict 10-year mortality for both men and women (using separate risk assessment tools). The component risk factors for the Framingham Risk Score are age range, total cholesterol (in mg/dl), smoking, HDL cholesterol (in mg/dl), and systolic blood pressure (in mmHg). The sum of the points attributed to the relevant categories/class intervals of the distribution of these risk factors is referred to risk of CHD categories. Where a risk scoring system is to be used in an entirely different setting from the one in which it was developed, it should be revalidated in context. For example, the Framingham Risk Score (WILSON *et al.*, 1998; updated in 2002) was shown to overestimate coronary risk in UK men aged 40–59 years (BRINDLE *et al.*, 2003). See also **classification, predictive model, calibration, discrimination, validation, prognostic index, severity of illness index**. See **TRIPOD statement** for reporting guidelines.

## Risk set

In the context of **survival analysis**, the particular set of individuals who are at risk for the event of interest at each exact time an event occurs over the course of follow-up. For example, when constructing the **Kaplan–Meier survival curve**, the occurrence of an event is represented by a step drop in the appearance of the curve, and the next step drop coincides with the occurrence of the next event. Between the two events, individuals who have just experienced the event, those lost to follow-up or withdrawn and those who experience the event due to a competing cause, will all leave the 'at-risk' group. The number at-risk (which is the denominator in the calculation of survival probabilities) is thus repeatedly reset over the course of follow-up. Nonetheless, cumulative survival probabilities must take account of the fact that at any given time a reset occurs, those individuals still at risk have already survived a given length of time, so the *cumulative* probability of survival at the relevant time points is given by the survival probability at that exact point in time multiplied by the cumulative probability of survival at the previous time point. These consecutively calculated cumulative probabilities of survival form the set of probabilities for the **survival function**, which is given on the **y-axis** of the Kaplan–Meier curve. The concept of risk set is relevant also in the context of **matched pairs designs** with a binary outcome, which are often analysed using **stratification** methods or **conditional logistic regression**. Here, each pair forms a risk set or stratum, and treatment and exposure effects are evaluated within each stratum.

## RMS error

Abbreviation for **root mean square error**.

## Robust method

A descriptive term for a method of **statistical inference** whose validity is not grossly affected by departures from usual **assumptions**. For example, the **t-test** is usually relatively robust to small departures from **normality**, though not so with regard to departures from the assumption of **homoscedasticity**. **Weighted least squares** (**WLS**) and **iteratively reweighted least squares** (**IRLS**) are regression methods often employed as alternatives to **ordinary least squares**. **Generalized estimating equations** are often employed to deal with correlated or **clustered** binary data and counts. Robust methods cannot, however, be employed to deal with problems such as **curvilinearity** and, in some cases, high **leverage** (HAMILTON, 1992). See HAMILTON (1992; 2012) for additional details. See also Huber–White or **sandwich variance estimate** (robust standard errors). Cf. **resistant estimate**, **nonparametric methods**. **Locally weighted regression** is an exploratory **smoothing** method that uses a downweighting procedure similar to IRLS in describing non-linear relationships.

## ROC curve

Acronym for 'receiver operating characteristic' curve. A graphical representation of the diagnostic accuracy of the range of test results for a **quantitative** (or ordinal) **diagnostic test**. The graph is a plot of **sensitivity** or detection rate *vs.* false-positive rate (100 − **specificity**%) for selected **cut-off points** of the quantitative variable. The choice of cut-off point above which (or sometimes, below which) disease is considered to be present is made by taking into account the trade-off between false-positive and false-negative rates. The most accurate cut-off point overall is the one closest to the top left-hand corner of the graph: high detection rate, low false-positive rate. The graph in Figure R.1 shows the comparative accuracy of fasting plasma glucose concentrations and the 50 g glucose challenge test in **screening** pregnant women for gestational diabetes, in a prospective population-based study in Switzerland (PERUCCHINI *et al.*, 1999). The analysis is based on 520 women of mixed ethnic backgrounds, with singleton pregnancies and no pre-existing diabetes. The screenings took place between the 24th and the 28th weeks of gestation, and all women were also given a diagnostic 3 h 100 g oral glucose tolerance test (the **gold standard**) within 1 week of the screening test. Fasting glucose concentrations' better overall performance or accuracy is clear from the fact that its curve is closest to the top left-hand corner of the graph, and for mostly all values for sensitivity it has higher specificity (i.e. lower false-positive rate) than the 50 g glucose challenge test. The values ascribed to each individual by a risk scoring or prognostic index may also be plotted in this way to determine best cut-off points for greater **discrimination** or classifying accuracy. Quantitative measurements need not always be dichotomized into disease present/absent, since the calculation of **likelihood ratios** permits a better use of the entire range of values obtained for the diagnostic (or screening) test. In the study by PERUCCHINI *et al.*, the authors conclude that "Measuring fasting plasma glucose concentrations using a cut off value of ≥4.8 mmol/l is an easier screening procedure for gestational diabetes than the 50 g glucose challenge test and allows 70% of women to avoid the challenge test. [...] The low sensitivity of the challenge test in our study might be explained by the fact that a high percentage of women reported food intake up to 2 hours before the test, which is known to reduce the test's sensitivity owing to the Staub–Traugott effect." See also **area under the curve** or **AUC, diagnostic threshold, diagnostic odds ratio, net benefit**; HANLEY & McNEIL (1982), MALLETT *et al.* (2012), HALLIGAN, ALTMAN & MALLETT (2015).

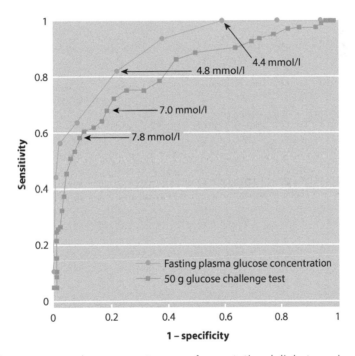

**Figure R.1** ROC curve: screening pregnant women for gestational diabetes using fasting plasma glucose concentration (AUC = 0.897) and plasma glucose concentration following the 1 h 50 g glucose challenge test (AUC = 0.815). Each data point is 0.2 mmol/l apart. Chosen cut-off point for fasting glucose is 4.8 mmol/l (81% sensitivity; 76% specificity, i.e. 24% false-positive rate). (Reproduced from Perucchini D *et al.* (1999). Using fasting plasma glucose concentrations to screen for gestational diabetes mellitus: prospective population based study. *Br Med J* **319**: 812–15 (with permission).)

## Root mean square error

Or RMS error. The square root of the residual or within-groups mean square (MS$_{residual}$ or **residual variance**), which in the context of **analysis of variance** gives an estimate of the common **standard deviation** among comparison groups, under the assumption of

**homoscedasticity** or equality of variances (the residual mean square gives an estimate of the common *variance*). Both may be used as overall measures of **goodness-of-fit** (**GoF**). In the context of **simple linear regression**, the RMS error is the average prediction error or **residual**. See **sum of squares**, **mean squares**.

## Rounding error

When performing arithmetic calculations, cumulative rounding errors will likely occur as a result of operating on numbers that have been rounded up. For instance, the sum of rounded-up percentages from the same frequency distribution might add up to over 100%. BLAND (2015) recommends keeping a sufficient number of **significant figures** through a sequence of statistical calculations so that the final reported result will not be distorted.

## RR

Abbreviation for **relative risk**, or, more specifically, for **risk** or **rate ratio**.

## RRI

Abbreviation for **relative risk increase**.

## RRR

Abbreviation for **relative risk reduction**.

# S

## S-shaped curve

See **sigmoid curve**.

## Safety

See **adverse reaction**.

## Sample

A group of individuals, or items, that are selected or sampled from a wider group or **population**. Samples are used in research studies to **estimate** population **parameters**, and to obtain estimates of **treatment** and **exposure effect**. Samples should be of adequate size in order for estimates to be calculated with the desired degree of **precision**. Samples should also be **unbiased**, i.e. representative of the **source population**, if used to estimate population parameters (the same applies to a random sample of controls from the source population in a case–control study). See also **sampling**, **sample size** (required), **sampling error**, sample **statistic**, **target population**.

## Sample estimate

See **estimate**, sample **statistic**.

## Sample size

Either the size of a **study sample** (that has been collected through selection or **sampling**) or the predetermined size of sample required to ensure desired statistical **power** and degree of **precision**. See **sample size** (required).

## Sample size (Required)

The number of individuals or **study units** required for a research study, so that **minimally important differences** (i.e. **clinically significant**), if real, may be detected as **statistically significant** (at a given level **alpha** of significance). Sample sizes may be calculated also for the purpose of **estimation**, in which case the issue is not statistical **power** but the **precision** (or width) of **confidence intervals** (POCOCK, 1983). Such calculations usually produce larger required sample sizes, as compared to 'power calculations'. BLAND (2015), and KIRKWOOD & STERNE (2003) give formulae for a number of estimates or **summary measures** for both power and precision calculations. In studies estimating or comparing

**rates**, required sample sizes are units of **person-time** (same as the denominator of the rate or rates). KIRKWOOD & STERNE give adjustment factors to be applied when the study design calls for unequal sample sizes between comparison groups, and discuss adjustments for losses to follow-up, confounding, interaction/subgroup analyses and clustered designs. BLAND (2015) also discusses unequal sample sizes, pointing out the resulting loss of **efficiency**, as well as requirements for **paired data**, and loss of power in **clustered designs**. HENNEKENS, BURING & MAYRENT (eds., 1987) give details regarding intervention and observational studies, and MACHIN & CAMPBELL (2005) give tables and formulae for a variety of study designs (observational, experimental, diagnostic and prognostic studies). COOK *et al.* (2014) review and discuss methodology for determining the minimally important or target difference in randomized controlled trials. For a comprehensive guide to sample size calculation see MACHIN *et al.* (2009). See also **design effect**, **effective sample size**, **sensitivity analyses**, **pilot study**.

## Sample statistic

See **statistic**, **estimate**.

## Sampling

The process of selecting a group of individuals from a population, with the aim to use the information provided by the **sample** to draw conclusions about a **source** or a **target population**. In **surveys** and **cross-sectional studies**, **random** and non-random sampling methods are used. Among the former, frequently used methods are **simple random sampling**, **stratified sampling**, **cluster sampling** and **multistage sampling**. **Systematic sampling** and quota sampling are examples of non-random methods frequently used in market research. The ability to generalize from sample to population relies on its representativeness or lack of **bias**. Sampling is not usually employed in **comparative studies** (with the exception of selection of **controls** in **case–control studies**, which may be carried out through sampling), where comparability and internal validity are the main concerns regarding avoidance of bias. See COCHRAN (1977) and LEVY & LEMESHOW (2009) for comprehensive guides to sampling techniques. See also **efficiency**.

## Sampling bias

A systematic error or distortion that affects **sample estimates**, and which is due to non-**random** methods of sample selection. See also **sampling**, **systematic sampling**, **selection bias**. Cf. **sampling error**.

## Sampling distribution

The **theoretical distribution** of sample **estimates**, for samples of a given size $n$. As sample size increases, the distribution of sample estimates may often be approximated by the **Normal distribution**, with **mean** equal to the (unknown) population mean, and **standard deviation** equal to the **standard error** of the estimate. This forms the basis of large sample methods of estimation and significance testing around a *single* sample estimate, i.e. given the value of the estimate and the size of the study sample, the spread of the sampling distribution may be inferred, and inferences may be made about the **precision** with which the estimate was calculated, and whether or not it is consistent with the **null value** being true. See also **sampling error, confidence interval, test statistic, central limit theorem.**

## Sampling error

A **random error** that affects **sample estimates** by virtue of being based on a sample, rather than ascertained from the entire **population** (whether this would actually be feasible, or simply a concept that recognizes that more precise and accurate results would be obtained if much greater numbers of individuals could be included in a research study). Thus, if a study could be repeated using a different study sample, it would be expected to yield a different result when compared to the initial study, due to random differences from sample to sample. However, both results would be expected to be in the vicinity (under or over) of the 'true' effect or 'true' parameter that is being estimated, provided **sample sizes** are sufficiently large and the assessments **unbiased**. This type of error is reflected in the magnitude of **standard errors** and the width of interval estimates. Greater **precision** may be achieved by increasing a study's sample size. See **sampling distribution.** Cf. **sampling bias.**

## Sampling frame

A list or enumeration of every single member of a given **source population**. Such a list is required for implementing a **simple random sampling** scheme, and for sampling a random **control series** from the relevant source population in a case–control study. Where sampling frames cannot be produced, alternative methods such as **cluster** and **multistage sampling** (or individual **matching** in a case–control study) may be employed.

## Sampling unit

The basic unit of **sampling**, which is usually either a single individual (as for example, in simple random sampling) or a group or collective of individuals (as in cluster sampling, or as in the first stage(s) of multistage sampling). See also **study unit, clustered designs**.

## Sampling variation

Synonym for **sampling error.**

## Sandwich variance estimate

Or Huber–White variance estimate. A **variance** estimate that takes account of observed variability (cluster-level or observation-level), rather than simply assume a **probability distribution** for the outcome variable. The square root of this quantity is a robust **standard error (SE)**. The Huber–White variance estimate finds an application in the analysis of **clustered designs** (for example, using **generalized estimating equations**), and in providing variance (or SE) estimates for regression models fitted through **weighted least squares**. See also **robust method, mean squared error (MSE)**. See KIRKWOOD & STERNE (2003) and HAMILTON (2012) for additional details and illustrative examples.

## Saturated model

A **model** that includes all possible **product terms** between its **predictor variables** and therefore provides **estimates** for all **main effects** and, in addition, for all possible first and higher order **statistical interactions** (i.e. product terms involving two or more predictor variables). A saturated model **fits** the observed data perfectly as it has as many parameters or coefficients as there are observations (HOSMER, LEMESHOW & STRURDIVANT, 2013). See also **nested model, goodness-of-fit (GoF)**, **deviance statistic, Pearson goodness-of-fit statistic, residual sum of squares**. Cf. **maximal model, null model**.

## SBM

Abbreviation for **science-based medicine**.

## Scale parameter

See **overdispersion**.

## Scatterplot

A **graphical display** of the relationship between two **ordinal** or **quantitative variables**. Scatterplots should be presented when measuring the **correlation** between any two given variables or when fitting a **regression model**, for a better assessment of the pattern of relationship (linear or otherwise) that is present. In addition, the presence of **outliers** may be detected by visual inspection of the scatterplot. In regression analysis, the **outcome variable** is plotted on the $y$-(vertical) axis, and the **predictor variable** on the $x$-(horizontal) axis. See Figure P.1 on p. 257.

## Scheffé's test

See **multiple-comparison procedures**.

## Science-based medicine

Also referred to by its abbreviation, SBM. A counterpoint, or, ideally, a complement to **evidence-based medicine (EBM)**, which stresses the crucial role of the basic medical sciences in determining the plausibility of research hypotheses in the medical field, and in translating the results from research studies into implementable measures and policies. Proponents of SBM hold the view that this has been a neglected aspect of EBM. Scientific plausibility may be regarded as a *prior belief,* which establishes an affinity between SBM and **Bayesian inference**. See also **cause–effect relationship**/biological plausibility.

## Scientific notation

A convenient way of expressing numbers (in the usual base 10) that are otherwise lengthy to write down in full, particularly if there are many zeros. For instance, it is convenient to express the speed of light in a vacuum, to three **significant figures**, as $300{,}000{,}000$ m s$^{-1} \equiv 3.00 \times 10^8$ m s$^{-1}$. Similarly, the charge on an electron, to three significant figures, is $0.000\ 000\ 000\ 000\ 000\ 000\ 160$ C $\equiv 1.60 \times 10^{-19}$ C.

## Score test

An alternative form of the **likelihood ratio test**.

## Scree plot

A plot of eigenvalues against the ordered orthogonal (i.e. uncorrelated) components in a **principal components analysis** (**PCA**). Components are combinations of individual items or variables, and the corresponding eigenvalues (the **variances** of the components) are a measure of a component's ability to encapsulate unique information. Eigenvalues are computed from the correlation coefficients (squared) between components and individual items, as displayed in a component matrix (see Table 3 in WU *et al.* [2013]). The graph in Figure S.1 is a scree plot from the population-based study by WU *et al.* (2013) to develop and validate a lifetime sunlight exposure questionnaire

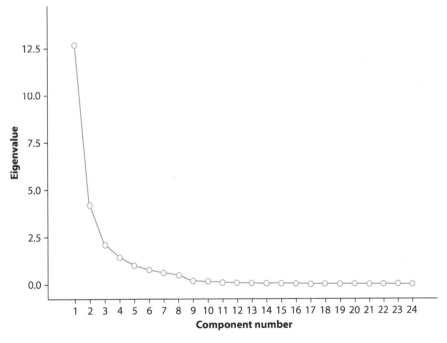

Figure S.1 Scree plot: eigenvalues *vs.* ordered components from a principal components analysis to evaluate the construct validity of a lifetime sunlight exposure questionnaire for Chinese women in Hong Kong. Four components are shown to have eigenvalues >1, with components 1 and 2 jointly explaining 70.4% of the variance in the data. (Reproduced from Wu SH *et al.* (2013). Development and validation of a lifetime exposure questionnaire for use among Chinese populations. *Sci Rep* **3**: 2793 (with permission).)

for use among Chinese women. Individual items in the questionnaire are a series of measurements that were found suitable for measuring lifetime exposure. A total of 650 premenopausal Chinese women in Hong Kong completed the questionnaire by telephone interview. By visual inspection, the 'elbow' of the plot divides the most important components from the least important ones; the former are retained as the key eigenvalues. Four components have eigenvalues >1, but in the end a two-component construct that used all the individual items was decided upon as appropriate, with the first component, labelled "frequency and duration worked in the sun in four respective seasons in life", explaining 52.9% (i.e. eigenvalue/no. of items*100%) of the variance in the data and the second component, "hours per day spent in the sun in summer and other 3 seasons in 4 life stages", 17.5%, for a cumulative 70.4%.

## Screening

Clinical, laboratory, radiological and other tests, which are performed on 'healthy' individuals in order to identify **risk factors** for disease, or detect disease at early, asymptomatic stages. For example, pregnant women may be screened for high hCG levels, which increase the risk of carrying a Down's syndrome fetus. Women with high hCG levels need to undergo further **diagnostic testing** (amniocentesis for chromosome typing) so that a conclusive Down's syndrome diagnosis may be made. Because screening tests target seemingly healthy individuals and are sometimes performed in settings with low **prevalence** of disease, the probability of **false-positive** results can be considerably high as the **predictive value** of positive test results will be low. Thus, when screening for less common disorders, it is particularly important that the screening test should have reasonable performance or accuracy, i.e. adequate detection (or sensitivity) and false-positive rates (WALD, 2004) (see **ROC curve**). Policy decisions, such as whether or not to implement wide-scale screening programmes, must balance these and other considerations. WALD (2004) also highlights **post-test odds**, also known as the 'odds of being affected given a positive result' or OAPR, as a valuable measure of performance, particularly when carrying out sequential testing (for example, a screening test followed by a diagnostic test) and comparing the performance of different tests. Post-test odds more readily reflect differences in diagnostic accuracy than the positive predictive value (also termed 'post-test probability of disease'). See also **lead-time bias**, **length-time bias**. WALD (2004) gives examples and requirements of worthwhile screening programmes, and WALD, HACKSHAW & FROST (1999) discuss the quantitative relation between risk factors and screening tests, and how strongly a risk factor needs to be associated with a disease before it is likely to be a useful screening test. See also HENNEKENS, BURING & MAYRENT (eds., 1987); Morrison, in ROTHMAN & GREENLAND (eds., 1998).

## SD

Abbreviation for **standard deviation**.

## SE

Abbreviation for **standard error**.

## Selection bias

A distortion of assessment that stems from the methods employed in selecting study partici-pants and from factors that influence study participation (ROTHMAN, 2012). In **surveys** and descriptive cross-sectional studies, selection bias commonly results from systematic differ-ences between a **sample** and its **source population**. This may be due to inappropriate **sam-pling** methods (**sampling bias**), or to systematic differences between those who volunteer to participate (for example, those who return a questionnaire that has been mailed to prospec-tive participants) and those who decline participation (**volunteer** or respondent **bias**). The bias resulting from the lack of representativeness of the study sample will be in the form of study results that underestimate or overestimate the parameters of interest in the population. In **comparative studies**, selection bias is usually due to factors that disrupt the comparabil-ity between exposure or treatment groups (or between cases and controls). For example, in **case–control studies**, cases that have higher levels of **exposure** are often more likely to be diagnosed in the first place and therefore more likely to be selected for inclusion in a study. This happens because their unusually high levels of exposure to a particular **risk factor** result in more intensive investigation (**detection bias**) when they present to a physician. Detection bias is likely to result in *overestimation* of exposure effect as exposure among cases is atypically high. Similarly, **matching** and **overmatching** of cases and controls may result in a control group with atypically high exposure, and therefore in the likely *underestimation* of exposure effect. **Berkson's fallacy** is another source of selection bias in case–control studies. Detection bias, overmatching and Berkson's fallacy all share a common feature in that selection of cases (or controls) is not independent of exposure status. In the context of **clinical trials**, selection or allocation bias may occur due to lack of **concealment** of **treatment allocation** (SCHULZ, 2000; ALTMAN & SCHULZ, 2001; SCHULZ & GRIMES, 2002b). Non-compliance with trial protocol (**drop-outs**, **'cross-overs'**, **withdrawals**, etc.) and **losses to follow-up** may also lead to selection bias and to underestimation or overestimation of treatment effects, in particular when these **protocol breaches** and losses to follow-up are both differential and informative. The latter may be an issue also in **cohort studies** (see also **censoring**). A particular type of selection bias may occur when occupational groups are compared to the general population. This is due to the **healthy worker effect**, which tends to result in underestimation of occu-pational exposure effects. Greenland & Lash, in ROTHMAN, GREENLAND & LASH (eds., 2012), make a distinction between selection biases that may be controlled like confounding ('selection confounding'), and selection biases that are uncontrollable. See also **bias, infor-mation bias, confounding**; GRIMES & SCHULZ (2002). Cf. **sampling error** or variation.

## SEM

Abbreviation for standard error of measurement (sometimes also, for **standard error** of the **mean**). See **repeatability, reliability**.

## Semi-interquartile range

A measure of **dispersion** or **variability** that is equal to one-half of the **interquartile range**.

## Semi-log plot

See **exponential curve, curvilinear regression**.

## Semi-parametric method

A method of statistical analysis that makes a limited number of **assumptions** regarding the data at hand. **Cox regression** is a well-known example: the model makes an assumption regarding the constancy of the hazard ratio over the period of follow-up, and models the effects of predictor variables, but no **distributional** assumptions are made with regard to the 'time-to-event' variable that records survival times. **Generalized estimating equations** (**GEEs**) are another example.

## Sensitivity

In the context of **diagnostic testing**, the sensitivity of a given test measures its ability to detect those individuals who are truly diseased or have some condition of interest (true positives). From Table 4 (p. 191):

$$Sensitivity = \frac{all\ testing\ positive\ and\ diseased}{all\ diseased} = \frac{a}{a+c}$$

The complement of sensitivity is the false-negative rate: $c/(a + c)$. Sensitivity relates to **specificity** in that increasing the former leads to a decrease in the latter. Like specificity, sensitivity is usually not affected by changes in **prevalence** of disease. However, **spectrum bias** may sometimes cause different studies to provide different estimates of accuracy (sensitivity and specificity) for a diagnostic test. Use of the term 'detection rate' is more intuitive and should perhaps be encouraged. See also **ROC curve**, **SnNout**, **diagnostic odds ratio** (**DOR**).

## Sensitivity analyses

The repetition of a particular statistical procedure or calculation under a number of different assumptions, in order to assess the impact each of these varying assumptions or scenarios would have on the conclusions of a study, or on logistic requirements. As an example, statistical analyses carried out at the end of a **follow-up study** will likely exclude data from individuals **lost to follow-up**. These analyses can then be repeated to include all subjects originally in the study. **Outcomes** for individuals lost to follow-up are **imputed**, allowing for best or worst case-scenarios, as appropriate to the aims of the study. This second round of data analyses may yield results that are not consistent with the initial analyses. In such cases, the results first obtained should be viewed with some caution. In terms of study requirements, sensitivity analyses may be used, for example, to calculate the **sample sizes** required given different scenarios, where any of the following may change: extent to which a **type I error** is allowed to occur; desired statistical **power**; ratio between number of unexposed and **exposed**; **minimally important difference** postulated to exist between treatment groups; degree of **variability** of measurements, etc. In the context of **systematic reviews**, where some individual studies may be of poorer quality than others, or where **publication bias** is suspected, sensitivity analyses can help assess the impact of removing such studies from the **meta-analysis**, (also referred to as 'influence analysis'), or the impact of assumed estimates of effect for studies that may be missing (known as 'trim and fill').

## Sequential designs

**Study designs** that allow for the conduct of **interim analyses**, which monitor the accumulating data in a **clinical trial** that is ongoing. The aim in using this type of design is to allow a trial to be stopped as soon as there is convincing evidence of clear benefit – or harm – of one of the treatments being compared. The algorithm to be followed, informed by the results of these analyses, constitutes the **stopping rules**, which are set in advance of conducting the trial. Sequential designs take place under two main modalities, *continuous*, after each patient's results become available, or *periodical*, after every few *x* number of patients. The latter is known as *group sequential design*, and is more commonly employed since it decreases the number of **multiple significance tests** to be carried out, while still retaining the chief feature of being able to detect a **treatment effect** early on. ALTMAN (1991) and POCOCK (1983) point out the suitability of the sequential design to situations in which the outcome is known relatively quickly. POCOCK (1983) further discusses the issue of how many interim analyses, and how many patients to evaluate between analyses, pointing out the need for overall larger sample sizes in sequential designs if a clear relative benefit does not emerge early on, a need that may nonetheless be obviated if indeed the early analyses also lead to early termination of the trial. Open and closed sequential plans and other issues pertaining to continuous sequential designs are also discussed. See also ARMITAGE, BERRY & MATTHEWS (2002), SENN (2008).

## Serial measurements

Data that are repeated measurements over a period of time. A distinction is often made between **time series**, where measurements are made at the group or population level, and over an extended period of time (typically, months, years or decades), and serial measurements, which are repeated measurements over time at the individual level. These tend to span a shorter period of time (commonly, a 24-hour period, 1 week, 1 month), although they may also be recorded over an extended follow-up period in **longitudinal studies**. The analysis of serial measurements evaluates the pattern of variation over time, including the presence of **cyclic variation**, in addition to providing estimates of relative activity or **treatment effect**, if of interest. Methods described under **longitudinal data** and **repeated measurements analysis** may be employed. Alternatively, a **summary measure** may be chosen that captures a pertinent feature of response over time (e.g. $C_{max}$, $T_{max}$, **AUC**), thus reducing the multiplicity of measurements for each individual to a single value. **Line graphs** showing individual trajectories over time offer the best visual representation for this type of data. This is illustrated in Figures S.2a–S.2d, from the study by PUKRITTAYAKAMEE *et al.* (2003) on the effects of adding rifampin (a tuberculostatic antibiotic) to quinine (QR *vs.* Q) in adults with uncomplicated falciparum malaria in Bangkok, Thailand. Although parasite clearance times were shorter with QR than Q alone, recrudescence rates were five times higher under the former, due to greater conversion of quinine to 3-hydroxyquinine (3-OH-Q), resulting in lower plasma levels of the drug (quinine). Serial drug concentration measurements (of Q and 3-OH-Q) show an overall *growth pattern* (ending in a plateau) for measurements in the Q alone group, and a *peak pattern* for measurements in the QR group. See also **area under the curve** (Figure A.2, p. 16); MATTHEWS *et al.* (1990), ALTMAN (1991).

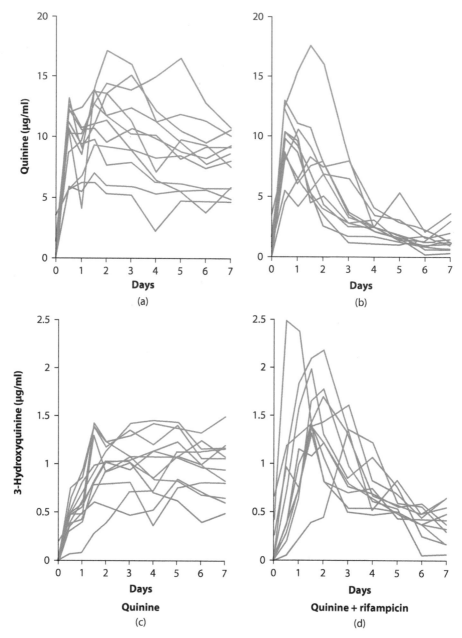

**Figures S.2a–S.2d** Serial measurements: concentrations of quinine (Q) and 3-hydroxyquinine (3-OH-Q) in the plasma of patients with *P. falciparum* malaria treated with Q (*n* = 12) or quinine plus rifampicin (QR) (*n* = 11). Each line represents serial drug concentration measurements of an individual patient. No patient had detectable levels on admission. The median $AUC_{0-7}$ of Q was significantly lower in patients treated with QR than in those given Q monotherapy, and this was attributable to significantly lower Q levels between the third and seventh days of treatment (median $AUC_{3-7}$: 11.7 versus 47.5 μg/ml*day; *P* < 0.004). (Reproduced from Pukrittayakamee S *et al.* (2003). Adverse effect of rifampin on quinine efficacy in uncomplicated falciparum malaria. *Antimicrob Agents Chemother* **47**: 1509–13 (with permission).)

## Severity of illness index

A rating tool that is used to assign a severity score to patients experiencing an acute, often critical episode of illness. A well-known example is the Glasgow Coma Scale (GCS), a neurological scale for measuring level of consciousness, reflecting the extent of brain injury in trauma patients and in patients undergoing acute medical conditions. Another example is the **APACHE score**. Both may be incorporated as an added component of other severity and **prognostic indices**. See also **classification**; TEASDALE & JENNETT (1974).

## Shapiro–Francia test

A **significance test** that is equivalent to the **Shapiro–Wilk test** and is also carried out to test the assumption of **normality** of distribution for interval/ratio data. The test statistic for the Shapiro–Francia test, $W'$, is the square of **Pearson's correlation coefficient**, $r$ (i.e. $r^2$), for the relationship between the values of the variable in question and the corresponding **z-** or Normal **scores** assuming a perfectly Normal distribution, as obtained when graphing a **Normal plot**. As the **null hypothesis** is that $W'$ ($r^2$) equals 1 (or 100%), high correlation and large **P-values** (as obtained from tables of the critical values of the S-F test statistic) are usually indicative of data that conform to a Normal distribution. See ALTMAN (1991) for an illustrative example. See also **goodness-of-fit (GoF)**.

## Shapiro–Wilk test

A **significance test** that is carried out to evaluate the extent to which the distribution of an **interval/ratio variable** departs from a **Normal distribution**. The assumption of normality is usually rejected if the Shapiro–Wilk test produces a small **P-value** (for example, <0.05). A statistic frequently reported, in addition to the **test statistic**, $W$, is $V$, which takes the value of 1 if a variable is normally distributed, or greater than 1 if not. The test should be interpreted with some caution as it may be too sensitive to departures from normality. It should preferably be used in conjunction with graphical methods, in particular, the **Normal plot**. An equivalent test is the **Shapiro–Francia test**. See also **goodness-of-fit (GoF)**.

## Sigmoid curve

A depiction of a **non-linear relationship** between two **continuous variables**, characterized by an initial slow or no growth phase, followed by growth acceleration in the form of a steeper segment, and a final deceleration or stagnant phase as an asymptotic upper value is approached. This is shown in Figure S.3 (MITCHELL & JAKUBOWSKI, 1999), which models the increasing complication rate with age, in a group of 1172 patients who underwent surgical treatment of unruptured intracranial aneurysms. As the negative exponential curve, this curve is characteristic of constrained population growth, although it differs in that it has an initial phase of slow growth. Sigmoid or S-shaped curves are fitted through **non-linear regression**. The specific curve obtained depends on the magnitude and direction of the parameters of a given model, and the values of the $x$-variable. Reverse sigmoid curves – in which there is a slow decline, followed by rapid decline, followed by a return to a slow decline – may also be obtained. HAMILTON (1992; 2012) describes logistic and Gompertz curves as examples of symmetrical and asymmetrical sigmoid curves. Sigmoid curves are also characteristic of **cumulative distribution functions** (for the Normal, $t$ and logistic **probability distributions**), and may be fitted to model cumulative response. See also **exponential curve, U-shaped curve, J-shaped curve, spline regression**.

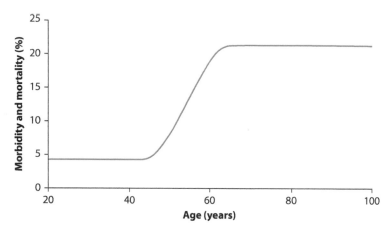

**Figure S.3** Sigmoid curve: operative morbidity and mortality (as % of individuals) as a function of age in 1172 patients who underwent surgical treatment of unruptured intracranial aneurysms. Morbidity refers to individuals requiring help with acts of daily living 1 year after surgery. (Reproduced from Mitchell P, Jakubowski J (1999). Risk analysis of treatment of unruptured aneurysms. *J Neurol Neurosurg Psychiatry* **68**: 577–80 (with permission).)

## Sign test

A basic test of **significance** that may be used with **paired data**. With paired interval/ratio and ordinal data, it is a simplified version of the **Wilcoxon signed rank test**, especially useful when the **assumption** of symmetry (for the distribution of paired differences) does not hold. With paired binary data, it is usually referred to as **McNemar's test**. It may also be used with paired ordered categorical (or nominal) data. See BLAND (2015), KIRKWOOD & STERNE (2003), ALTMAN (1991) and FLEISS (1999) for illustrative examples. See also POCOCK (2006).

## Significance level

In the context of **significance testing**, the significance level is the stipulated value for **alpha**, the **probability** of a **type I error**. The level of significance must be decided upon when calculating **sample size** requirements, as it expresses the degree of tolerance for a type I error when significance tests are later performed. Alpha ($\alpha$) is often set at 0.05 or 0.01 (that is, 5% or 1% probability, respectively). A significance level of 0.01 is considered *higher* than one of 0.05. Where **multiple significance tests** are to be performed on the same body of data, a useful strategy is the stipulation of **nominal significance levels** for each of the separate analyses to be carried out. This ensures the *overall* significance level remains at a given desired level, albeit lower than the stipulated nominal levels. The **P-value** is the significance level that is obtained *after* carrying out the actual significance test. See also **power, critical value**.

## Significance test

A statistical test that is performed to evaluate the plausibility of a given research hypothesis. Research hypotheses stem from questions such as 'are smokers at greater risk of having lung cancer?', 'is drug A better than drug B in treating asthma?', etc. The test evaluates the compatibility of data generated during the course of a research study with the **null hypothesis**. A **P-value** is produced, which gives the probability of a result of equal or greater magnitude as the result observed in the **study sample**, under the assumption that the null hypothesis is true. Although significance tests are widely used, it is often argued conclusions should be based on **estimation** rather than (or, at least, in addition to) significance testing. See also **test statistic, type I error, type II error, power**. The specific statistical test to be performed depends on the nature of the variable or variables involved and questions being asked. A comprehensive guide is given by BLAND (2015) and KIRKWOOD & STERNE (2003). See also **multiple significance testing**; comment under **hypothesis testing**.

## Significant figures

With the exception of leading zeros for numbers lying between zero and 1, these are the number of digits of accuracy to which given numbers are (to be) expressed. For instance, a plasma potassium level expressed as 4.3 mEq/l to two significant figures implies that the actual potassium level lies between the values of 4.25 mEq/l and 4.35 mEq/l. As a further example, 0.04865 = 0.0487 to three significant figures (ignoring the first leading zero after the decimal point and rounding up the 5). See also **precision, rounding error**.

## Simon-minimax design

A two-stage **Phase II trial** design that is similar to the **Simon-optimal design**. **Sample size** requirements for the two stages are calculated jointly so as to minimize the total number of patients recruited. MACHIN & CAMPBELL (2005) give details.

## Simon-optimal design

A two-stage **Phase II trial** design in which the number of responses showing treatment activity in the first stage determines whether the trial progresses into the second stage. The design is optimized to minimize further allocation of patients in Stage 1 to a treatment regimen without demonstrable activity. See also **sequential designs**. MACHIN & CAMPBELL (2005) give details.

## Simple random allocation

Synonym for **simple randomization**.

## Simple random sampling

A method for selecting a representative **sample** from a given **population**, in which the probability of being selected is the same for each individual. The method is carried out in a random fashion, so that the probability of an individual being selected from the population is also independent of his or her own characteristics. A **sampling frame** that enumerates each member of the population is necessary to carry out this sampling modality. Where the population cannot be enumerated, **cluster** and **multistage sampling** may provide an alternative way of carrying out **random sampling**. In addition to sample selection for **surveys** and **cross-sectional studies**, simple random sampling may also be employed to select the **controls** in a **case–control study** if the **source population** can be enumerated. Here, also, controls should be selected independently of their exposure status. See also **sampling**, **probability sampling**.

## Simple randomization

A treatment **allocation** scheme in which patients in a **clinical trial** or other intervention study are assigned to the different treatments under study with equal probability. As opposed to **cluster randomization**, individual patients are the **study units**. Unequal sized comparisons groups (cf. **restricted randomization**) and prognostic imbalances (cf. **stratified randomization**) may result from simple randomization, especially when study samples are small. See also **randomization**, **completely randomized design** (a study design that uses simple randomization), **randomization list**.

## Simple regression analysis

A **regression analysis** in which a single **predictor variable** is used to predict the value of the **outcome variable**. In simple **linear regression** both the outcome and predictor are **quantitative variables**, often **continuous**. A simple regression with a quantitative outcome and a **categorical** predictor produces results that are equivalent to one-way **analysis of variance**. Simple regression analysis is also referred to as univariable or univariate regression. Cf. **multiple** or multivariable (multiple predictors) **regression**, **multivariate** (multiple outcomes) **methods**.

## Simpson's paradox

An extreme type of **bias** that may occur when the evaluation of an exposure effect does not take into account an important **confounding factor**. Simpson's paradox may cause **crude estimates** of effect to show the *opposite* **direction** to that of **adjusted estimates** (which are obtained after **stratification**). The spurious association is due to the fact that a common cause creates the association between exposure and outcome. HERNÁN, CLAYTON & KEIDING (2011) commented that Simpson's intent in highlighting this phenomenon was less to point out the resulting confounding effect, and more to point out the fact that fallacies in defining a causal structure for the problem at hand will result in oddities and distortions. Box S.1 provides an illustrative example (although not conclusive regarding the effectiveness of the treatment in question). See JULIOUS & MULLEE (1994) for further illustration. Cf. **non-collapsibility**.

## BOX S.1

Based on Chan WK, Redelmeier DA (2012). Simpson's paradox and the association between vitamin D deficiency and increased heart disease. *Am J Cardiol* **110**: 143–4 (Abstract and Figure 1 reproduced with permission).

*From the abstract:* "Several recent investigations have highlighted a potential link between vitamin D deficiency and increased heart disease. Observational studies suggest cardioprotective benefits related to supplementation, but randomized trials remain to be conducted. This report adds a caution based on a statistical paradox that is rarely mentioned in formal medical training or in common medical journals. Insight into this phenomenon, termed Simpson's paradox, may prevent clinicians from drawing faulty conclusions about vitamin D deficiency and heart disease."

To illustrate this point, the authors present the results from a hypothetical cohort of 2600 patients. The aggregated results appear to indicate a significant association between vitamin D deficiency and risk of heart disease. When results are stratified according to levels of physical activity (sedentary *vs.* active), the association is reversed and vitamin D deficiency now seems to protect against heart disease (Figure 1, in CHAN & REDELMEIER, 2012).

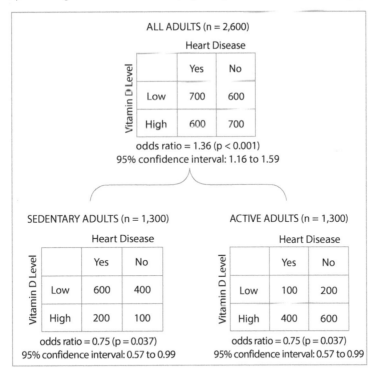

**Figure 1** When the full cohort of patients is analyzed as a whole, low levels of vitamin D are associated with increased heart disease (odds ratio 1.36, 95% confidence interval 1.16–1.59, p <0.001). When the study is stratified into sedentary and active patient subgroups, however, the effect reverses, and vitamin D deficiency seems to protect against heart disease (odds ratio 0.75, 95% confidence interval 0.57–0.99, p = 0.037).

*continued.....*

*continued.....*

*Interpretation:*

1  Low levels of vitamin D were more prevalent in the sedentary group (although in this stratum the odds of heart disease were *lower* among those with low vitamin D than among those with high levels of vitamin D, and the odds of low levels of vitamin D were *higher* among those *not* experiencing heart disease).

2  High levels of vitamin D were more prevalent in the active group (and the odds of heart disease were *higher* for high *vs.* low vitamin D; likewise, the odds of low vitamin D were higher among those *not* experiencing heart disease).

3  Because the sedentary group is more likely to experience heart disease, and because the active group is less likely to experience heart disease, when data were analysed in the aggregate, a larger number (600) of individuals with low vitamin D (from the sedentary group) and a smaller number (400) of individuals with high vitamin D (from the active group) found itself under the heart disease 'yes' column. The opposite occurred under the 'no' column, i.e. a smaller number (400) with low vitamin D (from the sedentary group), and a larger number (600) with high vitamin D (from the active group).

4  The possibility of occurrence of Simpson's paradox in observational studies also underscores the need for **randomized controlled trials** as the means to carry out a proper assessment of **treatment efficacy** and **effectiveness**. CATES (2002) and ALTMAN & DEEKS (2002) discuss the possibility of Simpson's paradox when carrying out **meta-analyses** of intervention studies in which there is imbalance in the number of patients in each **treatment arm** (in the individual **primary studies**). The 'treat-as-one-trial' method of combining results, based on raw totals, is particularly susceptible to bias.

## Single blind

See **blinding**.

## Skewness

The quality of a **distribution** that has a relatively long left (negatively skewed) or right (positively skewed) tail (Figures S.4a and S.4b). Positively skewed distributions can sometimes be converted into **Normal distributions** by **log transforming** their values. Such variables are said to have a **lognormal distribution**, with an arithmetic mean that is higher in value than the **geometric mean**, median and mode. The opposite is true for a negatively skewed distribution, the arithmetic mean being lower in value than the median and the mode. Negatively skewed variables may be normalised through a square or cubic **power transformation**. Alternatively, skewed data may be summarized using **resistant measures** such as the **median**, which, unlike the arithmetic mean, is not sensitive to **outliers**, and analysed using **non-parametric** and **robust methods**, which generally make no **assumptions** regarding the distribution of the variable(s) in question. See also **J-shaped** (and reverse J-shaped) **distribution**, **symmetry**, **kurtosis**, **Normal plot**.

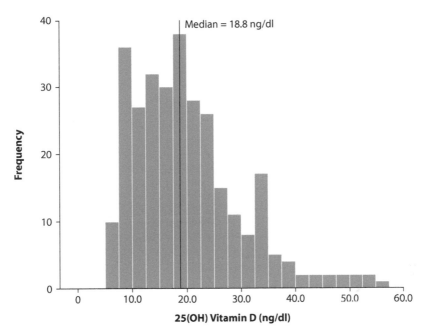

**Figure S.4a** Positively skewed distribution: distribution of serum 25(OH) vitamin D levels (in ng/dl) among asymptomatic adults (*n* = 300; 65% male; aged 30–80 years) in Karachi, Pakistan. Data are from a cross-sectional survey conducted in January 2011. The median 25(OH) vitamin D concentration was 18.8 ng/dl, and 84.3% of respondents had vitamin D levels <30 ng/dl. (Reproduced from Sheikh A *et al.* (2012). Vitamin D levels in asymptomatic adults – a population survey in Karachi, Pakistan. *PLoS One* **7**: e33452.)

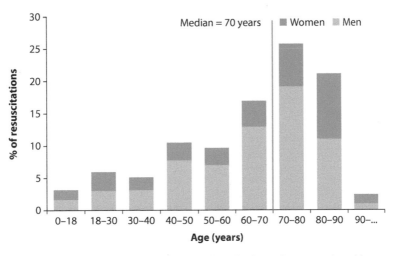

**Figure S.4b** Negatively skewed distribution: age distribution of cases of sudden cardiac death (SCD), based on 1212 EMS operations due to established SCD. Gender distribution in each age group is also shown. The median age at event was 69.5 years. Data is from an emergency medical service registry in Lower Saxony, Germany, and pertains to the period January 2002 to December 2009. (Adapted from Martens E *et al.* (2014). Incidence of sudden cardiac death in Germany: results from an emergency medical service registry in Lower Saxony. *Europace* **16**: 1752–8 (with permission).)

## Slope

Synonym for **regression coefficient**, in particular in the context of **simple linear regression**.

## Small area estimation

Or small area statistics. The range of techniques that may be employed in surveys and other studies, in order to shift estimation from the population to the subpopulation or local level. These techniques have been used, for example, to evaluate cancer clusters in connection with specific environmental exposures, such as the occurrence of leukaemia cases around the Sellafield (UK) nuclear plant. See ELLIOTT & WARTENBERG (2004) for an in-depth discussion of the analytical framework, types of studies, and methodological issues and challenges in carrying out small area estimation, with special focus on disease mapping and **clustering**, **ecological studies** (geographical correlation studies), and cluster detection and **surveillance**. See also **spatial epidemiology**.

## Smoothing

An **exploratory data analysis** technique for making the general shape of a data series apparent. Smoothed values may be obtained by calculating **moving averages**, for example, by taking **medians** (or some other location estimate) of each point in the original data and a few of the points around it. The number of points used is called the *span of the smoother*. Median smoothers are **resistant** to isolated outliers, so they are able to cope with spikes in the data. Because the median is also a non-linear operator, such smoothers are known as **robust** non-linear smoothers. Smoothing is usually applied to **time series**, but any variable with a natural order can be smoothed. For example, a smoother might be applied to birth rate recorded by maternal age (birth rate for 17-year-olds, birth rate for 18-year-olds, and so on). Additional smoothing methods include kernels and **locally weighted regression**. See HAMILTON (1990; 1992; 2012) and ARMITAGE, BERRY & MATHEWS (2002) for further details and illustrative examples. See also **spline regression**, **fractional polynomials**, **non-linear relationship**.

## SMR

Abbreviation for **standardized mortality ratio**.

## SND

Abbreviation for standard Normal deviate (**z-score**) and also **standard Normal distribution**.

## SnNout

In the context of **diagnostic testing**, a *negative* test result *rules out* the target disorder if both the **sensitivity** and the **likelihood ratio** for a positive test result are very high (Guyatt, Sackett & Haynes, in HAYNES *et al.* [eds., 2006]). See also **SpPin**.

## Source population

The carefully defined and identified **population** from which **samples** are to be drawn for **estimation** of population **parameters**. Often, in this type of study (surveys and other descriptive studies), source and **target population** are one and the same. The concept of source population is central also to estimation of **exposure effect**. For example, in **case–control studies**, specification of the source population allows the identification of cases within its confines, which in turn facilitates the identification of those who, had they developed the condition of interest, would also be identified as cases in this same population. Where the source population can be enumerated, a **random sample** of the non-diseased (or of the entire source population) provides an **unbiased** control series. The term **study population** is sometimes used as synonym for source population, i.e. a reasonably defined subset from a wider population from which study samples are selected through a given method.

## Spatial epidemiology

Defined by ELLIOTT & WARTENBERG (2004) as the description and analysis of geographically indexed health data with respect to demographic, behavioural, socioeconomic, genetic and infectious risk factors. The study of geographic correlations (**ecological studies**), disease mapping and **clustering**, and **surveillance** and detection of disease clusters are examples of studies that may be conducted. See also **epidemiology, small area estimation**.

## Spearman's rho

A **non-parametric** measure of **correlation**, which is calculated by computing **Pearson's correlation coefficient** ($r$) for the association between the **ranks** given to the values of each variable involved, as opposed to the actual data values. This coefficient may be calculated for **interval/ratio data** that do not meet the assumptions for Pearson's correlation, or for **ordinal data**. Spearman's rho ($\rho$) is not easily interpreted as a measure of the **strength of an association** (BLAND, 2015). Nevertheless, the **statistical significance** of the correlation may be assessed. See also **rank correlation, Kendall's tau**.

## Special exposure cohort

See **cohort study, control group**. Cf. general population cohort.

## Specificity

In the context of **diagnostic testing**, the specificity of a given test measures its accuracy at detecting those individuals who are not diseased or do not have some condition of interest (true negatives). From Table 4 (p. 191):

$$Specificity = \frac{all\ testing\ negative\ and\ non\text{-}diseased}{all\ non\text{-}diseased} = \frac{d}{b+d}$$

The **complement** of specificity is the false-positive rate (FPR): $b/(b+d)$ or $100 - specificity\%$. The concept of false-positive rate is more intuitive and more readily useful than that of specificity: one may not have a feel for the difference between a test that has 98% specificity and one that has 96%. However, when expressed as FPRs (2% *vs.* 4%), it is clear that one of the tests produces twice the number of false positives. Increasing the specificity of a test has the effect of decreasing its **sensitivity**. Like sensitivity, specificity is usually not affected by changes in **prevalence** of disease. However, **spectrum bias** may sometimes cause different studies to provide different estimates of accuracy (sensitivity and specificity) for a diagnostic test. See also **SpPin, diagnostic odds ratio (DOR), ROC curve**.

## Spectrum bias

A type of **bias** that occurs when estimating the **sensitivity** and **specificity** of a **diagnostic test** in groups with varying degrees of overall disease severity. Spectrum bias may explain why studies evaluating the same diagnostic tool sometimes produce different results. This type of bias is sometimes overlooked given the widespread belief that the sensitivity and specificity of a diagnostic test are immutable properties of the test. See Guyatt, Sackett & Haynes, in HAYNES *et al.* (eds., 2006).

## Spline regression

Also termed 'piecewise regression'. A method of **regression analysis** that uses linear or **polynomial** functions in order to describe complex **non-linear relationships**, with the analysis carried out for different intervals of the range of values of the **predictor variable**. The different segments of the resulting curve are joined at knots that correspond to the relevant interval boundaries of the predictor. Polynomial splines, cubic splines in particular, have greater flexibility than linear splines. See ARMITAGE, BERRY & MATHEWS (2002) for additional details. See also **smoothing**, **locally weighted regression**. Cf. **fractional polynomials**. See Figures J.1b (p. 176) and S.3 (p. 332) for illustrative examples.

## Split-plot design

Or more appropriately, 'split-unit' design in the context of medical rather than agricultural research. A **study design** for an **experimental study** in which the aim is to evaluate two different **factors**. A clinical trial employing this design would have patients randomly assigned to the different levels of factor A (the whole plot treatments), and patients within each level of factor A assigned to all the levels of factor B (the subplot treatments). The order of assignment of individuals to the levels of factor B is determined by **random permutations** (levels of factors A and B could be different treatment regimens and different modes of administration). This results in **repeated measurements** with regard to factor B, and *between-subject* comparisons on factor A and *within-subject* comparisons on factor B (HUITEMA, 2011). The **power** of the between-subject comparisons may be increased by including a covariate in the analysis (see **analysis of covariance**). The split-plot design can be viewed as an extension of the one-factor **randomized block design** with repeated measurements, on the one hand, and also of the **factorial design** (two factors, no repeated measurements). Mixed-design or split-plot **ANOVA** is appropriate for data analysis. When the different levels of factor B correspond to different time points in a **longitudinal study** (i.e. there is no randomization of order of assignment to the different levels of factor B), the analysis must factor in the correlation between repeated measurements over time. **Repeated measures ANOVA** and **linear mixed effects models** are employed in these situations. Additional details are given by FLEISS (1999), DIGGLE *et al.* (2002) and MITCHELL (2012b).

## SpPin

In the context of **diagnostic testing**, a *positive* test result *rules in* the target disorder if **specificity** is very high and the **likelihood ratio** for a negative test result is very low (Guyatt, Sackett & Haynes, in HAYNES *et al.* [eds., 2006]). See also **SnNout**.

## Square power transformation

See **transformations**, **polynomial regression**.

## Square root

A mathematical function, usually denoted by √. For example, the square root of 4 is 2, i.e. √4 = 2, and 4 equals the **square power** of 2, i.e. 4 = 2². See also **square root transformation**.

## Square root transformation

A **transformation** that may be applied to **quantitative variables** displaying a mild positive **skew**. The transformation is achieved by taking the **square root** (√) of the values of the variable in question, which has a **normalizing** and **variance-stabilizing** effect. It may be applied to **Poisson counts**, for which the variance is proportional to the mean. See FLEISS (1999) for an illustrative example. See also **logarithmic transformation, reciprocal transformation** (all transformations for positively skewed variables).

## S(t)

See **survival function**.

## Stacked bar chart

Also termed 'component bar chart'. A **graphical display** that may be used to show the relative **frequency distribution** of a **categorical variable** according to the categories of another variable. Figure S.5 shows the relative frequency distribution of causes of neonatal

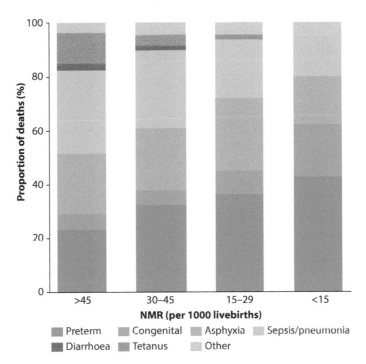

**Figure S.5** Stacked bar chart: relative frequency distribution of causes of neonatal death for 192 countries, according to degree of neonatal mortality (NMR) (2000). (Reproduced from Lawn JE *et al.* (2005). Neonatal survival 1: 4 million neonatal deaths: When? Where? Why? *Lancet* **365**: 891–900 (with permission).)

death for 192 countries, according to degree of neonatal mortality (year 2000), in the study by LAWN, COUSENS & ZUPAN (2005). It can be seen, for example, that in the countries with the lowest neonatal mortality rates (NMRs), preterm birth caused a larger proportion of neonatal deaths than sepsis & pneumonia, which were the leading causes of neonatal mortality in the countries with the highest NMRs.

## Standard deviation

A measure of the spread or **variability** of a set of quantitative measurements. Usually presented in conjunction with the **mean** to describe **interval** and **ratio data**. The standard deviation (SD) is a measure of the average distance individual observations are from the mean and is expressed in the same units as the measurements in question. A graphical assessment of the degree of symmetry of the variable's distribution aids in determining whether the standard deviation may be used to construct **central** and **reference intervals**. SD is the square root of the **variance**. The standard deviation of the **sampling distribution** of an estimate is given by the **standard error** of the sample estimate. See also **measures of dispersion**.

## Standard error

A statistic that reflects the degree of uncertainty around a sample **estimate**. The standard error may be interpreted as the **standard deviation** of a **sampling distribution**. **Sample size** and, with quantitative variables, the extent of **variability** of the measurements determine the magnitude of standard errors (SE). The larger the sample size and the narrower the range of variability, the smaller the standard error. Standard errors are more easily interpreted when used to construct **confidence intervals**. The **precision** of a confidence interval is *inversely* proportional to the magnitude of the standard error. See also **test statistic, inverse variance method, funnel plot**. See ALTMAN *et al.* (eds., 2000) for formulae and illustrative examples.

## Standard Normal deviate

Or its abbreviation, SND. Synonym for **z-score**. See also Table 6, p. 234 (**Normal distribution**). Cf. **inverse Normal**.

## Standard Normal distribution

See **Normal distribution**.

## Standard population

A **population** whose age structure or age-specific event rates are used as reference when evaluating **incidence** and **mortality rates** in a **study population**. See **standardization**.

## Standard score

See **z-score**.

## Standardization

A statistical method for comparing morbidity and mortality **rates** between different **populations**. The rationale for standardization is the potential for **confounding**, due to systematic differences in age and gender distribution, which **bias** the comparison of **crude** incidence and death rates. Standardization is usually performed to **adjust** for these differences in age/sex structure between the populations being compared. *Direct* and *indirect* standardization methods are employed. The former is used when studying large populations, and it involves the calculation of **standardized event rates** (commonly, age-standardized). These are calculated by applying the **age-specific rates** observed in the **study population** (for example, the population in a particular country, region or town) to the age structure (i.e. the proportion or relative frequency in each age group) of some prespecified **standard population** (for example, the population of England and Wales is often used as the standard population in studies looking at different regional health authorities). With the indirect method, the number of **expected events** in the study population is calculated, under the assumption that each age group in this population has experienced the same mortality or morbidity rates as in the standard population. The ratio between *observed* and *expected* number of events produces a standardized event ratio (e.g. **standardized mortality ratio** or **SMR**). The study population can now be compared either to the standard population, or to another study population (with similar structure) whose SMR has been computed with reference to the same standard population. The indirect method is especially indicated with small study populations, where event rates for the different age groups cannot be estimated with sufficient **precision** to allow the use of the direct method. With small populations, it is therefore preferable to work with the rates for the standard population. See BLAND (2015), and HENNEKENS, BURING & MAYRENT (eds., 1987).

## Standardized difference

A way of expressing a given difference in terms of the number of **standard deviations** this difference represents. Standardized differences are used in **meta-analyses** in order to combine **effect estimates** from the different **primary studies**, when these report different, albeit related, outcomes or endpoints. For **binary categorical data**, where a **proportion** (or risk) $p_0$ in calculated for group 0 (e.g. the control group) and $p_1$ for group 1 (the treatment group), the formula is given by:

$$\textit{Standardized difference between proportions} = (p_0 - p_1) / \sqrt{[p(1 - p)]}$$

where $p$ is $(p_0 + p_1)/2$, and $\sqrt{}$ stands for **square root**. For **continuous data** (or more generally, quantitative and ordinal data) relating to two **independent** groups, the formula is:

$$\textit{Standardized difference between means} = \textit{(difference between means)} / \textit{(standard deviation of the variable)}$$

where 'standard deviation of the variable' is given by the *pooled* estimate of standard deviation (see *t*-test). An illustrative example is shown in Figure S.6, from the meta-analysis by TAYLOR *et al.* (2014) of the effects of smoking cessation on mental health outcomes. See also **standardized measures of effect, Cohen's *d*, Glass's Delta, Hedge's adjusted *g*, effect size, weighted average, pooled estimate, nomogram**; BORENSTEIN *et al.* (2009). See HUITEMA (2011) and BLAND (2015) for illustrative examples.

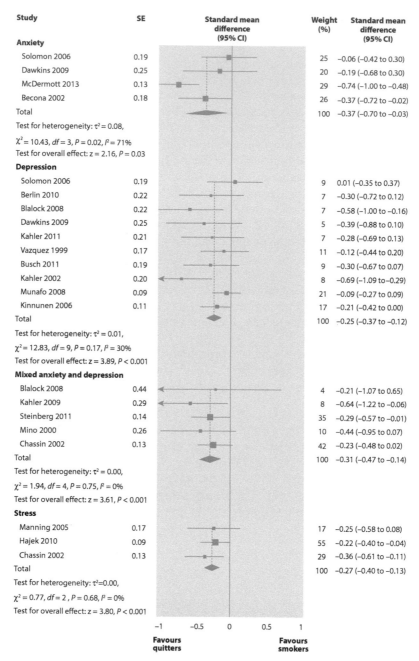

| Study | SE | Standard mean difference (95% CI) | Weight (%) | Standard mean difference (95% CI) |
|---|---|---|---|---|
| **Anxiety** | | | | |
| Solomon 2006 | 0.19 | | 25 | −0.06 (−0.42 to 0.30) |
| Dawkins 2009 | 0.25 | | 20 | −0.19 (−0.68 to 0.30) |
| McDermott 2013 | 0.13 | | 29 | −0.74 (−1.00 to −0.48) |
| Becona 2002 | 0.18 | | 26 | −0.37 (−0.72 to −0.02) |
| Total | | | 100 | −0.37 (−0.70 to −0.03) |

Test for heterogeneity: $\tau^2 = 0.08$,

$\chi^2 = 10.43$, $df = 3$, $P = 0.02$, $I^2 = 71\%$
Test for overall effect: $z = 2.16$, $P = 0.03$

| | | | | |
|---|---|---|---|---|
| **Depression** | | | | |
| Solomon 2006 | 0.19 | | 9 | 0.01 (−0.35 to 0.37) |
| Berlin 2010 | 0.22 | | 7 | −0.30 (−0.72 to 0.12) |
| Blalock 2008 | 0.22 | | 7 | −0.58 (−1.00 to −0.16) |
| Dawkins 2009 | 0.25 | | 5 | −0.39 (−0.88 to 0.10) |
| Kahler 2011 | 0.21 | | 7 | −0.28 (−0.69 to 0.13) |
| Vazquez 1999 | 0.17 | | 11 | −0.12 (−0.44 to 0.20) |
| Busch 2011 | 0.19 | | 9 | −0.30 (−0.67 to 0.07) |
| Kahler 2002 | 0.20 | | 8 | −0.69 (−1.09 to −0.29) |
| Munafo 2008 | 0.09 | | 21 | −0.09 (−0.27 to 0.09) |
| Kinnunen 2006 | 0.11 | | 17 | −0.21 (−0.42 to 0.00) |
| Total | | | 100 | −0.25 (−0.37 to −0.12) |

Test for heterogeneity: $\tau^2 = 0.01$,

$\chi^2 = 12.83$, $df = 9$, $P = 0.17$, $I^2 = 30\%$
Test for overall effect: $z = 3.89$, $P < 0.001$

| | | | | |
|---|---|---|---|---|
| **Mixed anxiety and depression** | | | | |
| Blalock 2008 | 0.44 | | 4 | −0.21 (−1.07 to 0.65) |
| Kahler 2009 | 0.29 | | 8 | −0.64 (−1.22 to −0.06) |
| Steinberg 2011 | 0.14 | | 35 | −0.29 (−0.57 to −0.01) |
| Mino 2000 | 0.26 | | 10 | −0.44 (−0.95 to 0.07) |
| Chassin 2002 | 0.13 | | 42 | −0.23 (−0.48 to 0.02) |
| Total | | | 100 | −0.31 (−0.47 to −0.14) |

Test for heterogeneity: $\tau^2 = 0.00$,

$\chi^2 = 1.94$, $df = 4$, $P = 0.75$, $I^2 = 0\%$
Test for overall effect: $z = 3.61$, $P < 0.001$

| | | | | |
|---|---|---|---|---|
| **Stress** | | | | |
| Manning 2005 | 0.17 | | 17 | −0.25 (−0.58 to 0.08) |
| Hajek 2010 | 0.09 | | 55 | −0.22 (−0.40 to −0.04) |
| Chassin 2002 | 0.13 | | 29 | −0.36 (−0.61 to −0.11) |
| Total | | | 100 | −0.27 (−0.40 to −0.13) |

Test for heterogeneity: $\tau^2 = 0.00$,

$\chi^2 = 0.77$, $df = 2$, $P = 0.68$, $I^2 = 0\%$
Test for overall effect: $z = 3.80$, $P < 0.001$

−1  −0.5  0  0.5  1

Favours quitters          Favours smokers

**Figure S.6** Standardized differences: unstandardized estimates of effect are the differences between mean change from baseline in mental health outcomes, as measured by a variety of scores (anxiety, depression, mixed anxiety and depression, stress), following smoking cessation (differences are between smokers who stopped *vs.* smokers who continued). **Standardized mean difference** is a standardized difference between two independent means. (Reproduced from Taylor G *et al.* (2014). Change in mental health after smoking cessation: systematic review and meta-analysis. *Br Med J* **348**: g1151 (with permission).)

## Standardized event rate

An **adjusted** mortality or morbidity **rate** (commonly age and sex adjusted), which is obtained using the direct **standardization** method. The adjusted event rate is calculated as follows: the *study population's* age/sex-specific rates are applied to the *standard population's* age/sex structure (i.e. the proportion or relative frequency in each age/sex stratum) by multiplying one by the other; this gives the contribution of each stratum which, when added up, produces a single overall measure of what the event rate would be in the **study population** if it had the same age/sex structure as the **standard population**. See BLAND (2015) for an illustrative example, and KIRKWOOD & STERNE (2003) for an alternative computation. Cf. **standardized mortality ratio**.

## Standardized measures of effect

A **measure of effect** that is standardized by rescaling it into units of standard deviation, or by expressing it as a proportion of total variability. *Unstandardized* effect measures are often used in the analysis of **primary studies**, and give estimates of **treatment** or **exposure effect** through measures such as differences between means, and risk and rate differences. *Standardized* measures, on the other hand, are particularly useful in the context of **meta-analysis**, where the individual studies included may have different, albeit related, **outcomes** (e.g. degree of flexibility and level of pain in patients with arthritis). For continuous outcomes, their calculation falls into two main 'families', *standardized differences* and *proportion-of-variance-explained* measures. Examples of the former are **Cohen's d**, **Glass's Delta (Δ)** and **Hedge's adjusted g**, which are generally calculated by dividing the estimated difference between means by a scale parameter, usually, the pooled **standard deviation**, or alternatively, the standard deviation in the control group. A **standardized difference** gives the difference between two groups in terms of number of standard deviations, as for example, 'the mean in group A is 2 standard deviations higher than in group B'. Standardized differences may also be calculated for binary outcomes (summarized as proportions or risks), with the pooled standard deviation calculated as $\sqrt{[p(1-p)]}$, where $p$ is the average of the two proportions or risks. Proportion-of-variance-explained measures relate to $r^2$, the square of **Pearson's correlation coefficient**, which in the context of correlation and simple linear regression analysis is interpreted as the proportion of the variability observed in a given variable that is explained by another. With linear regression and analysis of variance, $r$, **r-squared** ($r^2$), $R^2$ (**multiple correlation coefficient**, squared), $\eta^2$ (**eta squared**, also termed correlation ratio) and $\omega^2$ (**omega squared**) estimate the proportion of variability in the outcome variable that is explained by the effect or effects under study. Some of these measures are considered less **biased** ($R^2_{adjusted}$ and $\omega^2$). Partial measures (see **partial correlation coefficient**) may also be obtained. The square of the **intraclass correlation coefficient (ICC)** may be used with random effects models. For binary outcomes expressed as risks or odds, the **odds ratio** and the **risk ratio** may be better alternatives to proportion-of-variance-accounted-for measures. The **contingency coefficient**, $C$, and **Cramér's V** may be used with contingency tables. Standardized measures relate to the concept of *practical significance*, i.e. **clinical significance**, expressed in a manner that facilitates comparability between different studies. Methodological complexities and difficulties with correct interpretation should be kept in mind when evaluating standardized effects. The **magnitude of effect** is usually referred to as the **effect size**. Standardized differences may be calculated also for use with **nomograms** for **power** and **sample size** calculations (see Box P.6, Power, p. 276). See BLAND (2015) for an overview and further discussion, and BORENSTEIN *et al.* (2009) and ELLIS (2010) for a comprehensive presentation. HUITEMA (2011) gives illustrative examples for continuous outcomes. See also **weighted average, pooled estimate**.

## Standardized mortality ratio

Or its abbreviation, SMR. The ratio between the **observed** and **expected** numbers of an event (death if an SMR, but could be any other event), multiplied by 100:

$$SMR = \frac{observed\ number\ of\ events}{expected\ number\ of\ events} \times 100$$

SMRs are computed using the indirect **standardization** method. An SMR of 100 suggests the **rate** of occurrence of the event in the **study population** to be the same as in the **standard population**. HILLS (1974) shows internal SMRs for each group in a longitudinal study to be **weighted averages** of ratios across strata (stratum rates *over* pooled rate), with weights equal to the expected events in each group. The magnitude of an SMR is always lesser than the corresponding measure of relative risk (HENNEKENS, BURING & MAYRENT (eds.), 1987). Study populations with different age or age/sex structure should be compared via direct standardization rather than by comparing SMRs that were calculated with reference to the same standard population. See BLAND (2015) for an illustrative example. Cf. **standardized event rate, proportional mortality ratio (PMR)**.

## Standardized residual

The ratio of a **residual** to its **standard deviation**. In **linear regression**, for example, it is calculated as follows:

$$z_i = \frac{e_i}{s_e\sqrt{1-h_i}}$$

where the denominator is the standard deviation of the residual pertaining to the $i$th observation ($s_e$ is the standard deviation of the residuals and $h_i$ is the **leverage** of the same observation; the higher the leverage, the smaller the standard deviation, or variance, of the $i$th residual). The variance of the residuals ($s_e^2$) is given by the ratio of the **residual sum of squares** to its number of **degrees of freedom**. **Influential observations** tend to have high leverage and large standardized residuals (see **Cook's D**). With **generalized linear models**, measures of fit and influence are often based on standardized **deviance, Pearson** and other types of residuals (AGRESTI, 2007). See also **jackknifed** (or studentized) residual. HAMILTON (1992) makes reference also to scaled residuals, where the scale estimate is the common standard deviation or, alternatively, it may be computed on the basis of the 'median absolute deviation' or MAD when carrying out **robust** regression analysis.

## STARD statement

STARD (Standards for Reporting of Diagnostic Accuracy – BOSSUYT *et al.*, for the STARD Group, 2003; 2015) is a collaborative statement that sets out recommendations for reporting the rationale, methodology, results and conclusions of studies of diagnostic accuracy, in order to improve the accuracy and completeness of reporting, and facilitate the proper appraisal of the same (in particular, the assessment of potential for **bias** and variability of results in different studies, and the evaluation of **generalizability** of results). The set of recommendations comprises a 30-item checklist (updated in 2015 from the original 25-item checklist) and a flow diagram on which to provide details of the flow of participants through the study. See www.stard-statement.org for further details, supporting documentation, and extensions. See also **diagnostic test**, **EQUATOR Network**, **critical appraisal**, **TRIPOD statement**.

## Statistical interaction

Synonymous with **effect-measure modification**. See also **interaction**.

## Statistical significance

In the context of **significance testing**, whenever the resulting **P-value** is found to be below a predetermined (but arbitrary) cut-off point, conventionally set at 0.05. For correct interpretation, expressions such as '$P < 0.05$' or 'NS (non-significant)' should be avoided when reporting the results of a test. Instead, exact $P$-values should be quoted. In addition, **confidence intervals** should be calculated for a proper assessment of the **clinical significance** of study results. See also **type I error**, **positive study**, **negative study**, **multiple significance testing**.

## Statistical test

See **significance test**.

## Statistics

In a wider sense, this term refers to the collection, exploration, analysis, presentation and organization of **data** without seeking to draw any inferences about the larger population from which the sample is derived; this is **descriptive statistics**. In the context of inferential analysis, the term refers to quantities or summaries derived from **sample** data, from which the values of the corresponding **population parameters** may be inferred; the latter is **inferential** (or deductive) **statistics**. Sample statistics are usually denoted by Roman-alphabet letters ($\bar{x}$, SD, $p$), whereas population parameters are denoted by Greek-alphabet letters ($\mu$, $\sigma$, $\pi$). See also **estimate**, **test statistic**.

## Stem-and-leaf plot

A **graphical display** that is used to depict both the **frequency distribution** and the **raw data** values of a **quantitative variable**. Its construction gives the appearance of a sideways **histogram**. Here, each 'bar' of the 'histogram' is made up of a *stem*, which gives the first digit or digits of the relevant **class interval**, and one or more *leaves* (unless the frequency in the class interval is zero), which give the last digit of the data values, for each and every individual observation that falls in the class interval. Depending on **sample size**, stem-and-leaf plots provide a relatively quick way to display and tally the distribution of a variable. Where sample sizes are large, class intervals are usually further subdivided and the distribution in each class interval is given by two or more rows. Important data features such as **digit preference** are also easier to detect than on a histogram. Figure S.7 shows a stem-and-leaf plot for the age distribution of a hypothetical study sample of 105 individuals aged 5–<75 years. The count or frequency in each class interval is also shown, and a few data values are reconstructed for illustrative purposes (note that two of the class intervals, 5–<10; and 70–<75, are narrower, and the construction of a corresponding histogram would need to take this into consideration):

| Count | Stem | Leaves | Actual data values (age in years) |
|---|---|---|---|
| 07 | 0 | 5567899 | Class interval 5–<10 years old: 5, 5, 6, 7, 8, ... |
| 13 | 1 | 0112355678899 | Class interval 10–<20 years old: 10, 11, 11, 12, ... |
| 17 | 2 | 00122344456677789 | Class interval 20–<30 years old: 20, 20, 21, 22, ... |
| 21 | 3 | 012233334445555678999 | Class interval 30–<40 years old: 30, 31, 32, 32, ... |
| 17 | 4 | 12234566778887789 | Class interval 40–<50 years old: 41, 42, 42, 43, ... |
| 12 | 5 | 022445567789 | Class interval 50–<60 years old: 50, 52, 52, 54, ... |
| 11 | 6 | 12344566789 | Class interval 60–<70 years old: 61, 62, 63, 64, ... |
| 07 | 7 | 0112344 | Class interval 70–<75 years old: 70, 71, 71, 72, ... |

Figure S.7 Stem-and-leaf plot: age distribution for a hypothetical study sample of individuals aged 5–<75 years ($n$ = 105).

## Stepped wedge design

A **study design** that is often used in **cluster randomized trials**, in which randomization of clusters to the intervention under evaluation is carried out in a crossover (control to intervention) sequential manner, usually following a period of baseline assessments. This study design is well suited for evaluating the implementation of large-scale public health policies, and was developed for the phased introduction of hepatitis B (HBV) vaccination in infants in the Gambia in the 1980s (The Gambia Hepatitis Working Group, 1987). The new vaccine was introduced in a different geographical area every 10–12 weeks, with the aim of achieving national coverage within a period of 4 years. Important issues with this study design are **confounding** due to time trends, and a **design effect** due to the clustered nature of the design, among others. HEMMING *et al.* (2015) give a comprehensive overview of the rationale, design, analysis and reporting of stepped wedge trials.

## Stepwise regression

A method for selecting variables to be included as **predictors** in a **multiple** or **multivariable regression model**. Stepwise regression may be carried out as forward selection or backward elimination, and most statistical analysis software packages will perform the procedure in an automated way. The rationale behind the method is the need to find out which predictors relate independently to the **outcome variable**, and to simplify regression models, thus avoiding complex, unstable models, with highly correlated and redundant predictor variables. With forward selection, one begins by finding out which of the predictors is most strongly associated with the response variable (i.e. which predictor explains a larger proportion of the variability in the outcome variable). The **residuals** resulting from fitting a model with just this variable are then correlated with the other predictor variables in turn, the one most strongly correlated with the residuals (i.e. with the residual variance) being added to the model. These steps are repeated until no additional variables are found to make a **statistically significant** contribution to the model. It is usually recommended that a less stringent **P-value** than $P = 0.05$ be used as a cut-off for statistical significance, to prevent important predictors from being excluded. With backward elimination, all variables are initially included and subsequently dropped from the model if found not to make a significant contribution. **All-subsets regression** is possibly a better alternative to stepwise methods. Ideally, models fitted through stepwise methods should be **validated** against an independent data set, or against a random subset of the study data that has not been used in developing the model. Stepwise procedures are more adequate for fitting **predictive models** than for fitting models where the main purpose is **causal inference**. Greenland, in ROTHMAN, GREENLAND & LASH (eds., 2012), discusses strategies for **model selection** in epidemiology. Guyatt, Haynes & Sackett, in HAYNES *et al.* (eds., 2006), suggest retaining a hierarchy of predictors based on a plausible underlying biological model to ensure the final model reflects the causal relationships at play. See also ALTMAN (1991), BLAND (2015), KIRKWOOD & STERNE (2003), HAMILTON (1992).

## Stillbirth rate

The number of stillbirths occurring during a given time-period, in a given geographical region (such as a country), divided by the total number of births in the same region during the same given time-period. The stillbirth rate is often multiplied by 1000 to be given as a rate per 1000 births (births = stillbirths + live births), and the time-period chosen is usually 1 year. See also **perinatal mortality rate**, **neonatal mortality rate**, **infant mortality rate**.

## Stopping rules

A set of rules that constitute the algorithm to be followed in determining whether to bring a **clinical trial** to an end, following the results of **interim analyses** as stipulated under a given **sequential design**. This set of rules is usually a set of **statistical significance** thresholds that must be reached in the different interim analyses to be carried out, where the number of interim analyses is predetermined in advance as part of the study design. These statistical significance thresholds are selected in such a way as to ensure the *overall* significance level of the sequential interim analyses is kept at an acceptable level, due to the problem of **multiple significance testing**. To this aim, **nominal significance levels** are stipulated for the different tests, which set the required significance at a higher level (smaller **P-value**) than the chosen level for overall significance. Two approaches are commonly used with group sequential designs: *Pocock's* and *O'Brien–Fleming's*, which differ mainly in that under Pocock's approach the required nominal significance of the sequential interim analyses remains constant throughout the trial, while under O'Brien–Fleming's approach these levels vary as the trial progresses, starting with more stringent levels initially and relaxing the criteria at subsequent interim analyses (POCOCK, 1983). Whether or not nominal levels should vary or remain constant throughout a trial depends on statistical **power** – the greater the power, the less the need for nominal levels to vary from higher initial levels to lower levels at later analyses. Sackett, in HAYNES *et al.* (eds., 2006), refers to stopping rules as 'warning rules', in recognition of the "…additional information (clinical/biologic rationale) that will be used to interpret a statistical warning rule when it is triggered." (p. 133).

## Strata

The categories or levels of a **categorical variable** (or **categorized quantitative variable**, in which case the strata are also referred to as class intervals). Each stratum corresponds to a single level or to a combination of levels resulting from the cross-tabulation of two or more variables. Examples of strata are age and age/sex groups. See **stratification**.

## Stratification

A statistical technique that is employed to control for the effects of **confounding variables**, when assessing the relationship between an **exposure** and a given disease or **outcome**. Stratification divides the observations in a data set into groups (**strata**) according to the categories of the confounding variable(s). The association between exposure and disease is often presented for each stratum in a 2 × 2 table, and for each of these tables an estimate of **exposure effect** is computed. **Significance testing** may also be performed. This is illustrated with the example in Box C.2 (Confounding, p. 70). Stratum-specific estimates are generally viewed as unconfounded since there is little variation within strata with respect to the confounding variable, although some **residual confounding** may be present due to the categorization of quantitative confounders such as age (especially when categories are then collapsed to avoid non-informative strata), or due to **misclassification**. If the necessary **assumptions** hold, stratum estimates and test statistics may be summarized (or **pooled**) to produce a single **estimate** of effect and a single **test statistic** across all strata. The **Mantel–Haenszel method** is often used to this aim (see also **weighted average**). In doing this, the exposure effect is assumed to be constant across strata. Where there is **heterogeneity** of effects, summary estimates of exposure effect may be obtained through **standardization** (ROTHMAN, 2012). A drawback of stratification as compared to **generalized regression** methods that allow for multiple predictor variables (both quantitative and categorical) is that the effect of the confounding variable itself may not be estimated. In addition, comparisons are limited to just two exposure groups (KIRKWOOD & STERNE, 2003). Excessive stratification (by the strata of successive confounding variables) can lead to inflation of estimates of effect (Greenland & Rothman, in ROTHMAN, GREENLAND & LASH [eds., 2012]). Nonetheless, stratification allows for visualization of the data, and for this reason should be carried out when appropriate, even if just as **exploratory analysis**. In **cohort studies**, stratification by **matching** variable serves mainly to increase the **precision** of estimation, rather than to remove confounding effects (which is achieved by the matching). In **case–control studies**, stratification removes the **selection bias** that was introduced by matching (which is employed to increase the precision or **efficiency** of estimation) (ROTHMAN, 2012).

## Stratified randomization

See **allocation**, **randomization**.

## Stratified sampling

A **sampling** method that is employed when the aim is to produce a **study sample** that is representative of all **strata** in a given **population**. This is usually achieved by choosing the same proportion of individuals from each stratum (with regard to the factor of interest) so that the structure in the population is replicated in the sample. Contrary to **cluster sampling**, stratified sampling leads to greater **precision** of interval estimates (BLAND, 2015).

## Strength of association

The magnitude of a **measure of association**. It is important to note that the **P-value**, which results from the significance testing of the association, is not itself a measure of the strength of the association. In addition, the finding of a strong association that is also statistically significant does not by itself constitute proof of a **causal relationship** between exposure and disease. Measures of association commonly used in medical research are the **risk ratio**, the **rate ratio**, the **hazard ratio** and the **odds ratio**, sometimes also referred to as **relative risk** measures. **Cramér's *V*** and the **contingency coefficient** are additional measures for contingency tables. **Correlation coefficients** give a measure of the strength of linear relationship between any two quantitative or ordinal variables. See also **magnitude of effect**, **direction of effect**.

## STROBE statement

A collaborative statement published in 2007, the Strengthening the Reporting of Observational Studies in Epidemiology (STROBE) statement sets out standards and checklists for reporting the rationale, methodology, results and conclusions of **analytical observational studies**, namely, **cohort studies**, **case–control studies** and **cross-sectional studies**, in order to facilitate the proper appraisal of the same. von ELM *et al.* (for the STROBE initiative, 2007) detail the components of the 22-item checklist, 18 of which are common to all three study designs, while four are specific to each design. See also VANDENBROUCKE *et al.* (for the STROBE Initiative, 2007) for additional explanation and elaboration, and www.strobe-statement.org for further details, including proposed revisions and extensions. See also **PRISMA statement**, **CONSORT statement**, **EQUATOR Network**, **critical appraisal**.

## Stuart–Maxwell test

An extension of **McNemar's test**, which is carried out with larger tables, i.e. with a paired nominal variable, as opposed to a paired binary variable. As with McNemar's test, the **test statistic** follows a **chi-squared distribution** (but this time with more than one **degree of freedom**).

## Student's *t*-test

See **t-test**. 'Student' was the pseudonym used by William Gossett when publishing his findings in this field.

## Studentized residual

Synonym for **jackknifed residual**. See also **standardized residual**.

## Study design

The logistical and conceptual framework for collecting the necessary information in order to answer a particular research question. The choice of a study design involves decisions on, *inter alia*, whether to intervene actively (**clinical trial**) or simply describe what is observed (**observational study**), how to collect information on **exposure** and **outcome** (**follow-up** or **cross-sectional study**, **cohort** or **case–control study**), whom to choose as **controls** (**parallel**, **crossover** or **factorial design**, hospital or general population controls, **cumulative case–control** or **case–cohort study**), how to **allocate** patients to the alternative treatments in an experimental study (**simple randomization** or other method of random allocation; **minimization**), and **sample size** requirements. See also **clustered designs**, **matched pairs designs**, **adaptive designs**, **sequential designs**. See MACHIN & CAMPBELL (2005) for a comprehensive guide.

## Study population

This term is sometimes used as synonym for both **study sample** and **source population**, depending on the context. Under **standardization**, it refers to a defined population that is being compared to a given **standard population**, or to another study population via a comparison to the same standard population. See also **population**, **target population**.

## Study sample

The collection of **study units** (patients, healthy individuals, communities and other groups) that is the subject of a research study, and on whom measurements are taken and observations made, with the aim of generating data that will help answer the research question at hand. Study samples are usually derived from a reasonably defined **source** or study **population** (the term **study population** is sometimes used as a synonym for study sample). **Statistics** or sample **estimates** are commonly used to **infer** a parameter, or to infer a 'true' treatment or exposure effect, so that these same results may find application beyond the study sample with the source population, and possibly also with a wider still **target population**. See also **eligibility**, **sampling**, **sample size** (required), **generalizability**.

## Study unit

Or unit of analysis. Depending on **study design**, in research studies involving human subjects, the study unit may be an *individual* (as in a randomized controlled trial where treatment allocation is through **simple randomization**, or a survey utilizing **simple random sampling**), or a *group* or *community* (as in a community intervention trial in which **cluster randomization** is employed, or a cross-sectional study using **cluster sampling**). Combining features from the previous examples are studies in which **repeated measurements** are taken on each individual in the study group. Here, the study unit is the individual, not each separate measurement. Study designs in which the study unit is a group rather than an individual are termed **clustered designs**. **Design effects** must be taken into consideration in sample size calculations (see **effective sample size**) and choice of method of statistical analysis.

## Subcohort

Any given **exposure** group in a **cohort study**.

## Subgroup analyses

The testing of study hypotheses within subgroups of patients with certain characteristics (e.g. men only/women only, younger patients/older patients, patients with onset of acute myocardial infarction ≤12 h/onset >12 h, etc.), with the aim of assessing the magnitude and significance of **treatment effects** *within* those same subgroups, and sometimes making comparisons *between* subgroups. Although there is a justifiable clinical interest in doing so, such analyses are not always carried out in an appropriate way and study samples are often too small to offer reliable results when further divided into subgroups. In particular, the analyses should include adjustments for **multiple significance testing**, and comparisons between subgroups (for example, treatment effect among female patients *vs.* treatment effect among male patients) should not be based on the comparison of within-group **P-values**, but rather on the evaluation of a possible **biological interaction** between 'treatment' and the characteristic defining the subgroups (for example, gender or age group) (POCOCK, 1983). Thus, when subgroup analyses have been planned, the study design should require larger **sample sizes** (BLAND, 2015), and the comparisons to be made should be given thoughtful consideration prior to data collection. See also POCOCK *et al.* (2002).

## Sufficient cause of disease

See **causal mechanism**.

## Sum of squares

For a given set of measurements, the sum of squares (SS) or *total* sum of squares is the summation of the squared differences between each measurement or observation and the **mean**. Dividing the sum of squares by the total number of observations, $n$, *minus* 1, gives the **variance** for the set of measurements in question (i.e. SS is the numerator in the formula for calculating the variance; the denominator, $n - 1$, is the number of **degrees of freedom** for the variance estimate). In the context of **analysis of variance** (one-way), the total sum of squares (i.e. the total variability observed in the **outcome variable**) may be divided into two components: *between-groups* sum of squares and *within-groups* sum of squares. The latter is the **residual** variability that remains after taking differences between groups into account. These two components of variability are further divided by the corresponding number of degrees of freedom ($k - 1$, and $n - k$, where $k$ is the number of groups), which results in a between-groups mean square ($MS_{between-groups}$) and a within-groups or **residual mean square** ($MS_{residual}$). The ratio of these two quantities is the **test statistic** for the variance-ratio or **F-test** (see **mean squares** for additional information). In the context of **linear regression**, the variability observed in the outcome variable (about its mean value) may likewise be partitioned into a component that can be explained by the predictor(s) in the regression model, and a component that is left unexplained after all variables in the model have been taken into account. Again, dividing these components of variability by the appropriate number of degrees of freedom ($p - 1$, and $n - p$, where $p$ is the number of parameters or coefficients estimated by the model, including the constant or intercept) produces mean squares ($MS_{regression}$ and $MS_{residual}$) that may be used to evaluate the statistical significance of the predictor variable(s) in the model. See also **two-way ANOVA**.

## Summary measures

Or summary statistics, such as **means, proportions**, the **standard deviation, regression coefficients, relative risk** measures, etc., which reduce the information contained in several data values to a single value. Summary measures are frequently used in the analysis of **serial measurements** (see Figures A.2, p. 16, and S.2a–S.2d, p. 330). In this context, the choice of summary depends on the way the variable of interest changes with time. MATTHEWS *et al.* (1990) divide this broadly into 'peaked' and 'growth' patterns, and give summaries that are appropriate in each circumstance. The **area under the curve** (**AUC**) is one such measure, often used when the mean is unsuitable. See also $C_{max}$, $T_{max}$, **aggregate data, repeated measurements analysis**; ALTMAN (1991).

## Superiority trial

A **clinical trial** that seeks to demonstrate a given experimental treatment to be superior (by a clinically important amount) to a standard or established treatment for a given target disease, or to a placebo. This is in contrast to trials evaluating **equivalence** and **non-inferiority** of effect. Sackett, in HAYNES *et al.* (eds., 2006), argues in favour of **one-sided** significance testing and estimation to analyse results of superiority trials, as being more consistent with the clinical question at hand. **Two-sided** statistical significance and estimation are still, however, generally recommended for superiority and non-inferiority trials. See also **minimally important difference** (**MID**). Cf. **active control equivalence study** (equivalence and non-inferiority).

## Supported range

A range of likely values for a **parameter**, as estimated from sample data, the limits of which are given by the values of the parameter that correspond to a chosen cut-off point for the **likelihood ratio**. A likelihood ratio of 1 corresponds (under given conditions) to the ratio between the sample estimate and the value that would maximize the likelihood function for the parameter in question. The latter is also termed the **maximum likelihood estimate** (**MLE**) for the parameter. Any deviation from this estimate, i.e. a slightly lower value or a slightly higher value, results in a likelihood ratio that is less than 1. One may calculate likelihood ratios for values further and further from the MLE in this way, until the value for the likelihood ratio becomes too removed from its ideal value of 1, at which point the limits of the supported range have been identified. Supported ranges are analogous to **confidence intervals** and under certain conditions the two overlap precisely.

## Surrogate endpoint

See **surrogate marker**.

## Surrogate marker

In trials in which time to true endpoint may be too prolonged, the statistical analysis of the results may be based instead on a surrogate marker (also known as a surrogate endpoint). For example, in a clinical trial of a putative drug for HIV infection, rather than wait for and analyse the effects on an endpoint such as AIDS onset, it may be more expedient to use a surrogate biomarker such as the CD4+ count to determine the **effectiveness** of the drug for this infection. It is assumed such a biomarker is a **valid** surrogate for the **outcome** of interest, reflecting not only a strong statistical association with the same, but also a biological connection (Sackett, in HAYNES *et al.* [eds., 2006]) such as one would find where the surrogate biomarker is in the causal pathway between exposure or treatment and outcome (i.e. disease or adverse disease outcome). In cautioning against the use of surrogate endpoints (though useful to answer some early research questions), Sackett points out the fact that favourable treatment effects with regard to a surrogate marker cannot preclude the occurrence of harmful effects, at a later time, through different **causal mechanisms**.

## Surveillance

The continuous gathering of relevant information to the monitoring of disease occurrence, through established systems of data collection, analysis and dissemination, with the aim of detecting patterns and trends that would indicate changes in the susceptibility and risk factors of a given population. Ultimately, the goal of surveillance is the timely development and implementation of policies and programmes that will lead to health promotion and disease control and prevention. See BUEHLER, in ROTHMAN, GREENLAND & LASH (eds., 2012), for historical background and a comprehensive overview of the objectives and approaches to surveillance, components of surveillance systems, and analysis, interpretation and presentation of surveillance data. See also PORTA (ed., 2014); **spatial epidemiology, pharmacovigilance**.

## Surveillance bias

See **information bias**.

## Survey

An **observational study** that aims to describe one or more characteristics in a given population, such as the **prevalence** of a particular disease or the average value of a given measurement. Surveys are usually conducted by studying a cross-section of the **source** or **study population**. **Random sampling** is of particular importance in the conduct of surveys, as a means to ensure **sample** representativeness. See MACHIN & CAMPBELL (2005) and HAMILTON (2012) for an overview of survey methodology and data analysis. See also **descriptive study, cross-sectional study**.

## Survival analysis

The analysis of **survival times** (or length of survival), where the **outcome** is 'time to the event of interest'. The purpose of studies of survival is to estimate the probability of surviving to a given time, given a number of characteristics or **prognostic factors** (including 'treatment'), and to compare the survival experiences of two or more groups. Compared to Poisson-related methods, survival analysis allows for **rates** of events that do not remain constant over time. **Censoring** is a common occurrence in this type of study, whereby, for some individuals, the outcome remains unknown at the end of the study period. In addition, duration of **follow-up** often varies from person to person. Thus, methods for **risks** or **proportions** (e.g. 'what proportion of people died after 3 years?') or methods for **quantitative data** (e.g. 'what was the mean length of survival?') cannot usually be used. Instead, tests such as the **logrank test** are carried out to test for differences between groups, and **Cox regression** and other regression methods are employed to fit **predictive models** and to obtain estimates of relative hazard (**hazard ratios**). Other methods of analysis include **life tables** and the **Kaplan–Meier method**, both of which provide estimates of survival probability that are used to construct **survival curves**. The **power** of significance tests used in survival studies does not depend solely on sample size but also on the number of **observed events**. The rate at which these are expected to occur in the accrual and follow-up periods should be taken into consideration when determining the number of individuals to be followed up and the duration of follow-up (ALTMAN, 1991; MACHIN & CAMPBELL, 2005). See also BLAND (2015), KIRKWOOD & STERNE (2003), HAMILTON (2012), ARMITAGE, BERRY & MATHEWS (2002), HOSMER, LEMESHOW & MAY (2008), SINGER & WILLETT (2003), CLEVES, GOULD & MARCHENKO (2016). For the interested reader, PETO *et al.* (1976; 1977) give an overview of survival analysis methodology.

## Survival curve

A graphical representation of probability of survival over time. Estimates of survival probability (or, more precisely, *cumulative* probability of survival) at different points in time (what is known as the survivor or **survival function**) are given by the **Kaplan–Meier** (Figure K.1, p. 181) and **life table methods**. See also **logrank test**.

## Survival function

The set of estimates of cumulative probability of survival as obtained by the **life table** and **Kaplan–Meier methods**. The survival function, $S(t)$, may be illustrated graphically as a **survival curve**, from which estimates of **life expectancy** may be obtained. See also **baseline survival function** $[S_0(t)]$. Cf. **cumulative hazard function** $[H(t)]$.

## Survival times

The observed **outcome variable** in **survival analysis**, which measures, for any given individual, length of 'time to event' (where the event has occurred within the follow-up period for a research study), or, where the event is **censored**, 'duration of follow-up'. In survival analysis terminology, the occurrence of an event of interest is referred to as **failure**. Unlike **parametric survival models**, non-parametric (**Kaplan–Meier method**) and semi-parametric (**Cox regression**) methods make no assumptions regarding the **distribution** of survival times.

## Survivor function

Synonym for **survival function**.

## Symmetry

The quality of a **distribution**, often **unimodal**, which is symmetrical, as, for example, a **normally distributed** variable. Cf. **skewness**.

## Synergism

A type of **biological interaction** characterized by the joint effect of two factors being greater than the sum of their separate effects. Where the presence of both factors causes disease to occur, it is termed *causal synergism*. If, on the other hand, the presence of both factors leads to prevention of disease, it is termed *preventive synergism*. See also **antagonism**.

## Systematic error

As opposed to **random error**. See **bias, measurement bias**.

## Systematic review

A review of the methods, results and conclusions from all individual or **primary studies** that focus on a particular research question and conform to set criteria (see **PRISMA statement**). The term encompasses the entire review process, i.e. identification and selection of studies and avoidance of **publication bias**, assessment of study validity (see **CONSORT statement**) and summarization of results. Special statistical methods may be employed to obtain overall **estimates of effect** for a treatment, intervention or exposure, and also to summarize the results of studies evaluating **diagnostic accuracy**. The term **meta-analysis** is used with reference to systematic reviews when these quantitative methods are employed. CHALMERS & ALTMAN (eds., 1995), EGGER, DAVEY SMITH & ALTMAN (eds., 2001) and HIGGINS & GREEN (eds., 2008) give a broad discussion of issues around systematic reviews. Haynes, in HAYNES *et al.* (eds., 2006), offers a detailed overview of the rationale, principles and conduct of systematic reviews; a sample search strategy is appended.

## Systematic sampling

A **sampling** method that employs a systematic rather than a **random** approach to selecting individuals from a given **source** or **study population**. This type of sampling is often used in market research and when conducting exit or opinion polls. The method could be reasonably adequate (though rarely used in clinical or epidemiological research) provided no pattern is introduced in the sampling scheme that coincides with a systematic pattern in the population. An example could be where every tenth patient is selected in a practice-based study. Coincidentally, a fixed number of ten patients is seen at this same practice every weekday, the last consultation slot each day being reserved for the more severe cases of some disease of interest. The suggested sampling scheme would not result in a **sample** representative of patients seen at the practice, only of the most severe cases. Cf. **simple random sampling**.

# T

*t*

The **test statistic** for the ***t*-test**.

*T*

The **test statistic** for the **Wilcoxon signed rank test** or the **Wilcoxon rank sum test**.

## *t* distribution

The **probability distribution** followed by the **sampling distribution** of the *t* test statistic (i.e. the ratio of the **mean** of a set of normally distributed observations to its **standard error**), and which is used with small samples whose estimates of **variance** are usually considered not too reliable estimates of variance in the population. The distribution is defined by one **parameter**, the **degrees of freedom** (*df*), which are calculated as the sample size, *n*, *minus* 1 (see also calculation of *df* for the ***t*-test**). As the sample size increases, the shape of the *t* distribution approximates that of the **Normal distribution**. For smaller sample sizes, the distribution of *t* is less peaked than the Normal, so the probability in the tails is higher than in the tails of the Normal distribution (in other words, significance tests and confidence intervals will be more *conservative* when applied to small samples). Table 7 shows select percentage points (**critical values**) of the *t* distribution for **two-sided** significance. As may be seen, the threshold or critical value of *t* decreases with increasing number of degrees of freedom, and approaches that of the standard Normal distribution.

Table 7 Select percentage points of the *t* distribution: values in the body of the table are the critical values of *t*, at different levels of statistical significance, according to the number of degrees of freedom

| Degrees of Freedom | *P*-value or $\alpha$ (two-sided) | | | | |
|---|---|---|---|---|---|
| | 10% (0.1) | 5% (0.05) | 1% (0.01) | 0.5% (0.005) | 0.1% (0.001) |
| 1 | 6.31 | 12.71 | 63.66 | 127.32 | 636.62 |
| 2 | 2.92 | 4.30 | 9.92 | 14.09 | 31.60 |
| 5 | 2.02 | 2.57 | 4.03 | 4.77 | 6.87 |
| 10 | 1.81 | 2.23 | 3.17 | 3.58 | 4.59 |
| 30 | 1.70 | 2.04 | 2.75 | 3.03 | 3.65 |
| 60 | 1.67 | 2.00 | 2.66 | 2.92 | 3.46 |
| 120 | 1.66 | 1.98 | 2.62 | 2.86 | 3.37 |
| ∞ | 1.65 | 1.96 | 2.58 | 2.81 | 3.29 |

For one-sided significance, the critical value is approximately half the magnitude of the values shown for two-sided significance, at each level of statistical significance.

# *t*-test

A **significance test** that is carried out to compare **mean responses** with respect to some variable of interest. The **paired** or the **independent** samples *t*-test is indicated, depending on **study design**. The number of **degrees of freedom** for the independent samples test is $n - 2$, where $n$ is the total sample size in the two groups combined, $n_1 + n_2$ (see illustrative example in Box T.1). Both the **test statistic** and the corresponding degrees of freedom are referred to tables of the **$t$ distribution** for an assessment of **statistical significance**. An **assumption** of the independent samples *t*-test is that the variable of interest is **normally distributed** with similar variance (**homoscedasticity**) in the two groups being compared. A modification of the standard test (**Welch's test**) allows for unequal variances, or, alternatively, transformations, bootstrapping and non-parametric tests may be used. The *t*-test is somewhat **robust** to non-normality if the groups have similar size, but it might then lack the **power** to detect real differences as statistically significant. With large samples, the estimated **variance** is a good estimate of variability in the population, and the two-sample *t*-test is equivalent to the **z-test**. See also **paired *t*-test**, **analysis of variance** (one-way ANOVA), **Mann–Whitney *U* test**.

## BOX T.1

Adapted from Lucas A *et al*. (1998). Randomised trial of early diet in preterm babies and later intelligence quotient. *Br Med J* **317**: 1481–7.

The data below are the results from the randomized trial of early diet in preterm babies and later intelligence quotient (Trial A – infants not being breastfed, exclusively on one of the trial's formulas, standard or preterm nutrient-enriched; all infants weighed less than 1850 g at birth). The outcome variables are occurrence of cerebral palsy (binary) and overall IQ score at 7.5–8 years of age (quantitative – abbreviated Wechsler intelligence scale for children, revised). The $\chi^2$ test and the independent samples *t*-test are carried out below to analyse these data, for the 135 children (out of the 160 initially enrolled in Trial A) who were followed up (of which 133 were developmentally assessed):

| Diet | Cerebral palsy | No palsy | Mean IQ | (SE) | Total |
|---|---|---|---|---|---|
| Preterm | 1 | 66 | 97.0 | 1.8 | 67 (66) |
| Standard | 8 | 60 | 94.8 | 1.7 | 68 (67) |
| Total | 9 | 126 | | | 135 (133) |

*Chi-squared ($\chi^2$) test:*

$$X^2_{df} = \sum \frac{(O-E)^2}{E} = \frac{(1-4.47)^2}{4.47} + \frac{(66-62.53)^2}{62.53} + \frac{(8-4.53)^2}{4.53} + \frac{(60-63.47)^2}{63.47}$$

$X^2$ statistic = 5.681, 1 *df*, *P*-value* = 0.017 (**Fisher's exact test***: *P* = 0.033).

*Independent samples t-test:* Estimated difference in mean overall IQ score = 2.2 IQ units; SE of difference between the two means = 2.475; *t*-statistic = 2.2/2.475 = 0.889; *df* = 67 + 66 − 2 = 131; 95% CI = 2.2 ± 1.9782 × 2.475 = −2.70 IQ units to 7.10 IQ units; *P*-value* = 0.376. (*Calculations carried out using MedCalc.)

## Tan–Machin threshold designs

Two-stage **Phase II trial** designs that use a single or dual response rate threshold to determine whether the trial should proceed to a **Phase III trial**. MACHIN & CAMPBELL (2005) give details.

## Target population

The population to whom the results of a given study are to be generalized. In **survey**-type studies, sample **statistics** are often intended to give *unbiased estimates* of population **parameters**, and **generalizability** from sample to population depends on the representativeness of the former. In **analytical comparative studies**, the concept of target population may be more difficult to define and sample representativeness more difficult to achieve, as many practicalities determine who is included in a study sample. In these studies, *internal* **validity**, i.e. the ability to make an *unbiased comparison*, is the primary goal (and defining a **source population** is often an important prerequisite). *External* validity, i.e. the ability to extrapolate or generalize beyond the study sample, is also important. However, it cannot be concluded on the basis of statistical sampling and representativeness alone, but rather, an understanding of determinants of variability of biological response and their likely impact on treatment and exposure effects are the central factors. A distinction is usually made between the wider target population and the **study population** (used here as a synonym for source population), this being a subset of the former, from which the **study sample** is sampled or selected.

## Tau

See **Kendall's tau ($\tau$)**.

## Temporal relationship

See **cause–effect relationship**.

## Tertiles

The 1/3rd and 2/3rd **quantiles**. Tertiles divide the total number of observations in a given variable into three equal-sized groups. The 1st tertile, for example, is the observation value below which we find one-third or 33.33…% of all observations, when these are sorted in ascending order. See also **quartiles**, **quintiles**, **deciles**, **centiles**.

## Test statistic

The ratio of a sample **estimate** to its **standard error**, which is computed when carrying out **significance testing**. This value reflects the *strength of evidence* against the **null hypothesis**, which is the hypothesis being tested. Test statistics are referred to tables of the relevant **theoretical distributions** (which approximate their **sampling distributions** when the null hypothesis is true), from which a level of significance or **P-value** is obtained. For tests such as the *t*-test, the **chi-squared ($\chi^2$) test** and the *F*-test, **degrees of freedom** also need to be calculated, which in conjunction with the test statistic give the correct value of *P*. See also **critical value**, **statistical significance**, **significance level**. See BLAND (2015) for calculation of test statistics for a number of non-parametric tests.

## Theoretical distribution

As opposed to **empirical distribution**. A **distribution** whose values occur with probability determined by a mathematical model. Theoretical **probability distributions** fall into two broad categories, **discrete**, defined by a **probability mass function**, and **continuous**, defined by a **probability density function**. Examples of the former are the **binomial, geometric, hypergeometric, Poisson** and **negative binomial** distributions. Examples of the latter include the **Normal**, *t*, *F*, **chi-squared**, **lognormal** and **exponential** distributions. A specific theoretical distribution will result from the particular set of values given to the **parameters** of the probability distribution. The term theoretical distribution is also used with reference to the expected distribution of a **random variable**, i.e. **population** and **sampling distributions**. The latter refer to the distribution of **sample estimates**, and the distribution of **test statistics** when the null hypothesis is true. The precise mathematical equations defining these distributions are not usually known, but often may be **approximated** by a known theoretical probability distribution, especially when sample sizes are large (see **central limit theorem**).

## Threshold

See **cut-off point**, **diagnostic threshold**, **critical value**.

## Time series

Data that are repeated observations (typically, measurements and counts) over a period of time. A distinction is often made between time series, where measurements are usually made at the group or population level and over an extended period of time (typically, months, years or decades), and **serial measurements**, which are repeated measurements over time at the individual level. These tend to span a shorter period of time (commonly, a 24-hour period, 1 week, 1 month), although they may also be recorded over an extended follow-up period in **longitudinal studies**. The analysis of time series may be carried out to capture **trends** in mortality and disease occurrence. Time series are usually displayed as **line graphs**, which readily convey the pattern of variation over time, provided distortions in the representation of the data are avoided. **Smoothing** techniques are sometimes employed when **cyclic variation** or irregular fluctuation are present (see Figures T.1a and T.1b – HUANG *et al.*, 2011). When measuring the **association** between two variables (or series) that have both been measured at various points over the same period of time, a spurious correlation is to be expected due to the effect of time, i.e. due to an association between each of the series and some other factor which varies over time (ALTMAN, 1991). This **confounding** effect must be taken into account for an undistorted assessment of the relationship. Hertz-Picciotto, in ROTHMAN, GREENLAND & LASH (eds., 2012), points out meteorological factors, air pollutants, infectious agents and time trends in mortality as potential confounders in the context of environmental epidemiology. The relationship between a series and another variable is sometimes evaluated through the analysis of *interrupted* time series. The latter bear a resemblance to **before–after studies** in that the aim is to evaluate the effect of some wide-scaled intervention or policy change on the outcome of interest (see BLAND, 2015, for an illustrative example). Of interest is whether there is a 'before *vs.* after' change in level, whether a change in level is accompanied by a change in slope, or, more commonly, simply a change in slope in the trajectory of the series. 'Time' is included as an explanatory variable, together with a dummy variable to represent the 'intervention', i.e. the 'before *vs.* after' comparison. Confounding effects may also be at work here. **Autocorrelation** or time **dependence** between successive *observations* in the same series may sometimes be of interest for the purpose of **forecasting** or projecting trends, in which case special models for the analysis of time series (**autoregressive** and **moving average**) may be indicated. **Correlograms** are graphical tools that help assess the extent of correlation within (serial or auto) and between series (**cross-correlation**). When *exogenous* **predictor variables** (time, a second series, confounding variables, etc.) are included in the analysis, the errors produced by **ordinary least squares** regression may not conform to the **Normal i.i.d.** assumption. These errors, commonly termed 'disturbances', may be further decomposed into a random component (the true residual), and a systematic component due to the underlying autoregressive or moving average process. Models for autocorrelated *errors* may then be employed (see **correlogram**, this time, an autocorrelation function for the regression errors; **Durbin–Watson statistic**). When a series is count data over time, **Poisson regression** may be employed if the data conform to the necessary **assumptions**, but additional methods may be necessary due to data dependency. See CHATFIELD (2003) for a comprehensive presentation. See ARMITAGE, BERRY & MATHEWS (2002) and HAMILTON (1992; 2012) for an overview.

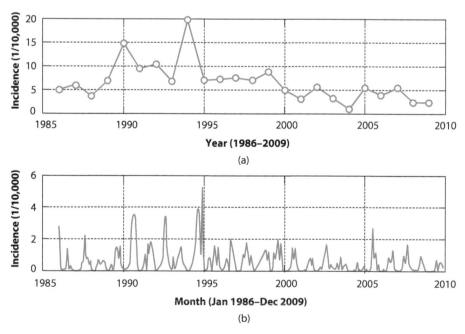

Figures T.1a and T.1b Time series: annual (a) and monthly (b) malaria incidence. Data are from the Motuo County in Tibet, for the period 1986–2009. Monthly malaria incidence was recalculated before further analysis was carried out, by smoothing and detrending to remove long-term fluctuations and trends that were not seen in the monthly meteorological factors (see Figures C.3a and C.3b, p. 85). (Reproduced from Huang F *et al.* (2011). Temporal correlation analysis between malaria and meteorological factors in Motuo County, Tibet. *Malar J* **10**: 54.)

## Time-varying covariate

A **covariate**, the value of which changes over time. An example is the age of a participant in a **longitudinal study**. Of note when conducting analyses with covariates that change over time, is that the hazard of the risk will change to coincide with the point in time when the value of the covariate changes, the underlying assumption being that anticipation and delay effects are negligible unless accounted for otherwise. See CLEVES, GOULD & MARCHENKO (2016) for an example of the analysis and interpretation in the context of **Cox regression**.

## $T_{max}$

The time at which the highest concentration of drug or $C_{max}$ (usually in the blood) for an individual subject is recorded, following the administration of a medical treatment or some other intervention. See also **serial measurements, repeated measurements analysis, summary measures, area under curve, bioequivalence study, Phase I trial**.

## Training set

A subsample that is used to build a **regression model** when **validation** is to be carried out through the method of cross-validation. This subsample is generated by randomly dividing the **study sample** into two subsamples, one of which is used for the model building exercise (the training set) and the other for the validation exercise (the **validation sample**).

## Transformations

Data manipulations that attempt to find, for a given variable $x$, the **measurement scale** that would facilitate and improve the validity of data analyses involving the same. Also, moving the data to a different measurement scale could make greater sense from a biological or other relevant stand point. Transformed variables ($x^*$) are often analysed using **parametric methods**. Transformations may be *linear* or *non-linear*. An example of the former is the conversion of a variable's values to **z-scores**, which changes the scale but not the shape of the variable's **distribution**. Non-linear transformations change both the scale and shape of the distribution, and are often applied for the purposes stated above (HAMILTON, 1990). **Logarithmic** and **power transformations** may be used. The former involves taking logs of the values of a variable [$x^* = \log(x)$], and the latter raising the values of the variable to a power $q < 0$ or $q > 0$ [$x^* = x^q$]. Conventionally, the logarithmic transformation is taken to be a power transformation where $q = 0$. A power 1 or identity transformation ($q = 1$) is equivalent to no transformation. Power transformations where $q < 1$ are used to make positively **skewed** variables more **symmetrical**, and transformations where $q > 1$ are used in a similar way with negatively skewed variables. Often, the goal is to attain a **Normal distribution** for the variable in question. The following 'ladder of powers' (MOSTELLER & TUKEY, 1977) gives the relative strength (weakest first) of different transformations. For positively skewed variables:

$$x \rightarrow x^{\frac{1}{2}} \rightarrow \ln x \rightarrow 1/x^{\frac{1}{2}} \rightarrow 1/x$$

i.e. if the logarithmic transformation does not succeed in adequately transforming the data, the **reciprocal root** and **reciprocal transformations**, $1/x^{\frac{1}{2}}$ or $x^{-\frac{1}{2}}$, and $1/x$ or $x^{-1}$, are the next rungs up on the transformation ladder. On the other hand, if a variable only displays a slight positive skew, the **square root transformation**, $x^{1/2}$ or $\sqrt{x}$, may achieve the desired effect. (Note: the reciprocal root and reciprocal transformations are also referred to as *negative* reciprocal root and *negative* reciprocal, as a negative sign must be attached to the transformed values [whenever $q < 0$] to preserve their relative order of magnitude.) For negatively skewed data, the square transformation is the weakest, and may be sufficient to deal with a moderate negative skew. If not, the cubic and quartic transformations may be used (higher powers are not commonly used):

$$x \rightarrow x^2 \rightarrow x^3 \rightarrow x^4, \text{ etc.}$$

Transformations are also effected to linearize a **non-linear relationship**, in order to meet **assumptions** for a given method of analysis, or to facilitate the data analysis (see **Tukey and Mosteller's bulging rule**; see also KIRKWOOD & STERNE, 2003, and HAMILTON, 1992). In addition, transformations for positively skewed variables may also achieve **homoscedasticity**, i.e. constant or stable **variance**. A transformation often used when modelling **binary outcomes** and **proportions** is the **logit**, the *predicted* outcome in **logistic regression**. Additional transformations for proportions are the **arcsine square root** transformation, the **complementary log-log** transformation and the **probit** transformation; for **rates** and speeds, the **reciprocal** transformation may be applied. Discrete **counts** may be normalized through the **square root** transformation, and the **Box–Cox transformation** may be applied to non-negative values. See also **back-transformation**, **exponentiation**, **Fisher's transformation**; BLAND & ALTMAN (1996a), BLAND (2015).

## Transition model

A **regression** model for the analysis of **longitudinal data**, in which past values of the **outcome variable** (at various time-lags) become predictors of present value. This type of model is sometimes referred to as *Markov chain* model. When the model includes additional **predictor variables**, the estimated effects of these are usually weaker as compared to estimates from a **marginal model**, given the conditioning of those effects on past outcome values (AGRESTI, 2007). Alternatively, **random effects** (or conditional) models may be fitted to longitudinal data, which assume within-subject or within-cluster **dependence** (i.e. between-subject or between-cluster **heterogeneity**), but not time dependence. Transition models are similar to **autoregressive models** for **time series**, and may be fitted to count and binary outcomes. See also DIGGLE *et al.* (2002); **antedependence model, forecast**.

## Treatment

In a wide sense, any experimental **exposure** thought to have the potential to bring about positive disease outcomes. In a narrow sense, a medical treatment, as opposed to a surgical, behaviour-change or other **intervention**.

## Treatment allocation

The process of allocating **study units** (usually patients) to the different treatments (including placebos, if any) in a **clinical trial**. See **allocation**.

## Treatment arm

Each of the **comparison groups** in a parallel or factorial design **clinical trial**, including the placebo or control group, if the trial is a placebo-controlled trial.

## Treatment effect

The *absolute* or *relative* difference in **outcome** between **treatment arms**. With categorical outcomes, in particular **binary responses**, treatment effect may be measured by **measures of association** (measures of **relative risk**), or, perhaps more appropriately, by **measures of impact** (both *net* and *proportional*). Examples of the latter are the absolute risk (or rate) difference, the relative risk reduction and the numbers needed to treat and to harm. With quantitative or **measurement outcomes**, **mean** differences between groups are usually calculated, with or without adjustments for **baseline measurements**. A special evaluation of treatment effect is the assessment of **dose–response relationships**. **Crossover trials** require application of methods for **paired data**. See also **adjusted treatment mean**, **measures of effect**, **standardized measures of effect**, **change** (study of).

## Treatment group

Synonymous with **treatment arm**, although use of the latter is more common in the context of pharmacological research, whereas the expression 'treatment group' usually has broader use as in 'intervention group'.

## Treatment–period interaction

In the context of **crossover trials**, this type of **interaction** is present when a **treatment effect** does not remain constant across trial periods. This is usually due to the treatment administered in a given period continuing to exert its effect (or being **carried-over**) into the following period. In planning crossover trials, it is important to allow for sufficiently long **wash-out periods** between treatments. See also **information bias**.

## Trend (Test for)

An extension of standard **significance tests**, which are indicated when the grouping variable is an **ordered categorical variable**, a **categorized continuous variable** or an **ordinal variable**. For example, the **chi-squared test** is commonly used to test for an **association** between **categorical variables**. If, however, one of the variables is binary and the other variable is ordered categorical ($r \times 2$ **contingency table**), it is of interest to test for the presence of a trend, i.e. whether the **proportions** with the **binary outcome** increase or decrease linearly, across levels of the ordered variable. This is accomplished with the **chi-squared test for trend**, which has just one **degree of freedom** regardless of the number of categories in the grouping variable. An example would be a cross-tabulation where chronic respiratory disease (yes/no) is the **outcome** and smoking (non-smoker, light smoker, moderate smoker, heavy smoker) represents **exposure**. The questions of interest are (a) is the risk of chronic respiratory disease *different* for different types of smokers, and (b) does the risk of chronic respiratory disease *increase steadily* from non-smokers to heavy smokers. The chi-squared trend statistic is always smaller than the standard chi-squared statistic for the same table. The difference between the two **test statistics**, with $r - 2$ degrees of freedom, tests the extent of departure from a linear trend (i.e. whether additional differences are present that are not explained by the linear trend). For **quantitative** or **ordinal outcomes**, **Cuzick's test**, **Kendall's correlation coefficient**, **analysis of variance** (with linear contrasts) and **regression analysis** may all be used. For a relationship involving two ordered categorical variables, the chi-squared test for trend and Kendall's tau may both be used (BLAND, 2015). **Non-linear** trends (U-shaped curves, for example) may be explored using **smoothing** techniques, and modelled using **regression** methods. See also **linear relationship**, **dose–response relationship**.

## TRIPOD statement

TRIPOD (Transparent Reporting of a Multivariable Prediction Model for Individual Prognosis or Diagnosis – COLLINS *et al.*, 2015) is a collaborative statement that sets out recommendations for reporting the rationale, methodology, results and conclusions of studies developing or validating multivariable prediction models, in order to facilitate the proper appraisal of the same. The set of recommendations comprises a 22-item checklist that applies to studies developing, validating or updating a prediction model, whether for diagnostic or prognostic purposes. See www.tripod-statement.org for further details and supporting documentation. See also **predictive model**, **prognostic index**, **risk score**, **validation**, **critical appraisal**, **STARD statement**.

## Tukey and Mosteller's bulging rule

A set of rules to guide the use of the 'ladder of powers' or 'ladder of re-expressions' (see **transformations**), in order to linearize a curved, monotonic relationship (MOSTELLER & TUKEY, 1977). Figure T.2 summarizes the transformations to be effected on either or both the *y*- and *x*-variable, depending on the shape of the curved relationship, i.e. depending on the direction of the bulge. A move 'up' for either variable requires a **power transformation** with powers >1 (e.g. a square or cubic power transformation). A move 'down' requires a power transformation with powers <1, which includes the **logarithmic transformation** (taken to be a power 0 transformation) and the **square root transformation** (power = ½). Note that negative-power transformations (**reciprocal transformations**) reverse the order of magnitude of the values of the variable in question (see transformations). See also **Box–Cox transformation**.

## Tukey–Kramer test

See **multiple-comparison procedures**.

## Tukey's Honestly Significant Differences test

See **multiple-comparison procedures**.

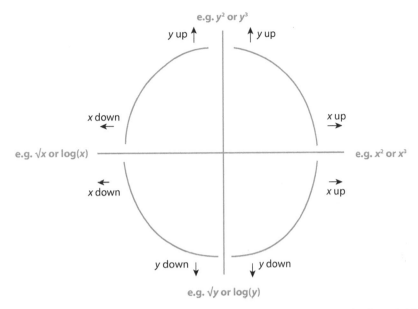

Figure T.2 Tukey and Mosteller's bulging rule for transforming the *y*, *x* or both variables in simple monotonic, non-linear relationships. (Reproduced from Mosteller F, Tukey JW (1977). *Data Analysis and Regression: A Second Course in Statistics*. Addison-Wesley (with permission).)

## Turn point

See **non-monotonic curve**.

## Two-by-two (2 × 2) table

A **contingency table** with two rows and two columns (i.e. four cells) (see Tables 2.a and 2.b, p. 72).

## Two-sided test

A **significance test** that explores both alternative directions from the **null hypothesis**. For example, when comparing mean serum cholesterol in vegetarians *vs.* meat-eaters, the null hypothesis states that the mean value is the same in the two comparison groups. The **alternative hypotheses**, as opposed to when a **one-sided test** is carried out, are that mean serum cholesterol in one of the groups could be *either* higher *or* lower than in the other group.

## Two-tailed test

Synonym for **two-sided test**.

## Two-way ANOVA

**Analysis of variance** of data classified according to two factors or characteristics (for example, (a) repeated measurements taken on different individuals under a number of different treatments; and (b) measurements taken on a group of individuals where the measurement for each individual falls under one of the cross-classifications between the two factors – ALTMAN, 1991). Two-way ANOVA may be carried out as a balanced or unbalanced design, depending on whether each cross-classification has the same number of observations. The **balanced design** *without* replication (for instance, as in example (a) above) is an extension of the **paired *t*-test**, where the pairing involves more than two sets of measurements (KIRKWOOD & STERNE, 2003). When repeated measurements are serial measurements over time, **repeated measures ANOVA** should be employed in the analysis of these data. With balanced designs with *replication* (as in example (b), where each cross-classification will have more than one individual observation – or replicates for the same individual), the total **sum of squares** for the **outcome variable** is partitioned into that due to the **main effects** (i.e. the *independent* effect of each of the factors), that due to an **interaction effect** (between the two factors) and a **residual** component reflecting the variability within each cross-classification. Individual replicates also allow for an assessment of interaction of effects under the scenario described in example (a). **Unbalanced designs** are usually analysed by carrying out **multivariable linear regression**. See BLAND (2015) for an illustrative example of a three-way analysis of variance. See also **mean squares**, **randomized block design** (parallel and repeated measurements designs), **factorial design**. Cf. **one-way ANOVA**.

## Type I error

A type of error that is incurred when evaluating the results of a **significance test**, whereby there is failure to accept the **null hypothesis** (**NH**) when in fact NH is true. The probability of incurring a type I error is **alpha** ($\alpha$), the value of which is stipulated when calculating sample size requirements. The **power** of a statistical test will decrease (and the probability of a **type II error** will increase) if the value of alpha is lowered (i.e. if the **significance level** is raised) without also increasing **sample size** (assuming variability remains unchanged). The **statistical significance** of the test, given by its ***P*-value**, is the probability that a type I error was incurred. See also **multiple significance testing**, **multiple-comparison procedures**.

## Type II error

A type of error that is incurred when evaluating the results of a **significance test**, whereby there is failure to reject the **null hypothesis** (**NH**) when the latter is false. The probability ($\beta$ or **beta**) of incurring a type II error decreases as the **power** of a test increases, and increases if tolerance for a **type I error** decreases (i.e. if the value of **alpha** decreases) without also increasing **sample size**.

## U-shaped curve

A depiction of a **non-linear relationship** that is either U-shaped, or the inverse, ∩-shaped. Such a curve might be best described with the inclusion of a **quadratic term** in a **curvilinear regression** model. Figure U.1a shows the U-shaped relationship between baseline haemoglobin levels and hazard ratio for incident Alzheimer disease (AD), and Figure U.1b the reverse U-shaped relationship between baseline haemoglobin levels and rate of annual cognitive decline, among a group of older community-dwelling individuals around the Chicago, Illinois area (SHAH *et al.*, 2011). Study participants were eligible for inclusion if there were no signs of dementia at the visit associated with the baseline haemoglobin measurement. Average length of follow-up for the 881 individuals included was 3.3 years. The curves show that higher and lower levels of haemoglobin were associated with higher risk of AD. See also **J-shaped curve**, **exponential curve**, S-shaped or **sigmoid curve**, **bathtub curve**.

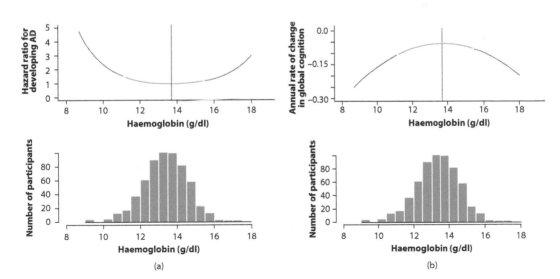

(a)  (b)

Figures U.1a and U.1b U-shaped and reverse U-shaped curve: hazard ratio for incident Alzheimer disease (AD) and rate of annual cognitive decline, both as a function of baseline haemoglobin level (in g/dl) among 881 older individuals. Mean age of study participants was 80.6 years (SD 7.4), and 75% were female. (Reproduced from Shah RC *et al.* (2011). Hemoglobin level in older persons and incident Alzheimer disease. *Neurology* **77**: 219–26 (with permission).)

## U-shaped distribution

A **frequency distribution** for a quantitative or ordinal variable with highest frequencies at both extremes of its range of values. See also **J-shaped distribution**, **exponential distribution**.

## Unbalanced design

A **two-way analysis of variance** in which there is an unequal number of observations in each cell. Data analysis of unbalanced designs is equivalent to **multiple** or **multivariable regression** analysis, where the effect of each **main factor** is estimated as an **adjusted estimate**, i.e. each main effect is adjusted for the presence of the other factor. Cf. **balanced design**.

## Unbiased

A procedure, method or assessment that is not affected by systematic distortions. The term is used to refer to **measurements**, **estimates** and **estimators**, methods of treatment **allocation**, **samples** and **sampling** schemes, and **comparisons** that are in fact unaffected by **bias**. Unbiased estimates are **valid**, although not necessarily **accurate** or **precise**.

## Underdispersion

The characteristic of a **discrete variable** that displays less **variability** than would be expected under an assumed **probability distribution** (e.g. **Poisson** or **binomial**). See also **overdispersion**.

## Uniform distribution

A **probability distribution** that assigns equal probability to each of the different values (or each of the different class intervals) of a given variable. An example is the expected distribution of the last digit of each of a set of measurements, in the absence of **digit preference**. Also, a string of **random numbers** can be generated as a random sample from a uniform distribution. The **mean** of a **discrete** or integer uniform distribution is $(a + b)/2$ with **variance** $[(b - a + 1)^2 - 1]/12$, where 'a' is the minimum value, and 'a + b' the maximum value. For **continuous** or rectangular uniform distributions, also bound between lower and upper limits, the variance is given by $(b - a)^2/12$. The uniform distribution may be used to generate **random samples** from other theoretical distributions, through what is known as the inverse transformation method.

## Unimodal distribution

A **distribution** with just one **mode** or peak, reflecting its highest **frequency** value(s). A unimodal distribution may be symmetrical or skewed. An example is shown in Figure H.2, p. 158. Cf. **bimodal distribution**, multimodal distribution.

## Unit of analysis

See **study unit**.

## Univariable analysis

See **univariate analysis**. Cf. multiple or **multivariable analysis**.

## Univariate analysis

A term that may be used to refer to the analysis of a *single* **variable** or characteristic (e.g. a 'univariate distribution'), and also to describe a **regression analysis** that includes only one **predictor variable** (i.e. as synonym for *simple* regression analysis). In recent years, the term 'univariable' has often been used to convey this meaning (and, likewise, the term 'multivariable' to signify the inclusion of two or more predictor variables, what is commonly known as 'multiple regression analysis'), while the terms 'univariate' and 'multivariate' may be used preferentially to refer to analyses including one or more (respectively) **outcome variables**.

# V

*V*

See **Cramér's V**.

## Validation

An assessment of the **goodness-of-fit** of a **regression model**, which has been specified and fitted. Validation is part of the process of **model checking**, which includes an assessment of goodness-of-fit using the sample data, and **regression diagnostics**. The aim now is to confirm the adequacy of the fit against an external sample (external validation) or against a random subset of the sample data not used in the model building exercise (cross-validation). **Jackknifing** is an alternative validation method that is employed when external samples or sample data subsets are not available. See also **validation sample, training set**; ALTMAN & ROYSTON (2000), ALTMAN *et al.* (2009). See **TRIPOD statement** for reporting guidelines for studies developing or validating multivariable **predictive models**.

## Validation sample

A subset of the study sample (or, sometimes, an external sample) that is used to make an independent assessment of a **model**'s **goodness-of-fit**, including its ability to make accurate predictions (**calibration**) and assign individuals to their correct categories (**discrimination**). The model itself is developed from a **training sample**. See **validation**.

## Validity

In the context of **clinical measurement**, this term refers to whether a particular variable does in fact measure the characteristic that is of interest (for example, does forced expiratory volume at 1 minute reflect lung function?). For many **diagnostic tests**, this is evaluated by measuring the test's accuracy against a **gold standard** test. A valid **measurement** must be **reliable** and **accurate** in order to be useful. These, however, are necessary but not sufficient conditions for validity: forced expiratory volume at 1 minute might be measured reliably and without error, but still not reflect lung function. This term is also used to refer to the quality of an assessment that is **unbiased**. In **surveys**, validity is mainly achieved through **random sampling**, and in **clinical trials**, through random assignment or **randomization**. Randomization ensures the *internal* validity of study results, whereas the composition of the study sample in surveys determines **generalizability** or *external* validity (JÜNI, ALTMAN & EGGER, 2001). It has been argued the latter is less crucial when evaluating research hypotheses in comparative studies than when estimating population parameters, as is often the case in surveys and cross-sectional studies.

## Variability

Variability is present when differences are observed *between* or *within* individuals, with respect to any characteristic or feature that may be measured or assessed. The main purpose of statistical methods is to unravel the underlying patterns that are obscured by natural and **random error** or variation. Commonly used **measures of** variability or **dispersion** are the **variance** or its square root, the **standard deviation**, and **central ranges** and **reference intervals** based on the standard deviation or constructed from ranked data, as the **interquartile range**. These measures are appropriate for **quantitative** and **ordinal variables**. The variability of a **categorical variable** is given by its relative **frequency distribution**.

## Variable

Any characteristic on which information may be collected and expressed as a **quantitative** or **qualitative** value. The term is also used to refer to a set of **observations** (measurements or assessments) on a given characteristic. Variables are classified according to their nature and expression as categorical (recorded), discrete quantitative (counted), continuous quantitative (measured); according to the **measurement scale** on which their values are recorded (e.g. ratio, ordinal, binary); according to the values taken as continuous or discrete; according to their function or role in data analyses (e.g. indicator, instrumental, surrogate, latent, confounding, outcome, predictor, offset); and according to the **probability distribution** that best describes their **frequency** and/or **sampling distribution** (e.g. Normal, binomial, Poisson, uniform, exponential). Variables may also result from **composite** sums or averages of a number of single items, and they may be rescaled (as in **z-scores**) or **transformed**. In comparative studies, such as clinical trials and observational studies, variables typically contain information on treatments and exposures, risk and prognostic factors, case–control status and outcome or disease status. See also **random variable**.

## Variance

A measure of the spread or **variability** of **quantitative measurements**. The variance is calculated as the *sum* of the squared differences between individual measurements and their **mean**, *divided* by the total sample size (*n*) *minus* 1:

$$s^2 = \frac{sum\ of\ all\ squared\ differences\ from\ the\ mean}{sample\ size - 1} = \frac{\sum (x_i - \bar{x})^2}{n-1}$$

where $x_i$ are the individual observations and $\bar{x}$ (read 'x bar') is the mean of all observations. The $n-1$ divisor gives a better estimate of the variability in the population (which is greater than in the sample). The square root of the variance is the **standard deviation**. (Note: $\sigma^2$ is used in reference to the **population parameter** and $s^2$ in reference to the **sample statistic**. The latter is used to estimate the former.) The term variance is also used with reference to the variance of sample **estimates** (see **sampling distribution**). The square root of this variance is the **standard error** of the estimate. See **measures of dispersion**.

## Variance-ratio test

Synonym for **F-test**.

## Variance-stabilizing transformation

A data **transformation** that achieves constancy of **variance** or **homoscedasticity**, as required by certain methods of analysis (see **assumptions**). Examples are the **arcsine square root** transformation for **proportions**, and the **logarithmic, square root** and **reciprocal** transformations. The latter are often employed as both **normalizing** and variance-stabilizing transformations for positively **skewed quantitative variables**. These typically display a non-independent relationship between variance (or **standard deviation**) and **mean**. For example, **Poisson counts** have *variance* proportional to the mean, and **lognormal distributions** have *standard deviation* proportional to the mean. The square root or the logarithmic transformation apply. The reciprocal transformation is indicated when the standard deviation is proportional to the square of the mean (BLAND, 2015).

## VAS

Abbreviation for **visual analogue scale**.

## Venn diagram

A diagrammatic representation of the logical relationships between different sets. In the Venn diagram shown in Figure V.1a, it can be seen that sets A and C are **mutually exclusive**, as are sets B and C. The cross-hatched area shows the overlap in set membership or *intersection* of sets A and B, which are clearly not mutually exclusive; this intersection is formally denoted as A ∩ B. The intersection between A and C may be denoted as A ∩ C = Ø, i.e. the *null set* that has no members.

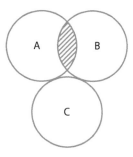

**Figure V.1a** A Venn diagram: intersection of sets A and B represented by cross-hatched area, while sets A and C (and B and C) are mutually exclusive.

Figure V.1b shows the global burden from cardiovascular disease (2005). The numbers attributed to two or more causes of disease may be gathered from the areas of intersection between the different causes. The total number of cardiovascular deaths, for example, due to either high blood pressure, high cholesterol or both, is given by the *union* of the two sets, which is denoted as 'high blood pressure deaths ∪ high cholesterol deaths'. Also, and unlike deaths due to overweight and obesity, all deaths due to high cholesterol were also classified as cardiovascular deaths – in other words, all deaths due to high cholesterol are *included* in the wider set of cardiovascular mortality ('high cholesterol deaths ⊆ cardiovascular deaths' or equivalently, 'cardiovascular deaths ⊇ high cholesterol deaths'):

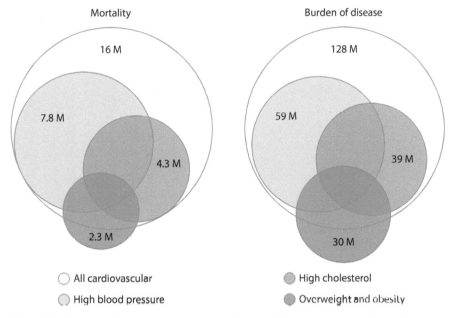

Figure V.1b Global burden from cardiovascular disease. The numbers attributed to two or more causes of disease may be gathered from the areas of intersection between the different causes (M, million). (Reproduced from (2005) Affluence and the worldwide distribution of cardiovascular disease risks. *PLoS Med* **2**: e148.)

## Visual analogue scale

A graphical tool that is used to measure subjective symptoms, attitudes, feelings and opinions. The scale is simply a straight line, along which the different possible outcomes are marked and **ranked** by degree of severity or intensity. Visual analogue scales (VAS) give rise to **ordinal data**, which are usually analysed using **non-parametric methods**. See also **Guttman scale**, **Likert scale**.

## Vital statistics

See **demographic indicators**.

## Volunteer bias

A type of bias that may occur in **cross-sectional studies** and **surveys**, when prospective participants are asked to provide information on a number of relevant variables. Typically, a given percentage of the above will decline participation or fail to respond. For example, in a study where questionnaires are sent to all residents in a particular area, or to all patients registered with a given general practice, some individuals will return the study question-naires (respondents or volunteers) and some will not (non-respondents). Volunteers tend to be different from non-respondents with respect to sociodemographic characteristics and **risk factors** for disease (and therefore, likely **outcomes**) (BLAND, 2015). A number of different strategies may be employed to keep non-response (and the ensuing **selection bias**) at a minimum in this type of study. Volunteer bias may also affect the results and conclusions of evaluations of **screening** programmes. See also **response rate**.

## W

*W*

See **coefficient of concordance**.

*W'*

See **Shapiro–Francia test**.

## Wald's $\chi^2$ test

A **significance test** based on a comparison of **log likelihoods**, as estimated by a theoretical approximation to the value of the log likelihood ratio at the value of the parameter of interest that corresponds to the null hypothesis. An alternative form of the test is as the **z-test**, the **test statistic** being equal to the square root of the likelihood ratio statistic. The Wald test is commonly used with **logistic**, **Poisson** and **Cox regression** to test the significance of single predictor variables. Where a predictor variable has a number of categories each included in the model (as **dummy variables**), the **likelihood ratio test** gives a better assessment of their overall significance (KIRKWOOD & STERNE, 2003). The test statistic ($X^2$) follows a **chi-squared** ($\chi^2$) **distribution** with 1 **degree of freedom**. The Wald test is also used to test the significance of predictor variables in **generalized estimating equations** (**GEEs**).

## Wash-out period

In the context of **crossover trials**, the length of time allowed between consecutive treatments, in order to prevent the effects of treatments given in any one period from being **carried over** into the following period, so that **treatment–period interactions** may be avoided. **Treatment effects** may then be assessed independently, without contamination.

## Weibull model

See **accelerated failure time models**, **proportional hazards models** (parametric survival models).

## Weighted average

An average measure, commonly the **mean**, which is computed by attributing different weights (relative importance) to the different observations in the variable of interest. This principle is often applied when estimating **pooled** or summary **measures of effect** across the **strata** of a **confounding variable**, or across the individual **primary studies** included in a **meta-analysis**. In the latter context, weights are usually inversely proportional to the variance (**inverse variance method**) of the individual estimates (or its square root, the standard error), so larger studies (or strata) tend to have greater weight. The use of weights increases the **precision** of summary estimates. **Mantel–Haenszel** weights are especially useful with sparse data (KIRKWOOD & STERNE, 2003). **Peto's method** of combining odds ratio estimates is particularly suitable for small study samples with similar numbers in each comparison group. For continuous outcomes, a *weighted mean difference* (WMD) may be calculated as the pooled estimate of a difference between means, or, alternatively, a **standardized mean difference** may be computed for each individual study, which then allows estimates of effect measured on different scales to be combined (using the inverse variance or the DerSimonian and Laird method, as appropriate). The **Der Simonian and Laird method** is commonly used to produce weighted averages if a **random effects model** is deemed more appropriate than a **fixed effect model**. See Deeks, Altman & Bradburn, in EGGER, DAVEY SMITH & ALTMAN (eds., 2001), for formulae, illustrative examples and further discussion. See also **standardized mortality ratio (SMR)**.

## Weighted least squares

Also referred to by its abbreviation, WLS. A type of **least squares** regression that seeks to minimize the *weighted* sum of the squared differences (i.e. **residuals**) between observed and predicted outcome, where a **robust method** of analysis is required to downweight **outlying** observations and reduce their influence on the results of data analyses. Weights are user-defined, often based on **Huber weights** or inversely proportional to the changing variance in case of **heteroscedasticity**. Robust **standard errors** must be computed for correct **inference**. Another application of WLS is in the analysis of continuous, **longitudinal data** (DIGGLE *et al.*, 2002). See HAMILTON (1992; 2012) for further details. Cf. **ordinary least squares (OLS)**. See also **iteratively reweighted least squares (IRLS)**.

## Weighted mean difference

Or its abbreviation, WMD. See **weighted average**. Cf. **standardized mean difference**.

## Weights

See **weighted average**.

## Welch's test

A variation of the independent samples *t*-test that allows for unequal **variances** or lack of **homoscedasticity**, a required **assumption** for the *t*-test to which it is sensitive.

## Wilcoxon matched pairs signed rank test

**A non-parametric significance test** that is carried out to compare paired interval/ratio variables when the **assumptions** for the **paired *t*-test** cannot be met. The **null hypothesis** is that there is no tendency for values under each paired variable to be higher or lower, whereas for the paired *t*-test the null hypothesis is that the mean difference between the variables is equal to zero. Paired observations for which the difference is zero do not contribute to the calculation of the **test statistic**, *T*, and therefore the **effective sample size** for the test may be smaller than the actual total sample size (in other words, the number of pairs contributing to the test may be smaller than the total number of pairs). The test statistic is referred to tables of the critical values of the *T* distribution. Contrary to most significance tests, the smaller the test statistic, *T*, the higher the **significance level** of the results (i.e. the smaller the ***P*-value** obtained). See also **sign test** (for paired ordinal data). See BLAND (2015) for further details and an illustrative example.

## Wilcoxon rank sum test

A **non-parametric significance test** that has the same purpose and is mathematically equivalent to the **Mann–Whitney *U*-test**.

## Williams mean

See **geometric mean**.

## Withdrawals

In the context of **clinical trials**, withdrawals are patients or individuals who are removed from trial participation after having been assigned to one of the treatments being compared. These decisions may be made by those conducting the investigation, or by the participants themselves who may thus choose to **drop-out**. Often, patient withdrawal is associated with treatment group membership, a high probability of an adverse outcome or both. **Intention-to-treat analysis** minimizes the **selection bias** that may result from these **protocol breaches**. See also **cross-overs**, **loss to follow-up**, **pragmatic trial**.

## Within-cluster variance

See **dependence**, **intraclass correlation coefficient (ICC)**. Cf. **between-cluster variance**.

## Within-groups variance

Or **residual mean square**. See **analysis of variance (ANOVA)**, ***F*-test**. Cf. **between-groups variance**.

## Within-subject variance

See **dependence**, **intraclass correlation coefficient (ICC)**, **repeatability**. Cf. **between-subject variance**.

## WLS

Abbreviation for **weighted least squares**.

## WMD

Abbreviation for weighted mean difference. See **weighted average**.

## Woolf's formula

A formula for calculating the **standard error (SE)** of the **logarithm** of an **odds ratio (OR)**. See **delta method, error factor (EF)**.

## Working correlation matrix

See **correlation structure, generalized estimating equations (GEEs)**.

# X

### $\bar{x}$

Symbol for **sample mean** (read 'x bar'), as opposed to **population** mean (μ or mu).

### x-axis

The horizontal axis on a two-dimensional graph. See **abscissa**.

### x-variable

Also termed independent, explanatory or **predictor variable**. In **scatterplots** and other bivariate plots, the x-variable is plotted on the horizontal axis (see **abscissa**).

# Y

### y-axis

The vertical axis on a two-dimensional graph. See **ordinate**.

### y-variable

Also termed dependent, response or **outcome variable**. In **scatterplots** and other bivariate plots, the $y$-variable is plotted on the vertical axis (see **ordinate**).

### Yates' continuity correction

A **continuity correction** that is applied to the **chi-squared test statistic** ($X^2$) when comparing **observed** ($O$) *vs.* **expected** ($E$) **frequencies** as displayed in a **two-by-two table**. This is achieved by subtracting ½ from the absolute value of the $O$ *vs.* $E$ difference in each cell of the table. The squares of these differences form the numerators of the addends of the $X^2$ statistic. The correction is necessary, especially with small samples, to improve the **approximation** of a **continuous** distribution (**chi-squared**) to a **discrete** distribution (**Poisson** or **multinomial**). The latter are the **sampling distributions** of the observed frequencies in each cell of the table, under the **null hypothesis** of **independence** or lack of association between the variables that are cross-tabulated.

# Z

## z-score

Also termed 'standard Normal deviate'. A z-score is a measurement from a **Normal distribution** that is expressed in units of **standard deviation** (**SD**), and not in the original units of the measurement. For example, if the **mean** height for a group of people is 172 cm with SD equal to 10 cm, a person measuring 182 cm has a z-score of 1 (i.e. is +1 SD away from the mean). z-scores are obtained through a linear **transformation**, by subtracting the mean from the individual measurements, and dividing the result by the SD. Thus, measurements are converted into a Normal distribution with mean = 0 and SD = 1 (i.e. the standard Normal distribution):

$$z\text{-}score = \frac{observation\ value - mean}{SD}$$

The values of a non-normal distribution may be converted into 'standard scores' through a similar transformation (HAMILTON, 1990). The resulting variable will not be normally distributed, but will have mean = 0 and SD = 1. When assessing normality of distribution using quantile-quantile plots (see **Normal plot**), z-scores are calculated for a **theoretical** Normal distribution (with the same **mean** and **standard deviation** as the variable in question). Each value of the observed distribution will have a corresponding **quantile** in the theoretical z-scores, i.e. a value with the same **cumulative probability**. Cf. **inverse normal**. See also **growth charts**.

## z-test

A **significance test** that is carried out to compare two groups with respect to a **mean** measurement, or with respect to the **proportion** in each group with a given binary outcome. In the latter case, the z-test is equivalent to the **chi-squared test** that is performed on the cross-tabulations of a two-by-two table. An **assumption** of the z-test is that **sample sizes** are sufficiently large. With smaller samples, the independent samples *t*-test and **Fisher's exact test** should be used. The z test statistic follows the standard Normal distribution when the null hypothesis is true, and therefore does not require the calculation of **degrees of freedom**. See also **Wald's test**, **large sample method**.

## Zelen's design

A **study design** for a **clinical trial** in which an attempt is made to deal with the difficulties of obtaining **informed consent** (ZELEN, 1979). Starting with all individuals **eligible** to enter the trial, they are often, but not necessarily, randomly divided into groups of equal size. The first group receives the standard treatment and is *not* informed of their participation in a trial. Individuals randomized to the second group *are* informed of their participation in a trial and offered the choice of receiving the experimental treatment. Should any of them refuse consent they are then allocated to receive the standard treatment. Clearly, for **selection bias** to be avoided, a large proportion of the second group must agree to receive the new treatment. Ethical arguments have been raised regarding the fact that individuals in the first group remain unaware of their participation in a trial. See ALTMAN (1991), POCOCK (1983) and MACHIN & CAMPBELL (2005) for further details.

## Zero-inflated Poisson regression

A regression method for **count variables**, in which the **distribution** of the variable of interest shows a high frequency of zero counts, and the distribution of the non-zero counts is **Poisson**. This type of data is often **overdispersed**, making the zero-inflated model preferable to **Poisson regression**. Alternatively, zero-inflated **negative binomial regression** may be used if overdispersion is due to unexplained between-subject heterogeneity and an excess of zero counts. **Clustered designs** may add variability to an already overdispersed count variable, and zero-inflated models with **random effects** may be indicated here. Both zero-inflated Poisson and zero-inflated negative binomial models are specified as two-part models, with a **logistic regression** part that models the proportion of zero count observations, and a Poisson or negative binomial part that models non-zero counts (but predicts zero counts also). See DWIVEDI *et al.* (2010) and ALEXANDER (2012) for further details and illustrative examples.

## ZINB model

See zero-inflated **negative binomial regression**.

## ZIP model

See **zero-inflated Poisson regression**.

# References

## Core references

Altman DG (1991). *Practical Statistics for Medical Research*. Chapman & Hall/CRC Press.
Bland M (2015). *An Introduction to Medical Statistics, 4th edition*. Oxford University Press.
Borenstein M, Hedges LV, Higgins JPT, Rothstein HR (2009). *Introduction to Meta-Analysis*. Wiley.
Egger M, Davey Smith G, Altman DG (eds., 2001). *Systematic Reviews in Health Care: Meta-analysis in Context, 2nd edition*. BMJ Books.
Hamilton LC (1992). *Regression with Graphics. A Second Course in Applied Statistics*. Duxbury Press.
Haynes RB, Sackett DL, Guyatt GH, Tugwell P (eds., 2006). *Clinical Epidemiology: How to do Clinical Practice Research, 3rd edition*. Lippincott Williams & Wilkins.
Hennekens CH, Buring JE, Mayrent SL (eds., 1987). *Epidemiology in Medicine*. Lippincott Williams & Wilkins.
Kirkwood BR, Sterne JA (2003). *Essential Medical Statistics, 2nd edition*. Blackwell.
Pocock SJ (1983). *Clinical Trials: A Practical Approach*. Wiley.
Rothman KJ (2012). *Epidemiology: An Introduction, 2nd edition*. Oxford University Press.
Wald NJ (2004). *The Epidemiological Approach: An Introduction to Epidemiology in Medicine, 4th edition*. Wolfson Institute of Preventive Medicine & The Royal Society of Medicine Press.

## Core and additional references

Afifi A, May S, Clark VA (2011). *Practical Multivariate Analysis, 5th edition*. Chapman & Hall/CRC Press.
Agresti A (2007). *An Introduction to Categorical Data Analysis, 2nd edition*. Wiley.
Agresti A (2013). *Categorical Data Analysis, 3rd edition*. Wiley.
Ajetunmobi O (2002). *Making Sense of Critical Appraisal*. Hodder Arnold.
Alexander N (2012). Review: analysis of parasite and other skewed counts. *Trop Med Int Health* **17**: 684–693.
Altman DG (1991). *Practical Statistics for Medical Research*. Chapman & Hall/CRC Press.

Altman DG (1993). Construction of age-related reference centiles using absolute residuals. *Stat Med* **12**: 917–924.

Altman DG, Deeks JJ (2002). Meta-analysis, Simpson's paradox, and the number needed to treat. *BMC Med Res Methodol* **2**: 3.

Altman DG, Machin D, Bryant TN, Gardner MJ (eds., 2000). *Statistics with Confidence, 2nd edition*. BMJ Books.

Altman DG, Royston P (2000). What do we mean by validating a prognostic model? *Stat Med* **19**: 453–473.

Altman DG, Schulz KF (2001). Concealing treatment allocation in randomised trials. *Br Med J* **323**: 446–447.

Altman DG, Vergouwe Y, Royston P, Moons KGM (2009). Prognosis and prognostic research: validating a prognostic model. *Br Med J* **338**: b605.

Andersen B (1990). *Methodological Errors in Medical Research*. Blackwell Scientific Publications.

Armitage P, Berry G, Mathews JNS (2002). *Statistical Methods in Medical Research, 4th edition*. Blackwell.

Barnett AG, van der Pols JC, Dobson AJ (2005). Regression to the mean: what it is and how to deal with it. *Int J Epidemiol* **34**: 215–220. (Correction in *Int J Epidemiol* 2015 **44**: 1748.)

Begg CB, Cho M, Eastwood S, *et al.* (1996). Improving the quality of reporting of randomized controlled trials. The CONSORT statement. *JAMA* **276**: 637–639.

Begg CB, Mazumdar M (1994). Operating characteristics of a rank correlation test for publication bias. *Biometrics* **50**: 1088–1101.

Bennett DA, Emberson JR (2009). Stratification for exploring heterogeneity in systematic reviews. *Evid Based Med* **14**: 162–164.

Bland JM. MSc Course Materials. University of York, Department of Health Sciences (accessed August 2016).

Bland JM, Altman DG (1986). Statistical methods for assessing agreement between two methods of clinical measurement. *Lancet* **327**: 307–310. (See end of http://www-users.york.ac.uk/~mb55/meas/ba.htm for corrections.)

Bland JM, Altman DG (1994a). Regression towards the mean. *Br Med J* **308**: 1499.

Bland JM, Altman DG (1994b). Some examples of regression towards the mean. *Br Med J* **309**: 780.

Bland JM, Altman DG (1996a). Transformations, means, and confidence intervals. *Br Med J* **312**: 1079.

Bland JM, Altman DG (1996b). The use of transformations when comparing two means. *Br Med J* **312**: 1153.

Bland JM, Altman DG (1996c). Measurements error proportional to the mean. *Br Med J* **313**: 106.

Bland JM, Altman DG (1999). Measuring agreement in method comparison studies. *Stat Methods Med Res* **8**: 135–160.

Bland JM, Altman DG (2011). Comparisons against baseline within randomised groups are often used and can be highly misleading. *Trials* **12**: 264.

Bland M (2015). *An Introduction to Medical Statistics, 4th edition*. Oxford University Press.

Blomqvist N (1977). On the relation between change and initial value. *J Am Stat Assoc* **72**: 746–749.

Blomqvist N (1987). On the bias caused by regression toward the mean in studying the relation between change and initial value. *J Clin Periodontol* **14**: 34–37.

Borenstein M, Hedges LV, Higgins JPT, Rothstein HR (2009). *Introduction to Meta-Analysis*. Wiley.

Bossuyt PM, Reitsma JB, Bruns DE, *et al.*, for the STARD Group (2003). Towards complete and accurate reporting of studies of diagnostic accuracy: the STARD initiative. *Br Med J* **326**: 41–44.

Bossuyt PM, Reitsma JB, Bruns DE, *et al.*, for the STARD Group (2015). STARD 2015: an updated list of essential items for reporting diagnostic accuracy studies. *Br Med J* **351**: h5527.

Box GEP, Cox DR (1964). An analysis of transformations (with discussion). *J Royal Stat Soc B* **26**: 211–252.

Bradburn MJ, Deeks JJ, Berlin JA, Localio AR (2007). Much ado about nothing: a comparison of the performance of meta-analytical methods with rare events. *Stat Med* **26**: 53–77.

Breslow NE, Day NE (1980). *Statistical Methods in Cancer Research: Vol I – The Design and Analysis of Case–Control Studies*. Lyon: International Agency for Research on Cancer.

Breslow NE, Day NE (1987). *Statistical Methods in Cancer Research: Vol II – The Analysis of Cohort Studies*. Lyon: International Agency for Research on Cancer.

Brindle P, Emberson J, Lampe F, *et al.* (2003). Predictive accuracy of the Framingham coronary risk score in British men: prospective cohort study. *Br Med J* **327**: 1267.

Campbell MJ, Machin D, Walters SJ (2007). *Medical Statistics: A Textbook for the Health Sciences, 4th edition*. Wiley.

Case LD, Morgan TM (2003). Design of Phase II cancer trials evaluating survival probabilities. *BMC Med Res Methodol* **3**: 6.

Cates CJ (2002). Simpson's paradox and calculation of number needed to treat from meta-analysis. *BMC Med Res Methodol* **2**: 1.

Chalmers I (1985). Proposal to outlaw the term 'negative' trial. *Br Med J* **290**: 1002.

Chalmers I, Altman DG (eds., 1995). *Systematic Reviews*. BMJ Publishing Group.

Chan A-W, Tetzlaff JM, Altman DG, *et al.* (2013). SPIRIT 2013 Statement: Defining standard protocol items for clinical trials. *Ann Intern Med* **158**: 200–207.

Chatfield C (2003). *The Analysis of Time Series: An Introduction, 6th edition*. Chapman & Hall/CRC Press.

Chiolero A, Paradis G, Rich B, Hanley JA (2013). Assessing the relationship between the baseline value of a continuous variable and subsequent change over time. *Front Public Health* **1**: 29.

Chow SC, Chang M (2008). Adaptive design methods in clinical trials – a review. *Orphanet J Rare Dis* **3**:11.

Chow SC, Chang M (2011). *Adaptive Design Methods in Clinical Trials, 2nd edition*. Chapman & Hall/CRC Press.

Clayton D, Hills M (1993). *Statistical Models in Epidemiology*. Oxford University Press.

Cleveland WS (1979). Robust locally weighted regression and smoothing scatterplots. *J Am Stat Assoc* **74**: 829–836.

Cleveland WS (1993). *Visualizing Data*. Hobart Press.

Cleveland WS (1994). *The Elements of Graphing Data, 2nd edition*. Hobart Press.

Cleveland WS, Devlin SJ (1988). Locally weighted regression: an approach to regression analysis by local fitting. *J Am Stat Assoc* **83**: 596–610.

Cleves M, Gould WW, Marchenko YV (2016). *An Introduction to Survival Analysis Using Stata, revised 3rd edition*. Stata Press.

Cochran WG (1957). Analysis of covariance: its nature and uses. *Biometrics* **13**: 261–281.

Cochran WG (1977). *Sampling Techniques, 3rd edition*. John Wiley & Sons.

Cole TJ (2012). The development of growth references and growth charts. *Ann Hum Biol* **39**: 382–394.

Coleman JJ, Ferner RE, Evans SJW (2006). Monitoring for adverse drug reactions. *Br J Clin Pharmacol* **61**: 371–378.

Collins GS, Reitsma JB, Altman DG, Moons KGM (2015). Transparent reporting of a multivariable prediction model for individual prognosis or diagnosis (TRIPOD): the TRIPOD Statement. *BMC Medicine* **13**: 1.

Cook JA, Hislop J, Adewuyi TE, *et al.* (2014). Assessing methods to specify the target difference for a randomised controlled trial: DELTA (Difference ELicitation in TriAls) review. *Health Technol Assess* **18**: 1–175.

Cook RJ, Sackett DL (1995). The number needed to treat: a clinically useful measure of treatment effect. *Br Med J* **310**: 452–454. (Erratum in *Br Med J* **310**: 1056.)

Cox DR (1972). Regression models and life tables. *J Royal Stat Soc B* **34**: 187–220.

Cox DR (1984). Interaction (with discussion). *International Statistical Review* **52**: 1–31.

Dawson B, Trapp RG (2004). *Basic & Clinical Biostatistics, 4th edition*. Lange Medical Books/McGraw-Hill.

de Brún C, Pearce-Smith N (2014). Heneghan C, Pereira R, Badenoch D (eds.). *Searching Skills Toolkit: Finding the Evidence, 2nd edition*. BMJ Books.

DerSimonian R, Laird N (1986). Meta-analysis in clinical trials. *Controlled Clinical Trials* **7**: 177–188.

Diggle PJ, Heagerty P, Liang KY, Zeger SL (2002). *Analysis of Longitudinal Data, 2nd edition*. Oxford University Press.

Drummond M (1994). *Economic Analysis alongside Controlled Trials. An Introduction for Clinical Researchers*. Department of Health (UK).

Drummond MF, Sculpher MJ, Claxton K, Stoddart GL, Torrance GW (2015). *Methods for the Economic Evaluation of Health Care Programmes, 4th edition*. Oxford University Press.

Dunn G, Everitt B (1995). *Clinical Biostatistics: An Introduction to Evidence-Based Medicine*. Hodder Education Publishers.

Dwivedi AK, Dwivedi SN, Deo S, Shukla R, Kopras E (2010). Statistical models for predicting number of involved nodes in breast cancer patients. *Health* (Irvine Calif.) **2**: 641–651.

Egger M, Davey Smith G, Altman DG (eds., 2001). *Systematic Reviews in Health Care: Meta-analysis in Context, 2nd edition*. BMJ Books.

Egger M, Davey Smith G, Schneider M, Minder C (1997). Bias in meta-analysis detected by a simple, graphical test. *Br Med J* **315**: 629–634.

Eldridge S, Kerry S (2012). *A Practical Guide to Cluster Randomised Trials in Health Services Research*. Wiley.

Elliott P, Wartenberg D (2004). Spatial epidemiology: current approaches and future challenges. *Environ Health Perspect* **112**: 998–1006.

Ellis PD (2010). *The Essential Guide to Effect Sizes: Statistical Power, Meta-analysis, and the Interpretation of Research Results*. Cambridge University Press.

Everitt BS (2006). *Medical Statistics from A to Z: A Guide for Clinicians and Medical Students, 2nd edition*. Cambridge University Press.

Everitt BS (2009). *Multivariable Modeling and Multivariate Analysis for the Behavioral Sciences*. Chapman & Hall/CRC Press.

Everitt BS, Palmer CR (eds., 2011). *Encyclopaedic Companion to Medical Statistics, 2nd edition*. Wiley.

Everitt BS, Skrondal A (2010). *The Cambridge Dictionary of Statistics, 4th edition*. Cambridge University Press.

Evidence-Based Medicine Working Group (1992). Evidence-based medicine: a new approach to teaching the practice of medicine. *JAMA* **268**: 2420–2425.

Fairfield Smith H (1957). Interpretation of adjusted treatment means and regressions in analysis of covariance. *Biometrics* **13**: 282–308.

Feinstein AR, Walter SD, Horwitz RI (1986). An analysis of Berkson's bias in case–control studies. *J Chronic Dis* **39**: 495–504.

Flanders WD, Boyle CA, Boring JR (1989). Bias associated with differential hospitalization rates in incident case–control studies. *J Clin Epidemiol* **42**: 395–401.

Fleiss JL (1999). *Design and Analysis of Clinical Experiments*. Wiley.

Freedman B (1987). Equipoise and the ethics of clinical research. *N Engl J Med* **317**: 141–145.

Frost C, Thompson SG (2000). Correcting for regression dilution bias: comparison of methods for a single predictor variable. *J Royal Stat Soc A* **163**: 173–189.

Galbraith RF (1988). A note on graphical presentation of estimated odds ratios from several clinical trials. *Stat Med* **7**: 889–849.

Gardner W, Mulvey EP, Shaw EC (1995). Regression analyses of counts and rates: Poisson, overdispersed Poisson, and negative binomial models. *Psych Bull* **118**: 392–404.

Ghosh M, Reid N, Fraser DAS (2010). Ancillary statistics: a review. *Statistica Sinica* **20**: 1309–1332.

Goldstein H (2010). *Multilevel Statistical Models, 4th edition*. Wiley.

Goodman S (2008). A dirty dozen: twelve p-value misconceptions. *Semin Hematol* **45**: 135–140. (Erratum in *Semin Hematol* 2011 **48**: 302.)

Goodman SN (1993). P values, hypothesis tests, and likelihood: implications for epidemiology of a neglected historical debate. *Am J Epidemiol* **137**: 485–496; 497–501.

Greenhalgh T (1997). How to read a paper: getting your bearings (deciding what the paper is about). *Br Med J* **315**: 243–246.

Greenhalgh T (2014). *How to Read a Paper: The Basics of Evidence-based Medicine, 5th edition*. BMJ Books.

Greenland S (2008). Bayesian interpretation and analysis of research results. *Semin Hematol* **45**: 141–149.

Greenland S, Senn SJ, Rothman KJ, *et al.* (2016). Statistical tests, *P* values, confidence intervals, and power: a guide to misinterpretations. *Int J Epidemiol* **31**: 337–350.

Grimes DA, Schulz KF (2002). Bias and causal associations in observational research. *Lancet* **359**: 248–252.

Guyatt G, Rennie D, Meade MO, Cook DJ (2014). *User's Guides to the Medical Literature: A Manual for Evidence-based Clinical Practice, 3rd edition*. JAMA & Archives Journals, McGraw-Hill.

Guyatt GH, Oxman AD, Vist GE, *et al.*, for the GRADE Working Group (2008). GRADE: an emerging consensus on rating quality of evidence and strength of recommendations. *Br Med J* **336**: 924–926.

Guyatt GH, Sackett DL, Sinclair JC, Hayward R, Cook DJ, Cook RJ, for the Evidence-based Medicine Working Group (1995). Users' guides to the medical literature. IX. A method for grading health care recommendations. *JAMA* **274**: 1800–1804.

Halligan S, Altman DG, Mallett S (2015). Disadvantages of using the area under the receiver operating characteristic curve to assess imaging tests: A discussion and proposal for an alternative approach. *Eur Radiol* **25**: 932–939.

Hamilton LC (1990). *Modern Data Analysis. A First Course in Applied Statistics*. Brooks/Cole Publishing Company.

Hamilton LC (1992). *Regression with Graphics. A Second Course in Applied Statistics*. Duxbury Press.

Hamilton LC (2012). *Statistics with STATA version 12, 8th edition*. Brooks/Cole, Cengage Learning.

Hanley JA, McNeil BJ (1982). The meaning and use of the area under a receiver operating characteristic (ROC) curve. *Radiology* **143**: 29–36.

Hayes RJ (1988). Methods for assessing whether change depends on initial value. *Stat Med* **7**: 915–927.

Haynes RB, Sackett DL, Guyatt GH, Tugwell P (eds., 2006). *Clinical Epidemiology: How to do Clinical Practice Research, 3rd edition*. Lippincott Williams & Wilkins.

Heneghan C, Badenoch D (2006). *Evidence-based Medicine Toolkit, 2nd edition*. BMJ Books.

Hennekens CH, Buring JE, Mayrent SL (eds., 1987). *Epidemiology in Medicine*. Lippincott Williams & Wilkins.

Hernán MA, Clayton D, Keiding N (2011). The Simpson's paradox unravelled. *Int J Epidemiol* **40**: 780–785.

Higgins JPT, Altman DG, Gøtzsche PC, *et al.*, Cochrane Bias Methods Group, Cochrane Statistical Methods Group (2011). The Cochrane Collaboration's tool for assessing risk of bias in randomised trials. *Br Med J* **343**: d5928.

Higgins JPT, Green S (eds., 2008). *Cochrane Handbook for Systematic Reviews of Interventions*. Wiley.

Higgins JPT, Thompson SG, Deeks JJ, Altman DG (2003). Measuring inconsistency in meta-analyses. *Br Med J* **327**: 557–560.

Higgins JPT, Thompson SG, Spiegelhalter DJ (2009). A re-evaluation of random-effects meta-analysis. *J Royal Stat Soc A* **172**: 137–159.

Hills M (1974). *Statistics for Comparative Studies*. Chapman & Hall.

Hosmer DW, Lemeshow S, May S (2008). *Applied Survival Analysis: Regression Modelling of Time to Event Data, 2nd edition*. Wiley.

Hosmer DW, Lemeshow S, May S (2008). *Applied Survival Analysis: Regression Modelling of Time-to-Event Data, 2nd edition*. Wiley.

Hosmer DW, Lemeshow S, Sturdivant RX (2013). *Applied Logistic Regression, 3rd edition*. Wiley.

Huitema BE (2011). *The Analysis of Covariance and Alternatives: Statistical Methods for Experiments, Quasi-experiments, and Single-case Studies, 2nd edition*. Wiley.

Hutton JL (2000). Number needed to treat: properties and problems. *J Royal Stat Soc A* **163**: 403–419.

Jüni P, Altman DG, Egger M (2001). Assessing the quality of controlled clinical trials. *Br Med J* **323**: 42–46.

Kirkwood BR, Sterne JA (2003). *Essential Medical Statistics, 2nd edition*. Blackwell.

Knaus WA, Draper EA, Wagner DP, Zimmerman JE (1985). APACHE II: a severity of disease classification system. *Crit Care Med* **13**: 818-829.

Knaus WA, Wagner DP, Draper EA, *et al.* (1991). The APACHE III prognostic system. Risk prediction of hospital mortality for critically ill hospitalized adults. *Chest* **100**: 1619–1636.

L'Abbé KA, Detsky AS, O'Rourke K (1987). Meta-analysis in clinical research. *Ann Intern Med* **107**: 224–233.

Last JM (ed., 2001). *A Dictionary of Epidemiology, 4th edition*. Oxford University Press.

Lau J, Ioannidis JPA, Terrin N, Schmid CH, Olkin I (2006). The case of the misleading funnel plot. *Br Med J* **333**: 597–600.

Levy PS, Lemeshow S (2009). *Sampling of Populations: Methods and Applications, 4th edition*. Wiley.

Liang KY, Zeger SL (1986). Longitudinal data analysis using generalized linear models. *Biometrika* **72**: 13–22.

Liberati A, Altman DG, Tetzlaff J, *et al.* (2009). The PRISMA statement for reporting systematic reviews and meta-analyses of studies that evaluate health care interventions: explanation and elaboration. *PLoS Med* **6**: e1000100.

Machin D, Campbell MJ (2005). *Design of Studies for Medical Research*. Wiley.

Machin D, Campbell MJ, Tan SB, Tan SH (2009). *Sample Size Tables for Clinical Studies, 3rd edition*. Wiley-Blackwell.

Mallett S, Halligan S, Thompson M, Collins GS, Altman DG (2012). Interpreting diagnostic accuracy studies for patient care. *Br Med J* **345**: e3999.

Matthews JN, Altman DG, Campbell MJ, Royston P (1990). Analysis of serial measurements in medical research. *Br Med J* **300**: 230–235.

Michels KB, Rothman KJ (2003). Update on unethical use of placebos in randomized trials. *Bioethics* **17**: 188–204.

Miettinen O (1976). Estimability and estimation in case-referent studies. *Am J Epidemiol* **103**: 226–235.

Mitchell MN (2012a). *A Visual Guide to Stata Graphics, 3rd edition*. Stata Press.

Mitchell MN (2012b). *Interpreting and Visualizing Regression Models using Stata*. Stata Press.

Moher D, Cook DJ, Eastwood S, Olkin I, Rennie D, Stroup DF (1999). Improving the quality of reports of meta-analyses of randomised controlled trials: the QUOROM statement. Quality of Reporting of Meta-analyses. *Lancet* **354**: 1896–1900.

Moher D, Liberati A, Tetzlaff J, Altman DG, The PRISMA Group (2009). Preferred Reporting Items for Systematic Reviews and Meta-Analyses: The PRISMA Statement. *PLoS Med* **6**: e1000097.

Moher D, Schulz KF, Altman D (2001). The CONSORT statement: revised recommendations for improving the quality of reports of parallel-group randomized trials. *JAMA* **285**: 1987–1991.

Moons KGM, Royston P, Vergouwe Y, Grobbee DE, Altman DG (2009). Prognosis and prognostic research: what, why, and how? *Br Med J* **338**: b375.

Mosteller F, Tukey JW (1977). *Data Analysis and Regression: A Second Course in Statistics*. Addison-Wesley.

Moyé LA, Tita ATN (2002). Defending the rationale for the two-tailed test in clinical research. *Circulation* **105**: 3062–3065.

Muscatello DJ, Searles A, Macdonald R, Jorm L (2006). Communicating population health statistics through graphs: a randomised controlled trial of graph design interventions. *BMC Medicine* **4**: 33.

Naggara O, Raymond J, Guilbert F, Roy D, Weill A, Altman DG (2011). Analysis by categorizing or dichotomizing continuous variables is inadvisable: an example from the natural history of unruptured aneurysms. *AJNR Am J Neuroradiol* **32**: 437–440.

Oldham PD (1962). A note on the analysis of repeated measurements of the same subjects. *J Chronic Dis* **15**: 969–977.

Olejnik S, Algina J (2003). Generalized eta and omega squared statistics: measures of effect size for some common research designs. *Psych methods* **8**: 434–447.

Peto R, Pike MC, Armitage P, *et al.* (1976). Design and analysis of randomized clinical trials requiring prolonged observation of each patient. Part I: Introduction and design. *Br J Cancer* **34**: 585–612.

Peto R, Pike MC, Armitage P, *et al.* (1977). Design and analysis of randomized clinical trials requiring prolonged observation of each patient. Part II: Analysis and examples. *Br J Cancer* **35**: 1–39.

Piaggio G, Elbourne DR, Altman DG, Pocock SJ, Evans SJW (2006). Reporting of noninferiority and equivalence randomized trials: an extension of the CONSORT statement. *JAMA* **295**: 1152–1160.

Pocock SJ (1983). *Clinical Trials: A Practical Approach*. Wiley.

Pocock SJ (2006). The simplest statistical test: how to check for a difference between treatments. *Br Med J* **332**: 1256–1258.

Pocock SJ, Assmann SE, Enos LE, Kasten LE (2002). Subgroup analysis, covariate adjustment and baseline comparisons in clinical trial reporting: current practice and problems. *Stat Med* **21**: 2917–2930.

Porta M (ed., 2014), Greenland S, Hernán M, dos Santos Silva I, Last JM (associate eds.), Burón A (assistant ed.). *A Dictionary of Epidemiology, 6th edition*. Oxford University Press.

Rabe-Hesketh S, Skrondal A (2012). *Multilevel and Longitudinal Modeling using Stata, volumes I and II, 3rd edition*. Stata Press.

Riley RD, Higgins JPT, Deeks JJ (2011). Interpretation of random effects meta-analyses. *Br Med J* **342**: d549.

Rothman KJ (1974). Synergy and antagonism in cause–effect relationships. *Am J Epidemiol* **99**: 385–388.

Rothman KJ (1986). *Modern Epidemiology*. Little, Brown & Co.

Rothman KJ (2012). *Epidemiology: An Introduction, 2nd edition*. Oxford University Press.

Rothman KJ, Greenland S (eds., 1998). *Modern Epidemiology, 2nd edition*. Lippincott Williams & Wilkins.

Rothman KJ, Greenland S, Lash TL (eds., 2012). *Modern Epidemiology, revised 3rd edition*. Lippincott Williams & Wilkins.

Rothman KJ, Michels KB (1994). The continuing unethical use of placebo controls. *N Engl J Med* **331**: 394–398.

Royston P, Altman DG (1994). Regression using fractional polynomials of continuous covariates: parsimonious parametric modelling. *Appl Stat* **43**: 429–467.

Royston P, Altman DG, Sauerbrei W (2005). Dichotomizing continuous predictors in multiple regression: a bad idea. *Stat Med* **25**: 127–141.

Royston P, Ambler G, Sauerbrei W (1999). The use of fractional polynomials to model continuous risk factors in epidemiology. *Int J Epidemiol* **28**: 964–974.

Royston P, Moons KGM, Altman DG, Vergouwe Y (2009). Prognosis and prognostic research: developing a prognostic model. *Br Med J* **338**: b604.

Sackett D (1979). Bias in analytical research. *J Chron Dis* **32**: 51–63.

Schlesselman JJ (1982). *Case–control Studies: Design, Conduct, Analysis*. Oxford University Press.

Schulz KF (2000). Assessing allocation concealment and blinding in randomized controlled trials: why bother? *ACP J Club* **132**: A11–A13.

Schulz KF, Grimes DA (2002a). Generation of allocation sequences in randomised trials: chance, not choice. *Lancet* **359**: 515–519.

Schulz KF, Grimes DA (2002b). Allocation concealment in randomised trials: defending against deciphering. *Lancet* **359**: 614–618.

Sedgwick P (2013). What is the number needed to treat? *Br Med J* **347**: f4605.

Senn S (2011). Francis Galton and regression to the mean. *Significance* **8**: 124–126.

Senn SJ (1995). In defence of analysis of covariance: a reply to Chambless and Roeback (letter; comment). *Stat Med* **14**: 2283–2285.

Senn SJ (2002). *Cross-over Trials in Clinical Research, 2nd edition*. Wiley.

Senn SJ (2006). Change from baseline and analysis of covariance revisited. *Stat Med* **25**: 4334–4344.

Senn SJ (2008). *Statistical Issues in Drug Development, 2nd edition*. Wiley.

Siler W (1979). A competing-risk model for animal mortality. *Ecology* **60**: 750–757.

Simera I, Moher D, Hoey J, Schulz KF, Altman DG (2010). A catalogue of reporting guidelines for health research. *Eur J Clin Invest* **40**: 35–53.

Singer JD, Willett JB (2003). *Applied Longitudinal Data Analysis: Modelling Change and Event Occurrence*. Oxford University Press.

Skrondal A, Rabe-Hesketh S (2004). *Generalized Latent Variable Modelling: Multilevel, Longitudinal, and Structural Equation Models*. Chapman & Hall/CRC Press.

Smith PG, Morrow RH (eds., 1991). *Methods for Field Trials of Interventions against Tropical Diseases: a Toolbox*. Oxford University Press.

Snoep JD, Morabia A, Hernández-Diaz S, Hernán MA, Vandenbroucke JP (2014). A structural approach to Berkson's fallacy and a guide to a history of opinions about it. *Int J Epidemiol* **43**: 515–521.

Spiegelhalter DJ, Abrams KR, Myles JP (2004). *Bayesian Approaches to Clinical Trials and Health-Care Evaluation*. Wiley.

Stata Online Manual @ www.stata.com. StataCorp.

Sterne JAC, Sutton AJ, Ioannidis JPA, *et al.* (2011). Recommendations for examining and interpreting funnel plot asymmetry in meta-analyses of randomised control trials. *Br Med J* **343**: d4002.

Straus SE, Richardson WS, Glasziou P, Haynes RB (2010). *Evidence-based Medicine: How to Practice and Teach It, 4th edition*. Churchill Livingstone.

Teasdale G, Jennett B (1974). Assessment of coma and impaired consciousness. A practical scale. *Lancet* **2**: 81–84.

Thompson SG (1994). Systematic reviews: why sources of heterogeneity should be investigated. *Br Med J* **309**: 1351–1355.

Thompson SG, Barber JA (2000). How should cost data in pragmatic randomised trials be analysed? *Br Med J* **320**: 1197–1200.

Thompson SG, Higgins JPT (2002). How should meta-regression analyses be undertaken and interpreted? *Stat Med* **21**: 1559–1574.

Thompson SG, Smith TC, Sharp SJ (1997). Investigating underlying risk as a source of heterogeneity in meta-analysis. *Stat Med* **16**: 2741–2758.

Tukey JW (1977). *Exploratory Data Analysis*. Addison-Wesley.

Turner L, Boutron I, Hróbjartsson A, Altman DG, Moher D (2013). The evolution of assessing bias in Cochrane systematic reviews of interventions: celebrating methodological contributions of the Cochrane Collaboration. *Systematic Reviews* **2**: 79.

Vandenbroucke JP, von Elm E, Altman DG, *et al.*; STROBE Initiative (2007). Strengthening the Reporting of Observational Studies in Epidemiology (STROBE): explanation and elaboration. *PLoS Med* **4**: e297.

Vickers AJ (2001). The use of percentage change from baseline as an outcome in a controlled trial is statistically inefficient: a simulation study. *BMC Med Res Methodol* **1**: 1–6.

Vickers AJ, Altman DG (2001). Analysing controlled trials with baseline and follow up measurements. *Br Med J* **323**: 1123–1124.

Vincent JL, Moreno R (2010). Clinical review: Scoring systems in the critically ill. *Critical Care* **14**: 207.

von Elm E, Altman DG, Egger M, Pocock SJ, Gøtzsche PC, Vandenbroucke JP; STROBE Initiative (2007). The Strengthening the Reporting of Observational Studies in Epidemiology (STROBE) statement: guidelines for reporting observational studies. *PLoS Med* **4**: e296.

Wald NJ (2004). *The Epidemiological Approach: An Introduction to Epidemiology in Medicine, 4th edition*. Wolfson Institute of Preventive Medicine & The Royal Society of Medicine Press.

Wald NJ, Hackshaw AK, Frost CD (1999). When can a risk factor be used as a worthwhile screening test? *Br Med J* **319**: 1562–1565.

Waller PC, Evans SJW (2003). A model for the future conduct of pharmacovigilance. *Pharmacoepidemiol Drug Saf* **12**: 17–19.

Wilson PW, D'Agostino RB, Levy D, Belanger AM, Silbershatz H, Kannel WB (1998). Prediction of coronary heart disease using risk factor categories. *Circulation* **97**: 1837–1847.

Zelen M (1979). A new design for randomized clinical trials. *N Engl J Med* **300**: 1242–1245.

## Illustrative examples

(2005) Affluence and the worldwide distribution of cardiovascular disease risks. *PLoS Med* **2**: e148.

Adam I, Ahmed S, Mahmoud MH, Yassin MI (2002). Comparison of HemoCue® hemoglobin-meter and automated hematology analyser in measurement of hemoglobin levels in pregnant women at Khartoum hospital, Sudan. *Diagn Pathol* **7**: 30.

Almohmeed Y, Avenell A, Aucott L, Vickers MA (2013). Systematic review and meta-analysis of the sero-epidemiological association between Epstein Barr virus and multiple sclerosis. *PLoS One* **8**: e61110.

Argos M, Rathouz PJ, Pierce BL, *et al.* (2010). Dietary B vitamin intakes and urinary total arsenic concentration in the Health Effects of Arsenic Longitudinal Study (HEALS) cohort, Bangladesh. *Eur J Nutr* **49**: 473–481.

Bax L, Ikeda N, Fukui N, Yaju Y, Tsuruta H, Moons KG (2009). More than numbers: the power of graphs in meta-analysis. *Am J Epidemiol* **169**: 249–255.

Binnian W, Blount BC, Xia B, Wang L (2016). Assessing exposure to tobacco-specific carcinogenic NNK using its urinary metabolite NNAL measured in US population: 2011–2012. *J Expo Sci Environ Epidemiol* **26**: 249–256.

Brenner DR, McLaughlin JR, Hung RJ (2011). Previous lung diseases and lung cancer risk: A systematic review and meta-analysis. *PLoS One* **6**: e17479.

Caraguel CGB, Vanderstichel R (2013). The two-step Fagan's nomogram: *ad hoc* interpretation of a diagnostic test result without calculation. *Evid Based Med* **18**: 125–128.

Cesaroni G, Forastiere F, Stafoggia M, *et al.* (2014). Long term exposure to ambient air pollution and incidence of acute coronary events: prospective cohort study and meta-analysis in 11 European cohorts from the ESCAPE Project. *Br Med J* **348**: f7412.

Chan WK, Redelmeier DA (2012). Simpson's paradox and the association between vitamin D deficiency and increased heart disease. *Am J Cardiol* **110**: 143–144.

Chatellier G, Zapletal E, Lemaitre D, Menard J, Degoulet P (1996). The number needed to treat: a clinically useful nomogram in its proper context. *Br Med J* **312**: 426–429, 563.

Chaturvedi N, Jarrett J, Morrish N, Keen H, Fuller JH (1996). Differences in mortality and morbidity in African Caribbean and European people with non-insulin dependent diabetes mellitus: results of a 20 year follow up of a London cohort of a multinational study. *Br Med J* **313**: 848–852.

Cox SE, Makani J, Newton CR, Prentice AM, Kirkham FJ (eds. Lavelle D, Lawrie CH, Liang D-C, 2013). Hematological and genetic predictors of daytime hemoglobin saturation in Tanzanian children with and without sickle cell anemia. *ISRN Hematol* **2013**: 472909.

Das M, Ghose M, Borah NC, Choudhury N (2010). A community based study of the relationship between homocysteine and some of the life style factors. *Indian J Clin Biochem* **25**: 295–301.

Davey Smith G, Song F, Sheldon TA (1993). Cholesterol lowering and mortality: the importance of considering initial level of risk. *Br Med J* **306**: 1367–1373.

di Castelnuovo A, Costanzo S, Bagnardi V, Donati MB, Iacoviello L, de Gaetano G (2006). Alcohol dosing and total mortality in men and women. And updated meta-analysis of 34 prospective studies. *Arch Intern Med* **166**: 2437–2445.

Doll R, Peto R, Wheatley K, Gray R, Sutherland I (1994). Mortality in relation to smoking: 40 years' observations on male British doctors. *Br Med J* **309**: 901–911.

Drummond GB, Vowler SL (2011). Show the data, don't conceal them. *Br J Pharmacol* **163**: 208–210.

Engelman M, Caswell H, Agree EM (2014). Why do lifespan variability trends for the young and old diverge? A perturbation analysis. *Demogr Res* **30**: 1367–1396.

Ermers MJJ, Rovers MM, van Woensel JB, Kimpen JL, Bont LJ; on behalf of the RSV Corticosteroid Study Group (2009). The effect of high dose inhaled corticosteroids on wheeze in infants after respiratory syncytial virus infection: randomised double blind placebo controlled trial. *Br Med J* **338**: b897.

Fagan TJ (1975). Nomogram from Bayes' theorem. *N Engl J Med* **293**: 257.

Findley I, Chamberlain G (1999). ABC of labour care: Relief of pain. *Br Med J* **318**: 927.

Gore S, Altman D (eds., 1982). *Statistics in Practice.* BMJ Publishing.

Hackshaw AK, Law MR, Wald NJ (1997). The accumulated evidence on lung cancer and environmental tobacco smoke. *Br Med J* **315**: 980.

Hemming K, Haines TP, Chilton PJ, Girling AJ, Lilford RJ (2015). The stepped wedge cluster randomized trial: rationale, design, analysis, and reporting. *Br Med J* **350**: h391.

Huang F, Zhou S, Zhang S, Wang H, Tang L (2011). Temporal correlation analysis between malaria and meteorological factors in Motuo County, Tibet. *Malar J* **10**: 54.

Ishinaga M, Ueda A, Mochizuki T, Sugiyama S, Kobayashi T (2005). Cholesterol intake is associated with lecithin intake in Japanese people. *J Nutr* **135**: 1451–1455.

ISIS Collaborative Group (1988). Randomized trial of streptokinase, oral aspirin, both, or neither among 17,187 cases of suspected acute myocardial infarction: ISIS-2. *Lancet* **332**: 349–360.

Joseph DV, Jackson JA, Westaway J, Taub NA, Petersen SA, Wailoo MP (2007). Effect of parental smoking on cotinine levels in newborns. *Arch Dis Child Fetal Neonatal Ed* **92**: F484–F488.

Julious SA, Mullee MA (1994). Confounding and Simpson's paradox. *Br Med J* **309**: 1480–1481.

Kahigwa E, Schellenberg D, Sanz S, *et al.* (2002). Risk factors for presentation to hospital with severe anaemia in Tanzanian children: a case–control study. *Trop Med Int Health* **7**: 823–830.

Lawn JE, Cousens S, Zupan J (2005). Neonatal Survival 1: 4 million neonatal deaths: When? Where? Why? *Lancet* **365**: 891–900.

Leclercq PD, Murray LS, Smith C, Graham DI, Nicoll JAR, Gentleman SM (2005). Cerebral amyloid angiopathy in traumatic brain injury: association with apolipoprotein E genotype. *J Neurol Neurosurg Psychiatry* **76**: 229–233.

Lowe AJ, Carlin JB, Bennett CM, *et al.* (2010). Paracetamol use in early life and asthma: prospective birth cohort study. *Br Med J* **341**: c4616.

Lucas A, Morley R, Cole TJ (1998). Randomised trial of early diet in preterm babies and later intelligence quotient. *Br Med J* **317**: 1481–1487.

Maclean H, Dhillon B (1993). Pupil cycle time and human immunodeficiency virus (HIV) infection. *Eye* **7**: 785–786.

Maeda SS, Saraiva GL, Hayashi LF, *et al.* (2013). Seasonal variation in the serum 25-hydroxyvitamin D levels of young and elderly active and inactive adults in São Paulo, Brazil – The São PAulo Vitamin D Evaluation Study (SPADES). *Dermatoendocrinol* **5**: 211–217.

Martens E, Sinner MF, Siebermair J, *et al.* (2014). Incidence of sudden cardiac death in Germany: results from an emergency medical service registry in Lower Saxony. *Europace* **16**: 1752–1758.

Midlöv P, Calling S, Memon AA, Sundquist J, Sundquist K, Johansson S-E (2016). Women's health in the Lund area (WHILA) – Alcohol consumption and all-cause mortality among women – a 17-year follow-up study. *BMC Public Health* **16**: 22.

Mitchell P, Jakubowski J (1999). Risk analysis of treatment of unruptured aneurysms. *J Neurol Neurosurg Psychiatry* **68**: 577–580.

Morioka TY, Lee AJ, Bertisch S, Buettner C (2015). Vitamin D status modifies the association between statin use and musculoskeletal pain: A population based study. *Atherosclerosis* **238**: 77–82.

Mould RF, Hearnden T, Palmer M, White GC (1976). Distribution of survival times of 12,000 head and neck cancer patients who died with their disease. *Br J Cancer* **34**: 180–190.

National Center for Health Statistics. Health, United States, 2008 With Chartbook. Hyattsville, MD: 2009.

Nijman RG, Thompson M, van Veen M, Perera R, Moll HA, Oostenbrink R (2012). Derivation and validation of age and temperature specific reference values and centile charts to predict lower respiratory tract infection in children with fever: prospective observational study. *Br Med J* **345**: e4224.

Ostovar A, Haghdoost AA, Rahimiforoushani A, Raeisi A, Majdzadeh R (2016). Time series analysis of meteorological factors influencing malaria in south eastern Iran. *J Arthropod Borne Dis* **10**: 222–236.

Owen CG, Whincup PH, Cook DG (2005). Are early life factors responsible for international differences in adult blood pressure? An ecological study. *Int J Epidemiol* **34**: 649–654.

Patel KV (2008). Epidemiology of anemia in older adults. *Semin hematol* **45**: 210–217.

Pérez Gutthann S, Garcia Rodriguez LA, Castellsague J, Duque Oliart A (1997). Hormone replacement therapy and risk of venous thromboembolism: population based case–control study. *Br Med J* **314**: 796–800.

Perucchini D, Fischer U, Spinas GA, Huch R, Huch A, Lehmann R (1999). Using fasting plasma glucose concentrations to screen for gestational diabetes mellitus: prospective population based study. *Br Med J* **319**: 812–815.

Pukrittayakamee S, Prakongpan S, Wanwimolruk S, Clemens R, Looareesuwan S, White NJ (2003). Adverse effect of rifampin on quinine efficacy in uncomplicated falciparum malaria. *Antimicrob Agents Chemother* **47**: 1509–1513.

Radwan G, Hecht SS, Carmella SG, Loffredo CA (2013). Tobacco-specific nitrosamine exposure in smokers and nonsmokers exposed to cigarette or waterpipe tobacco smoke. *Nicotine Tob Res* **15**: 130–138.

Roberts M, Alexander F, Anderson T, *et al.* (1984). The Edinburgh randomised trial of screening for breast cancer: description of method. *Br J Cancer* **50**: 1–6.

Royston P, Ambler G, Sauerbrei W (1999). The use of fractional polynomials to model continuous risk factors in epidemiology. *Int J Epidemiol* **28**: 964–974.

Scherpbier-de Haan N, van der Wel M, Schoenmakers G, *et al.* (2011). Thirty-minute compared to standardized office blood pressure measurement in general practice. *Br J Gen Pract* **61**: e590–e597.

Sempos CT, Durazo-Arvizu RA, Dawson-Hughes B, *et al.* (2013). Is there a reverse J-shaped association between 25-hydroxyvitamin D and all-cause mortality? Results from the U.S. nationally representative NHANES. *J Clin Endocrinol Metab* **98**: 3001–3009.

Shah RC, Buchman AS, Wilson RS, Leurgans SE, Bennett DA (2011). Hemoglobin level in older persons and incident Alzheimer disease. *Neurology* **77**: 219–226.

Sheikh A, Saeed Z, Jafri SAD, Yazdani I, Hussain SA (ed. Burdmann EA, 2012). Vitamin D levels in asymptomatic adults – a population survey in Karachi, Pakistan. *PLoS One* **7**: e33452.

Shroff R, Egerton M, Bridel M, *et al.* (2008). A bimodal association of vitamin D levels and vascular disease in children on dialysis. *J Am Soc Nephrol* **19**: 1239–1246.

Sodemann M, Nielsen J, Veirum J, Jakobsen MS, Biai S, Aaby P (2008). Hypothermia of newborns is associated with excess mortality in the first 2 months of life in Guinea-Bissau, West Africa. *Trop Med Int Health* **13**: 980–986.

Stanner SA, Bulmer K, Andrès C, *et al.* (1997). Does malnutrition in utero determine diabetes and coronary heart disease in adulthood? Results from the Leningrad siege study, a cross-sectional study. *Br Med J* **315**: 1342.

Straus SE, Richardson WS, Glasziou P, Haynes RB (2010). *Evidence-based Medicine: How to Practice and Teach It, 4th edition*. Churchill Livingstone.

Sumner DJ, Meredith PA, Howie CA, Elliot HL (1988). Initial blood pressure as a predictor of the response to antihypertensive therapy. *Br J Clin Pharmacol* **26**: 715–720.

Sureda X, Martínez-Sanchéz JM, Fu M, *et al.* (ed. Behrens T, 2014). Impact of the Spanish smoke-free legislation on adult, non-smoker exposure to secondhand smoke: cross-sectional surveys before (2004) and after (2012) legislation. *PLoS One* **9**: e89430.

Tait R, Voepel-Lewis T, Brennan-Martinez C, McGonegal M, Levine R (2012). Using animated computer-generated text and graphics to depict the risks and benefits of medical treatments. *Am J Med* **125**: 1103–1110.

Taylor G, McNeill A, Girling A, Farley A, Lindson-Hawley N, Aveyard P (2014). Change in mental health after smoking cessation: systematic review and meta-analysis. *Br Med J* **348**: g1151.

The Gambia Hepatitis Study Group (1987). The Gambia Hepatitis Intervention Study. *Cancer Res* **47**: 5782–5787.

van Crevel H, Habbema J, Braakman R (1986). Decision analysis of the management of incidental intracranial saccular aneurysms. *Neurology* **36**: 1335–1339.

van der Mei J, Volmer M, Boersma ER (2000). Growth and survival of low birthweight infants from 0 to 9 years in a rural area of Ghana. Comparison of moderately low (1501–2000g) and very low birthweight (1000–1500g) infants and a local reference population. *Trop Med Int Health* **5**: 571–577.

Vespa J, Watson F (1995). Who is nutritionally vulnerable in Bosnia-Hercegovina? *Br Med J* **311**: 652–654.

Vickers AJ, Altman DG (2001). Analysing controlled trials with baseline and follow up measurements. *Br Med J* **323**: 1123–1124.

Vincze B, Kapuvári B, Udvarhelyi N, *et al.* (2015). Serum estrone concentration, estrone sulphate/estrone ratio and BMI are associated with human epidermal growth factor receptor 2 and progesterone receptor status in primary postmenopausal breast cancer patients suffering invasive ductal carcinoma. *SpringerPlus* **4**: 387–397.

Wald NJ (2004). *The Epidemiological Approach: An Introduction to Epidemiology in Medicine, 4th edition.* Wolfson Institute of Preventive Medicine & The Royal Society of Medicine Press.

Weinshenker B, Penman M, Bass B, Ebers G, Rice G (1992). A double-blind, randomized crossover trial of pemoline in fatigue associated with multiple sclerosis. *Neurology* **42**: 1468–1471.

Wilson IB, Landon BE, Marsden PV, *et al.* (2007). Correlations among measures of quality in HIV care in the United States: cross sectional study. *Br J Med* **335**: 1085–1091.

Wu SH, Ho SC, Lam TP, Woo J, Yuen PY, Qin L, Ku S (2013). Development and validation of a lifetime exposure questionnaire for use among Chinese populations. *Sci Rep* **3**: 2793.

## Other dictionaries of medical statistics, epidemiology and research methodology

Armitage P, Colton T (eds., 2005). *Encyclopedia of Biostatistics, 2nd edition.* Wiley.

Bégaud B (2000). *Dictionary of Pharmacoepidemiology.* Wiley.

Day S (2007). *Dictionary for Clinical Trials, 2nd edition.* Wiley.

Dodge Y (ed., 2003). *The Oxford Dictionary of Statistical Terms, 6th edition.* Oxford University Press.

Everitt BS (2006). *Medical Statistics from A to Z: A Guide for Clinicians and Medical Students, 2nd edition.* Cambridge University Press.

Everitt BS, Palmer CR (eds., 2011). *Encyclopaedic Companion to Medical Statistics, 2nd edition.* Wiley.

Everitt BS, Skrondal A (2010). *The Cambridge Dictionary of Statistics, 4th edition.* Cambridge University Press.

Gail MH, Benichou J (eds.), Armitage P, Colton T (series eds.) (2000). *Encyclopedia of Epidemiologic Methods.* Wiley.

Indrayan A, Holt MP (2016). *Concise Encyclopedia of Biostatistics for Medical Professionals.* Chapman & Hall/CRC Press.

Li Wan Po A (1998). *Dictionary of Evidence-based Medicine.* Radcliffe Medical Press.

Marriott FHC (1990). *Dictionary of Statistical Terms, 5th revised edition.* Longman Scientific.

Meinert CL (2012). *Clinical Trials Dictionary: Terminology and Usage Recommendations, 2nd edition.* Wiley.

Porta M (ed., 2014), Greenland S, Hernán M, dos Santos Silva I, Last JM (associate eds.), Burón A (assistant ed.). *A Dictionary of Epidemiology, 6th edition.* Oxford University Press.

Upton G, Cook I (2014). *A Dictionary of Statistics, 3rd edition.* Oxford University Press.

Vogt WP, Johnson RB (2015). *The Sage Dictionary of Statistics & Methodology: A Nontechnical Guide for the Social Sciences, 5th edition.* Sage Publications.

## Further reading

BMJ Statistical Notes series. *Br Med J.* (http://www-users.york.ac.uk/~mb55/pubs/pbstnote.htm)

Perera R, Heneghan C, Badenoch D (2008). *Statistics Toolkit.* BMJ Books.

## Links and websites

- Cochrane Handbook for Systematic Reviews of Interventions:
  http://handbook.cochrane.org/front_page.htm

- Confidence Interval Analysis software (Statistics with Confidence):
  http://www.som.soton.ac.uk/research/sites/cia/

- CONSORT statement:
  http://www.consort-statement.org/

- Critical Appraisal Skills Programme (CASP):
  http://www.casp-uk.net/

- EQUATOR Network:
  http://www.equator-network.org/

- GLLAMM (Generalized Linear Latent and Mixed Models) Stata programs and other resources:
  http://www.gllamm.org/

- GRADE approach (to grading evidence for clinical guidelines):
  http://www.gradeworkinggroup.org/

- MedCalc Statistical Software:
  https://www.medcalc.org/ (MedCalc version 16.8.4)

- Missing data website at the London School of Hygiene and Tropical Medicine:
  http://www.missingdata.org.uk/

- PRISMA statement:
  http://www.prisma-statement.org/

- STARD statement:
  http://www.stard-statement.org/

- Stata Online Manual:
  http://www.stata.com/features/documentation/

- STROBE statement:
  http://www.strobe-statement.org/

- TRIPOD statement:
  http://www.tripod-statement.org/

- The WHO Multicentre Growth Reference Study (MGRS):
  http://www.who.int/childgrowth/mgrs/en/